# RESEARCH REGULATORY COMPLIANCE

# RESEARCH
# REGULATORY
# COMPLIANCE

*Edited by*

MARK A. SUCKOW
*University of Notre Dame, Office of Research Notre Dame, IN, USA*

BILL J. YATES
*University of Pittsburgh, Department of Otolaryngology Pittsburgh, PA, USA*

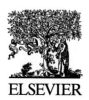

ELSEVIER

AMSTERDAM • BOSTON • HEIDELBERG • LONDON
NEW YORK • OXFORD • PARIS • SAN DIEGO
SAN FRANCISCO • SINGAPORE • SYDNEY • TOKYO
Academic Press is an imprint of Elsevier

Academic Press is an imprint of Elsevier
125 London Wall, London EC2Y 5AS, UK
525 B Street, Suite 1800, San Diego, CA 92101-4495, USA
225 Wyman Street, Waltham, MA 02451, USA
The Boulevard, Langford Lane, Kidlington, Oxford OX5 1GB, UK

**Notices**
Knowledge and best practice in this field are constantly changing. As new research and experience broaden our
understanding, changes in research methods, professional practices, or medical treatment may become necessary.

Practitioners and researchers must always rely on their own experience and knowledge in evaluating and using
any information, methods, compounds, or experiments described herein. In using such information or methods
they should be mindful of their own safety and the safety of others, including parties for whom they have a
professional responsibility.

To the fullest extent of the law, neither the Publisher nor the authors, contributors, or editors, assume any liability
for any injury and/or damage to persons or property as a matter of products liability, negligence or otherwise, or
from any use or operation of any methods, products, instructions, or ideas contained in the material herein.

ISBN: 978-0-12-420058-6

**British Library Cataloguing-in-Publication Data**
A catalogue record for this book is available from the British Library

**Library of Congress Cataloging-in-Publication Data**
A catalog record for this book is available from the Library of Congress

For information on all Academic Press publications
visit our website at http://store.elsevier.com/

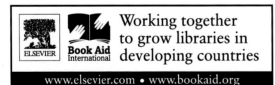

Working together
to grow libraries in
developing countries

www.elsevier.com • www.bookaid.org

*Publisher:* Janice Audet
*Acquisition Editor:* Janice Audet
*Editorial Project Manager:* Mary Preap
*Production Project Manager:* Caroline Johnson
*Designer:* Mark Rogers

Typeset by TNQ Books and Journals
www.tnq.co.in

Printed and bound in the United States of America

# Contents

Contributors      ix
Preface      xi

## 1. Human Subjects Research Protections

JOHN R. BAUMANN, HEATHER MULLINS-OWENS,
DAVID RUSSELL AND AMY WALTZ

1. Introduction      1
2. Historical Perspectives      2
3. Key Regulatory Agencies and Mandate      7
4. Common Challenges      14
5. Current Influences Shaping the Future
   of Human Research Subject Protection      17
   References      20

## 2. Investigational New Drug and Device Exemption Process

DENNIS P. SWANSON

1. Introduction      21
2. Historical Perspectives      21
3. Relevant Regulatory/Oversight
   Agencies, Regulations, and Guidance
   Documents      23
4. Regulatory Mandates      35
5. Key Personnel and University Committees
   Designated to Implement Regulatory
   Mandates      38
6. Common Compliance Challenges      39
7. Addressing Noncompliance      39
   References      40

## 3. The Institutional Animal Care and Use Committee

JERALD SILVERMAN

1. Introduction      41
2. Regulatory History      42
3. Relevant Regulatory and Oversight Laws,
   Regulations, and Guidance Documents      44

4. Key Regulatory Mandates for the
   Institutional Animal Care and
   Use Committee      49
5. Key Personnel and Committees
   Designated to Implement Regulatory
   Mandates      58
6. Common Compliance Challenges      65
7. Addressing Noncompliance      71
8. Final Comments      75
   References      76

## 4. Biological Hazards and Select Agents

MOLLY STITT-FISHER

1. Introduction      79
2. Historical Perspectives      79
3. Relevant Regulatory/Oversight Agencies,
   Regulations, and Guidance Documents      85
4. Key Regulatory Mandates      89
5. Key Personnel and University Committees
   Designated to Implement Regulatory
   Mandates      100
6. Common Compliance Challenges      103
7. Addressing Noncompliance      108
   References      108

## 5. Radiological Hazards and Lasers

MICHAEL SHEETZ

1. Introduction      113
2. Historical Perspectives      119
3. Relevant Regulatory/Oversight Agencies,
   Regulations, and Guidance Documents      125
4. Key Regulatory Mandates      131
5. Key Personnel and University Committees
   Designated to Implement Regulatory
   Mandates      139
6. Common Compliance Challenges      147
7. Addressing Noncompliance      153
8. Conclusion      155
   References      156

### 6. Controlled Substances: Maintaining Institutional Compliance

PATRICK A. LESTER, KATHERINE A. SHUSTER,
PORTIA S. ALLEN, GERALD A. HISH Jr. AND
DANIEL D. MYERS Jr.

| | |
|---|---|
| 1. Introduction | 159 |
| 2. Historical Perspectives | 160 |
| 3. Relevant Regulatory/Oversight Agencies, Regulations, and Guidance Documents | 166 |
| 4. Key Regulatory Mandates | 168 |
| 5. Key Personnel and University Committees Designated to Implement Regulatory Mandates | 177 |
| 6. Common Compliance Challenges | 181 |
| 7. Addressing Noncompliance | 184 |
| References | 184 |

### 7. Export Controls and US Research Universities

GRETTA ROWOLD AND JENNIFER A. PONTING

| | |
|---|---|
| 1. Summary | 187 |
| 2. Key Definitions | 187 |
| 3. Introduction | 188 |
| 4. Historical Perspectives | 188 |
| 5. Relevant Regulatory/Oversight Agencies, Regulations, and Guidance Documents | 195 |
| 6. Regulatory Mandates | 195 |
| 7. Key Personnel and University Committees | 199 |
| 8. Common Compliance Challenges | 203 |
| 9. Addressing Noncompliance | 204 |
| References | 206 |

### 8. Data Management and Research Integrity

SHANNON WAPOLE AND DAVID A. STONE

| | |
|---|---|
| 1. Introduction | 209 |
| 2. Historical Perspectives | 210 |
| 3. Relevant Regulatory/Oversight Agencies, Regulations, and Guidance Documents | 212 |
| 4. Key Regulatory Mandates | 222 |
| 5. Key Personnel and University Committees Designated to Implement Regulatory Mandates | 225 |
| 6. Common Compliance Challenges | 227 |

| | |
|---|---|
| 7. Addressing Noncompliance | 235 |
| References | 240 |

### 9. Intellectual Property

JAMES H. BRATTON

| | |
|---|---|
| 1. Summary | 243 |
| 2. Key Personnel and University Committees Designated to Implement Regulatory Mandates | 243 |
| 3. Common Compliance Challenges | 248 |
| 4. Addressing Noncompliance | 250 |
| References | 251 |

### 10. Financial Conflicts of Interest in Research

JULIE D. GOTTLIEB

| | |
|---|---|
| 1. Introduction | 253 |
| 2. Historical Perspectives | 254 |
| 3. Relevant Regulatory/Oversight Agencies, Regulations, and Guidance Documents | 261 |
| 4. Key Regulatory Mandates of the 2011 Public Health Service Regulation | 263 |
| 5. Key Personnel and University Committees Designated to Implement Regulatory Mandates | 269 |
| 6. Common Compliance Challenges | 272 |
| 7. Addressing Noncompliance | 274 |
| 8. End-of-Chapter Notes | 275 |
| References | 275 |

### 11. Good Laboratory Practices (GLPs)

ANNE M. BROOKS, MICHAEL A. KOCH,
ASHELEY B. WATHEN AND TIM VALLEY

| | |
|---|---|
| 1. Introduction | 277 |
| 2. Historical Perspectives | 279 |
| 3. Relevant Regulatory/Oversight Agencies | 281 |
| 4. Key Regulatory Mandates | 287 |
| 5. Key Personnel | 287 |
| 6. Common Compliance Challenges | 290 |
| 7. Addressing Noncompliance | 294 |
| References | 295 |

12. Human Embryonic Stem Cell Research Oversight: A Confluence of Voluntary Self-Regulation and Shifting Policy Initiatives

MELINDA ABELMAN, MELISSA LOPES AND
P. PEARL O'ROURKE

1. Introduction                                             297
2. Historical Perspectives                                  299
3. Relevant Regulatory Agencies and
   Oversight Laws, Regulations, and
   Guidance Documents in Effect Today                       303

4. Key Regulatory Mandates                                  312
5. Key Personnel and University Committees
   Designated to Implement Regulatory
   Mandates                                                 313
6. Common Compliance Challenges                             314
7. Addressing Noncompliance and Anticipating
   Emerging Compliance Issues                               316
   References                                               318

**Index                                                     321**

# Contributors

**Melinda Abelman**   Partners HealthCare System, Boston, MA, USA

**Portia S. Allen**   Unit for Laboratory Animal Medicine, University of Michigan, Ann Arbor, MI, USA

**John R. Baumann**   Indiana University, Indianapolis and Bloomington, IN, USA

**James H. Bratton**   Office of Technology Development, University of Oklahoma, Norman, OK, USA

**Anne M. Brooks**   WuXi AppTec, Inc., Shanghai, China

**Julie D. Gottlieb**   Johns Hopkins University, Baltimore, MD, USA

**Gerald A. Hish Jr.**   Department of Comparative Medicine, University of Washington, Seattle, WA, USA

**Michael A. Koch**   Covance, Inc., NJ, USA

**Patrick A. Lester**   Unit for Laboratory Animal Medicine, University of Michigan, Ann Arbor, MI, USA

**Melissa Lopes**   Harvard University, Cambridge, MA, USA

**Heather Mullins-Owens**   Indiana University, Indianapolis and Bloomington, IN, USA

**Daniel D. Myers Jr.**   Unit for Laboratory Animal Medicine, University of Michigan, Ann Arbor, MI, USA; Conrad Jobst Vascular Research Laboratories, University of Michigan, Ann Arbor, MI, USA

**P. Pearl O'Rourke**   Partners HealthCare System, Boston, MA, USA

**Jennifer A. Ponting**   Office for Sponsored Programs, Harvard University, Cambridge, MA, USA

**Gretta Rowold**   Office of Legal Counsel, University of Oklahoma, Norman, OK, USA

**David Russell**   Indiana University, Indianapolis and Bloomington, IN, USA

**Michael Sheetz**   University of Pittsburgh, Graduate School of Public Health, Pittsburgh, PA, USA

**Katherine A. Shuster**   Safety Assessment and Laboratory Animal Resources, Merck, Kenilworth, NJ, USA

**Jerald Silverman**   University of Massachusetts Medical School, Worcester, MA, USA

**Molly Stitt-Fisher**   University of Pittsburgh, Pittsburgh, PA, USA

**David A. Stone**   Northern Illinois University, DeKalb, IL, USA

**Dennis P. Swanson**   University of Pittsburgh, Pittsburgh, PA, USA

**Tim Valley**   Covance, Inc., NJ, USA

**Amy Waltz**   Indiana University, Indianapolis and Bloomington, IN, USA

**Shannon Wapole**   Northern Illinois University, DeKalb, IL, USA

**Asheley B. Wathen**   Covance, Inc., NJ, USA

# Preface

As the complexity of scientific inquiry has increased in recent history, so has the oversight and regulation of research. The increased focus on oversight arises from societal expectation that experimentation be conducted in a sound and responsible manner. In addition, the public's confidence in the scientific process periodically has been eroded by rare but noteworthy examples of lapses in oversight. Concerns that experiments on human and animal subjects are conducted ethically and studies incorporating chemical, biological, or radiological hazards are performed safely led to a number of oversight committees and bodies and the requirement for a thorough review of proposed studies before they are initiated. As new technologies developed, such as the use of stem cells in biomedicine, additional regulatory mandates evolved in parallel.

Increased interactions between academic institutions and industry, and global collaborations between scientists, have also necessitated new oversight mechanisms, including those related to intellectual property, export control, conflict of interest, and data management. In some cases the evolution of these oversight mechanisms was directed by regulatory requirements, and in other cases by best practices.

The introduction of new and complex regulatory requirements by many different oversight bodies is daunting for most investigators and research administrators, who often struggle in understanding and implementing the mandates. The goal of this book is to provide an overview of the issues commonly encountered in research regulatory compliance. Topics are presented to provide perspective, but are not exhaustively reviewed. Because specific regulations and best practices can be expected to evolve and change, readers are directed to the appropriate sources of information for further guidance. It is our hope that this book will serve as a tool to aid scientists, research compliance professionals, and academic administrators in developing strategies to ensure sound practices in accordance with ethical, legal, and regulatory expectations.

**Mark A. Suckow, DVM, DACLAM**
Associate Vice President for Research Compliance
University of Notre Dame

**Bill J. Yates, PhD**
Professor, Department of Otolaryngology
University of Pittsburgh

# Human Subjects Research Protections

*John R. Baumann, Heather Mullins-Owens,*
*David Russell, Amy Waltz*
Indiana University, Indianapolis and Bloomington, IN, USA

## 1. INTRODUCTION

A researcher from the school of business seeks to enroll students in a study to assess variables that might influence levels of risk tolerance and aversion.

An anthropologist proposes an ethnographic study of disruptions in a local market in a Mexican community on the opening of a "big box" store in the near vicinity.

An oncologist proposes a study to test the safety of an investigational new drug (drug C) in patients with multiple myeloma. Patients participating in the study will receive either Treatment Arm 1 (drugs O, L, and D) or Treatment Arm 2 (drugs O, C, and D). The chances of being assigned to either treatment are approximately 50/50.

A sociologist proposes a mixed methods study to assess the impact of a recent hurricane on the city's pattern of illegal drug use and illegal drug markets. Similar research will take place in two surrounding communities to which residents were re-located.

A physician-researcher proposes to access the electronic medical records of all patients undergoing a new presurgical preparation procedure to determine whether they have better outcomes than patients who do not undergo the procedure.

A school of education professor seeks to explore the relative effectiveness of three pedagogical approaches for teaching language arts to elementary school students.

A psychologist is funded to investigate and further develop a new approach for reducing "burn out" among the professional and paraprofessional staff of substance abuse and mental health service agencies.

The research studies summarized above are all very different from one another: different subject populations, different academic disciplines, different procedures, different methodologies, operating from different paradigms, and so on. However, they share one crucial factor: They are each an example of human subject research that requires the research team to submit their project to their institution's human research protection program (HRPP) for review and approval in advance of initiation.

*Research Regulatory Compliance*
http://dx.doi.org/10.1016/B978-0-12-420058-6.00001-0

The aim of this chapter is to present an overview of the history, processes, and selected issues related to the institutional oversight of human subjects research. Our beginning point is the HRPP. An HRPP encompasses all aspects and components of an institution involved in conduct and oversight of human subject research—in other words, more than just the institutional review board (IRB) or research ethics committee (REC) itself. The organization perhaps most in the forefront of developing the idea of an HRPP is the Association for the Accreditation of Human Research Protection Programs (AAHRPP). AAHRPP describes an HRPP (http://www.aahrpp.org/learn/accreditation/goals-principles-standards) as consisting of:

- The organization. By organization, AAHRPP is referring to more than the office that receives studies for IRB review,sometimes named the IRB office, human subjects office, or compliance office. It refers, rather to a host of administrative components and features of organizational culture and practice in addition to that office. This may include, but is not limited to: the institutional official, other compliance committees (such as conflict of interest and radiation safety), grant/contracts office, pharmacy, and a host of activities beyond the review of individual studies.
- The IRB or REC itself. This is the specific group of individuals that has the responsibility and authority to review and approve, disapprove, or table human subject research studies.
- The researchers. These are researchers and research staff who are responsible for, and involved, in the design, conduct, and reporting of human subject research.

This chapter begins with a historical perspective—a discussion of some of the practices and processes that gave rise to our contemporary principles of, and processes for, human subject research protections. An overview of the regulatory context follows: review of the major regulatory mandates, the regulatory agencies, and committees empowered to oversee and implement those mandates. The chapter concludes with a discussion of common challenges, mechanisms for addressing or preventing noncompliance issues, and, finally, a discussion of some of the issues that may shape the future directions of human subject protection.

## 2. HISTORICAL PERSPECTIVES

### 2.1 Recognition of Need

The practice of research on humans is, of course, long standing. Even a quick review of medical history reveals countless examples of this. However, the formal idea and regulation of "human subjects research" is recent and was, like many such reforms, generated by a controversy. Serious ethical issues arising from the Tuskegee syphilis experiments in 1972 caused a moral outrage [1–3]. Congress was moved to act and in 1974 passed the National Research Act, which established the National Commission for the Protection of Human Subjects of Biomedical and Behavioral Research. From 1974 to 1978, the commission issued several reports related to biomedical and behavioral research with human subjects, culminating in 1979 with their final, formal report known as the Belmont Report, named after the conference room in which they met [4]. The Belmont Report summarized the basic ethical principles and corresponding guidelines that the commission recognized for the conduct of human experimentation. Principles and codes addressing the conduct of human subject research have existed in various forms and have been followed by a variety of organizations since the mid 1940s, but the Belmont Report has arguably had the greatest effect on human subject research protections in the United States.

The Belmont Report's ethical principles and guidelines address key areas of concern following the aforementioned Tuskegee syphilis study. Officially known as the Tuskegee Study of Untreated Syphilis in the Negro Male, the study was sponsored by the United States Public Health Service and was conducted between 1932 and 1972. As the title suggests, the study aimed to follow the progression of untreated syphilis in the human body with a target study population of black males. Subjects infected with syphilis, and some who were not infected, were recruited into the study with the promise of medical care, free food, and burial insurance. The subjects were not informed of the true nature of the procedures to which they agreed and were told only that they were being treated for "bad blood" [1–3]. The researchers deliberately withheld penicillin and other treatments that were developed during the course of the study from the subjects so they could monitor and document the progression of the disease. As both a direct and indirect consequence, subjects experienced psychological/cognitive distress, physical deficiencies, and even death. Further, the disease may well have been transmitted to sexual partners and children born to research participants.

The core principles and practices identified in the Belmont Report were central to the public outcry regarding the overall conduct of this research and the treatment of the research subjects: patient autonomy, lack of informed consent, the direct harm done to subjects due to withholding medical care, and the unequal/inequitable distribution of research risks on one segment of the population. The Belmont Report identified three key ethical principles for the practice of human subject research: respect for persons, beneficence, and justice. Emerging from these three principles were three guidelines for their implementation or actualization: informed consent, assessment of risk and benefit, and equitable sharing of the burdens and benefits of research [4,5].

*Respect for persons* specifically addresses patient autonomy and requires that, as autonomous beings, subjects should be afforded the right to be informed of the procedures being performed in the research in which they are asked to participate and that their participation be voluntary. The Belmont Report describes an autonomous human being as one capable of self-determination and consideration of a variety of choices based on information provided to them. The full application of this principle, through informed consent, involves the provision of all relevant information, the confirmation that this information is comprehended and understood, and the ensuring of voluntary participation, or not, based on the potential subject's choice.

Just as the autonomy of each person is recognized, the commission also recognized the necessity of protections for persons with diminished autonomy. Individuals who are incapacitated, ill, mentally disabled, immature, or are otherwise vulnerable to undue influence or coercion may have diminished autonomy requiring special care when including them in research—known as "vulnerable populations." This care involves ongoing evaluation of their awareness of the consequences of participation, assessment of the subjects' voluntariness, and protections to prevent coercion. It is the responsibility of the researchers to ensure patient autonomy is preserved and potentially to remove a subject from research if this cannot be established.

*Beneficence* refers to the prospective risks and harms that a research subject may face by participating in a study with the prospective benefits that may arise from the research for either the subject or, more generally, society with the development of new knowledge. For the Belmont committee, it addressed the direct harm done to the subjects in the Tuskegee syphilis study. By withholding medical care, specifically penicillin, the participants in this study were denied care that otherwise would have been available to them were they not research subjects. Penicillin was established as the standard treatment for syphilis in 1947, approximately 15 years after the initiation of this study; however, the subjects were denied this treatment, and the study continued for another 25 years. For these subjects, participation was actually maleficent, which is contrary to the very precepts of the practice of medicine and the principle of beneficence. The Belmont Report extends this precept of medicine into human subject research with the two prongs of beneficence: 1) to do no harm to subjects; and 2) if harm/risk is unavoidable, to maximize benefit while minimizing possible harm. The report acknowledged that individual research subjects may not directly benefit from their participation, but their inclusion in the study must still be justifiable in consideration of the benefits to be gained and possible risks. An evaluation should be made of the ratio of potential risks to potential benefits. There is, of course, some tension between this and the principle implicit in respect for persons. Respect for persons and autonomy require that researchers do not treat subjects as "means" to an "end," but the assessment of risks/harm against possible benefits implies some dimension of this, especially when there is no direct benefit for the subjects and the only benefits are advancement of knowledge. The practice of informed consent, however, is designed to mitigate this tension.

The principle of *justice* addresses the unequal distribution of the burdens and risks of participation in research on subject populations in general, as illustrated by the inequitable inclusion of only the black male population in the Tuskegee syphilis study. This principle seeks to address the fairness of the distribution of research risks and possible benefits and to prevent injustice. There is no question that the rural black male population was exploited and manipulated in this study. Similarly, prisoners, the poor, and institutionalized individuals have been exploited in various other research studies throughout the last 100 years. The Belmont Report breaks down the equal treatment of human research subjects using five prongs: (1) to each person an equal share; (2) to each person according to individual need; (3) to each person according to individual effort; (4) to each person according to societal contribution; and (5) to each person according to merit. By evaluating the subject population in this way, the burdens of research can be distributed in an equitable manner, with no single population being exploited to address a medical condition that affects all populations or even specific other populations, as may have been the case with testing of medicines for human immunodeficiency virus/acquired immune deficiency syndrome among African populations that probably would not have had access to such medicines even if proved effective.

## 2.2 Broader History of Unethical Research

In much the same way, other research studies conducted since the early twentieth century raised ethical questions and influenced the regulatory environment for the conduct of human subject research [6–8]. Surgical experiments were conducted on inmates at San

Quentin Prison from 1913 to 1951, including experimental transplantation and sterilization. The medical staff of the prison believed that the prison population was "appropriate" for research because they lived in a controlled environment where variables could be controlled, much like a research laboratory. While the prisoners did receive adequate medical care, they were also made to participate in surgical experiments without consent. Similar studies were conducted throughout the prison system in the United States in the first half of the twentieth century, and concerns related to such experimentation on prisoners has influenced much of the discourse related to human research ethics [6]. However, this history of the use of prisoners in the United States was ignored and, when it did arise, denied during trials of the Nazi medical doctors [6,9].

Perhaps most well-known are the experiments conducted by the Nazis throughout World War II. The Nazis used concentration camp prisoners as research subjects in a wide range of studies aimed at determining everything from the physical limitations of the human body to how best to multiply the German race. Most infamous was the research of Dr. Josef Mengele. Among his studies were experiments at Auschwitz on twins in an effort to garner knowledge that could assist the Germans in exponentially growing their population. Over 80 percent of the pairs of twins were executed on conclusion of the experiments [6,9,10].

Many of the Nazi's experiments were conducted for purposes of advancing their military interests [9,10]. These included experiments at Dachau in which physicians carried out high altitude tests in pressure chambers on prisoners in an effort to determine the altitude limitations for air force crews to parachute from airplanes. Experiments were also conducted to develop treatment for, and understand the progression of, hypothermia, with prisoners stripped naked and either left outside in the cold or thrown into ice water. In an effort to develop treatments for battlefield injuries, many prisoners were deliberately injured and then infected with bacteria and other material. Other experiments included artificial insemination, sterilization, and transplantation procedures at many of the Nazi concentration camps. All of these experiments were done without consent of individuals, and most of them caused severe pain, disfigurement, and death of the participants.

Many of the physicians responsible for these experiments were prosecuted for war crimes and crimes against humanity during the Nuremberg trials after the conclusion of World War II. Following these trials, the Counsel for War Crimes issued in 1947 10 points that defined legitimate medical research. These 10 points became known as the Nuremberg Code, were specifically borne out of the Nazi human experiments, predating the Belmont Report, and were the first international effort to establish guidelines for human experimentation. The 10 points for guiding legitimate research include: (1) voluntary consent; (2) experiments should yield fruitful results; (3) research should be designed based on animal experimentation; (4) researchers should avoid suffering and injury to subjects; (5) experiments should not be conducted when it is believed death or disabling injury will occur; (6) risks should be limited and should not exceed the benefit or humanitarian importance of the problem the research seeks to solve; (7) adequate facilities and proper preparations are necessary; (8) scientifically qualified personnel should conduct the research; (9) subjects have a right to end their participation at any time; and (10) researchers should be prepared to discontinue the experiment at any time if subject safety is at risk. The Nuremberg Code was, basically, a statement of outrage and principle without any regulatory enforceability [11].

In 1964, the World Medical Association developed and adopted the Declaration of Helsinki to provide ethical principles for human subject research and research involving identifiable data (www.wma.net). The Declaration of Helsinki marks what can be described as the modern era of research ethics and regulation, and the World Medical Association continues to amend and update the declaration, most recently in October 2013 [12].

Many of the principles of the Declaration of Helsinki overlap with the principles discussed previously in the Nuremberg Code and the Belmont Report, but it introduced several new essential principles and provided greater detail for some of the more generalized principles. The Declaration of Helsinki provided, for the first time, the requirement that human experiments should be reviewed by a REC. In the United States, this concept is carried out by IRBs; in other nations, such committees are known as RECs. These committees are responsible for the review, deliberation, guidance, and approval of studies before they are initiated. These committees should also provide ongoing monitoring of the studies they approve and pay particular attention to serious adverse events.

The Declaration of Helsinki provided, for the first time, specific protections and considerations for vulnerable populations. The declaration did not mention specific groups that were considered to be vulnerable (such as children), but did state that certain groups of individuals are vulnerable and may be more likely to be harmed when participating in research. Such groups should be included in research only when the research is in response to a particular health need or priority of that population that cannot be addressed in the general population. These principles were adopted as subparts to the regulations in the United States.

The requirements for informed consent were expanded considerably as well. The declaration required participation in research to be voluntary and for informed consent to be obtained from those subjects who are capable of providing it. The importance of consulting family members and other trusted individuals was recognized and encouraged, but it is essential that individuals provide consent for their own participation under their own free will. When an individual is incapable of providing his own consent, a legally authorized representative is permitted to consent on behalf of the individual.

Specific procedures were outlined in the declaration for the process of obtaining informed consent and the types of information that should be provided to subjects. This included the aims and methods of the study, the funding sources, possible conflicts of interest or other affiliations the researcher may have, the benefits and risks of the study and any discomforts the subject may experience, and the subject's right to refuse to participate at any time. The process of obtaining consent must be formally documented and witnessed.

Other important considerations outlined in the Declaration of Helsinki include requirements for ongoing education and training of researchers, adherence of the study to a preapproved and peer-reviewed protocol that is guided by generally accepted scientific principles, the researcher's duty to promote and safeguard health, welfare, and rights of subjects with the goal of the research never overtaking the rights of the individual research subjects, protections for the privacy and confidentiality of subjects, and the registration of clinical trials and the dissemination of their results.

Neither the Nuremberg Code nor the Declaration of Helsinki is law in the United States. They both, as well as the experience of unethical research conducted here in the United States by federal, state, and university- or hospital-based researchers, were influential in the codification of the human subject research regulations in the Common Rule (described in 3.2).

# 3. KEY REGULATORY AGENCIES AND MANDATE

## 3.1 Agencies: OHRP, FDA, and VA

The Belmont Report, released in 1979 by the National Commission for the Protection of Human Subjects of Biomedical and Behavioral research, was the primary basis for the regulations guiding human subject research in the United States. The Belmont Report does not directly mandate the treatment for human subjects in the United States and does not have regulatory authority. Its three benchmark principles: respect for persons, beneficence, and justice; and their accompanying guidelines of informed consent, assessment of risk and benefit, and equity in the selection of subject, were influential in the framing and drafting of the regulations and guidance of all federal agencies: Department of Health and Human Services (DHHS; Office of Human Research Protections (OHRP), and Food and Drug Administration (FDA)), Veterans Administration (VA), and the Departments of Defense, Justice and Education.

The Office of Human Research Protections (OHRP), formerly Office for Protection from Research Risks, provides guidance and regulatory oversight on issues related to human subject participation for research conducted or supported by the DHHS. In 1981, its primary regulation guiding the conduct of human subject research, "Protection of Human Subjects" (Code of Federal Regulations 45 Part 46 (45 CFR 46) (http://www.hhs.gov/ohrp/humansubj ects/guidance/45cfr46.html), was enacted. This regulation was further revised in 2005. Additional federal departments and agencies adopted it as well. These include the Department of Agriculture, Consumer Product Safety Commission, Department of Housing and Urban Development, Department of Defense, Department of Education, Department of Veterans Affairs, and Environmental Protection Agency. The Central Intelligence Agency, Department of Homeland Security, and Social Security Administration also comply with 45 CFR 46 subparts, but did not promulgate it into regulations. It has become known as the "Common Rule." While formally mandated for federally supported research, it has emerged as the "gold standard" for all research regardless of funding source. Most institutions engaged in human subject research in the United States have adopted it as the fundamental foundation for overseeing all human subject research, whether funded by federal agencies or not. OHRP requires institutions to develop a policy statement that sets forth procedures used to protect human research subjects and has the ability to grant institutions Federal Wide Assurance (FWA), as described in more detail below.

The FDA regulates (see http://www.accessdata.fda.gov/scripts/cdrh/cfdocs/cfcfr/CFR Search.cfm?CFRPart=50) research involving drugs, biological products, and medical devices pursuant to 21 CFR 50 (protection of human subjects), 21 CFR 56 (IRBs), 21 CFR 312 (investigational new drug application, IND), and 21 CFR 812 (investigational device exemptions, IDE). The Office of Good Clinical Practice is an office within the FDA that manages issues related to human subject protections and good clinical practices. A separate chapter on the IND and IDE processes provides more information regarding FDA procedures, particularly related to the testing of new drugs and devices.

All human subject research conducted or supported by the VA must comply with the common rule, as codified at 38 CFR part 16. Title 38 CFR 16.103(a) provides that (http://www1.va.gov/vhapublications/ViewPublication.asp?pub_ID=2531):

1. Each VA facility engaged in human subject research must provide a written assurance, acceptable to the secretary of Veterans Affairs, committing the facility to comply with 38 CFR part 16.
2. Each non-VA institution engaged in human subject research conducted or supported by VA must provide a written assurance, acceptable to the secretary of Veterans Affairs, committing the institution to comply with 38 CFR part 16.
3. VHA Handbook 1200.5 stipulates that the VA Medical Center director or chief executive officer is the VA institutional official responsible for ensuring that the VA facility conducting research involving human subjects or biological specimens applies through the Office of Research Oversight to the DHHS, OHRP, for an assurance.

The VHA handbook requirements apply to all research involving human subjects or human biological specimens conducted or supported by the VA. VA requirements provide some additional stringent rules for VA research, such as the storage of study-related documents and prompt review of adverse events that may be related to research.

## 3.2 Regulations

### 3.2.1 Common Rule

The common rule has played an important role in guiding human subject research since it was published in 1991. It is also sometimes referred to as OHRP regulations. The common rule offers requirements for informed consent, IRBs, and assurances of compliance [13]. The common rule must be followed for all research supported by a federal agency that has adopted it. An institution may decide whether to apply the common rule to non-federally funded research through institutional FWAs. Regardless of whether or not an institution commits to applying the common rule to all research (known as checking or unchecking the box), most institutions apply the regulation in principle.

The common rule contains subparts which include protections for pregnant women, fetuses, and neonates; prisoner protections; protections for children; and registration of IRBs. It is now codified by 15 federal departments and agencies as separate regulations. The common rule is enforced by OHRP, which can conduct site visits to ensure compliance; OHRP may also conduct investigations. If noncompliance is determined by an OHRP investigation, then determination letters are sent to the sites and posted publicly on the OHRP website. Once compliance is obtained, that will also be noted on the OHRP website. Although exceedingly uncommon, OHRP has the authority to suspend the conduct of federally funded human subject research at an institution. Institutions also self-report a variety of actions, such as determinations of noncompliance, unanticipated problems involving risks to subjects, and suspensions and terminations of approvals to OHRP with a statement outlining their planned corrective action.

Research is defined by the common rule as "a systematic investigation, including research development, testing and evaluation, designed to develop or contribute to generalizable knowledge" [14]. Human subject refers to "a living individual about whom an investigator (whether professional or student) conducting research obtains either (1) data through intervention or interaction with the individual or (2) identifiable private information."

Some research activities may be deemed exempt from the regulation if they are of no more than minimal risk (as defined by 45 CFR 46.102(i)) and the only human subject involvement is within the parameters of the following six exemptions:

1. Research conducted in established or commonly accepted educational settings, involving normal educational practices, such as (a) research on regular and special educational instructional strategies, or (b) research on the effectiveness of or the comparison among instructional techniques, curricula, or classroom management methods.

2. Research involving the use of educational tests (cognitive, diagnostic, aptitude, achievement), survey procedures, interview procedures or observation of public behavior, unless all of the following are true:
   a. Information obtained is recorded in such a manner that the human subjects can be identified, directly or through identifiers linked to the subjects; and
   b. Any disclosure of the subjects' responses outside the research could reasonably place the subjects at risk of criminal or civil liability or be damaging to the subjects' financial standing, employability, insurability, or reputation.

3. Research involving the use of educational tests (cognitive, diagnostic, aptitude, achievement), survey procedures, interview procedures, or observation of public behavior that is not exempt under category two above, if either:
   a. The human subjects are elected or appointed public officials or candidates for public office; or
   b. Federal statute(s) require(s) without exception that the confidentiality of the personally identifiable information will be maintained throughout the research and thereafter.

4. Research involving the collection or study of existing data, documents, records, pathological specimens, or diagnostic specimens, if these sources are publicly available or if the information is recorded by the investigator in such a manner that subjects cannot be identified, directly or through identifiers linked to the subjects. To qualify for this exemption, data, documents, records, or specimens must exist at the time the research is proposed and not prospectively collected.

5. Research and demonstration projects that are conducted by, or subject to, the approval of department or agency heads and which are designed to study, evaluate, or otherwise examine:
   a. public benefit or service programs;
   b. procedures for obtaining benefits or services under those programs;
   c. possible changes in or alternatives to those programs or procedures; or
   d. possible changes in methods or levels of payment for benefits or services under those programs.

6. Taste and food quality evaluation and consumer acceptance studies,
   a. if wholesome foods without additives are consumed; or
   b. if a food is consumed that contains a food ingredient at or below the level and for a use found to be safe, or agricultural, chemical, or environmental contaminant at or below the level found to be safe, by the FDA or approved by the Environmental Protection Agency or the Food Safety and Inspection Service of the US Department of Agriculture.

Human subject research determined not to be exempt may be reviewed by either an IRB or by means of expedited review by one or more IRB members. Research that poses "greater than minimal risks" to subjects must be reviewed by an IRB at a formally convened meeting. Minimal risk is defined as: the probability or magnitude of harm or discomfort anticipated in the research is not greater, in and of itself, than that ordinarily encountered in daily life or during the performance of routine physical or psychological examinations or tests. There is some latitude in the application of this standard. For instance, in whose daily life should risks be "ordinarily encountered?" For a study to be determined eligible for initial expedited review, it must both be no greater than minimal risk and meet one of the criteria for expedited review (see below).

The IRB must include a minimum of five members with backgrounds that promote complete and adequate review of research activities commonly conducted at the institution; members of more than one profession; at least one scientific member and one nonscientific member; and at least one member unaffiliated with the institution.

Not all research must be reviewed at a convened meeting of an IRB. It may be reviewed by means of expedited review. This consists of one or more IRB member(s), depending on institutional policy, reviewing the research outside of a convened meeting. To be eligible for expedited review, the research must pose no more than minimal risk and meet one of the following nine criteria:

1. Clinical studies of drugs and medical devices only when condition (a) or (b) is met.
   a. Research on drugs for which an IND application (21 CFR part 312) is not required. (Note: Research on marketed drugs that significantly increases the risks or decreases the acceptability of the risks associated with the use of the product is not eligible for expedited review.)
   b. Research on medical devices for which (1) an investigational device exemption application (21 CFR part 812) is not required, or (2) the medical device is cleared/approved for marketing and the medical device is being used in accordance with its cleared/approved labeling.
2. Collection of blood samples by finger stick, heel stick, ear stick, or veinipuncture as follows:
   a. from healthy, nonpregnant adults who weigh at least 110 pounds. For these subjects, the amount drawn may not exceed 550 ml in an 8-week period, and collection may not occur more frequently than two times per week; or
   b. from other adults and children, considering the age, weight, and health of the subjects, the collection procedure, the amount of blood to be collected, and the frequency with which it will be collected. For those subjects, the amount drawn may not exceed the lesser of 50 ml or 3 ml per kg in an 8-week period, and collection may not occur more frequently than two times per week.
3. Prospective collection of biological specimens for research purposes by noninvasive means.

Examples: (1) hair and nail clippings in a nondisfiguring manner; (2) deciduous teeth at time of exfoliation or if routine patient care indicates a need for extraction; (3) permanent teeth if routine patient care indicates a need for extraction; (4) excreta and external secretions (including sweat); (5) uncannulated saliva collected either in an unstimulated fashion or stimulated by chewing gumbase or wax or by applying a dilute citric solution to the tongue;

(6) placenta removed at delivery; (7) amniotic fluid obtained at the time of rupture of the membrane prior to or during labor; (8) supragingival and subgingival dental plaque and calculus, provided the collection procedure is not more invasive than routine prophylactic scaling of the teeth and the process is accomplished in accordance with accepted prophylactic techniques; (9) mucosal and skin cells collected by buccal scraping or swab, skin swab, or mouth washings; and (10) sputum collected after saline mist nebulization.

4. Collection of data through noninvasive procedures (not involving general anesthesia or sedation) routinely used in clinical practice, excluding procedures involving X-rays or microwaves. When medical devices are used, they must be cleared/approved for marketing. (Studies intended to evaluate the safety and effectiveness of the medical device are not generally eligible for expedited review, including studies of cleared medical devices for new indications.)

5. Research involving materials (data, documents, records, or specimens) that have been collected or will be collected solely for nonresearch purposes (such as medical treatment or diagnosis). Note: Some research in this category may be exempt from the HHS regulations for the protection of human subjects. 45 CFR 46 101 (b)(4).

6. Collection of data from voice, video, digital, or image recordings made for research purposes.

7. Research on individual or group characteristics or behavior (including, but not limited to, research on perception, cognition, motivation, identity, language, communication, cultural beliefs or practices, and social behavior) or research using survey, interview, oral history, focus group, program evaluation, human factors evaluation, or quality assurance methodologies. Note: Some research in this category may be exempt from the HHS regulations for the protection of human subjects. 45 CFR 46.101(b)(2) and (b)(3).

8. Continuing review of research previously approved by the convened IRB as follows:
   a. When (1) the research is permanently closed to the enrollment of new subjects, (2) all subjects have completed all research-related interventions, and (3) the research remains active only for long-term follow-up of subjects; or
   b. When no subjects have been enrolled and no additional risks have been identified; or
   c. When the remaining research activities are limited to data analysis.

9. Continuing review of research, not conducted under an investigational new drug application or investigational device exemption in which categories two through eight do not apply, but the IRB has determined and documented at a convened meeting that the research involves no greater than minimal risk and no additional risks have been identified.

Regardless of whether a study is reviewed by a convened board or by expedited review, it must meet the following criteria in order to be considered for approval (see common rule):

- that risks to subjects are minimized;
- that risks are reasonable in relation to anticipated benefits;
- that the selection of subjects is equitable;
- that the procedures for obtaining informed consent are appropriate or are appropriately waived;
- that informed consent will be appropriately documented or appropriately waived;

- that, when appropriate, the research plan makes adequate provision for monitoring the data collected to ensure the safety of subjects;
- that, when appropriate, there are adequate provisions to protect the privacy of subjects and to maintain the confidentiality of data;
- that the appropriate additional safeguards are in place to protect, if included in the research, the rights and welfare of subjects likely to be vulnerable to coercion or undue influence.

At a convened meeting, IRBs have the authority and responsibility to approve or disapprove research by majority vote. They may also require modifications for approval of research. Expedited reviewers may not disapprove research; they may approve, require modifications, or refer to a convened meeting. Once research has been approved, the IRB must conduct continuing review, investigate subject complaints, and review any adverse events as they occur. IRB approval may be suspended or terminated if appropriate for the protection of subjects.

The common rule also offers guidelines for informed consent, requiring that subjects receive such information as:

- an explanation of the research, the purpose of the research, and what procedures will be performed;
- risks involved;
- potential benefits;
- whether compensation will be offered;
- alternatives to participation in research;
- how confidentiality will be maintained;
- what costs may be associated with their participation;
- contact information for questions;
- an explanation of unforeseeable risks;
- how they may withdraw from the study (at any time);
- how many subjects are expected to participate.

While it is presumed that all subjects' informed consent will be formally documented, there are provisions for its waiver. Waiver of documentation of informed consent may be permissible if the research has no more than minimal risk to subjects and the research includes no procedures for which consent is normally required or the principal risk is harm from loss of confidentiality when the only document linking the subject to research is the consent form. Not only documentation of informed consent, but the process of informed consent itself may, in fact, be waived as well. While generally rare to do so, there are certain research studies for which this is appropriate, such as and most commonly, research involving only the review of medical records. The bar, however, for granting a waiver of consent is rather high. The research must meet the following criteria: be no more than minimal risk; the granting of such a waiver will not adversely affect the rights and welfare of the subjects; and the research could not practicably be conducted without the waiver.

### 3.2.2 FDA Regulations

If research involves a biologic product or device under FDA jurisdiction, both the FDA regulations and the common rule are applicable. Relevant FDA regulations include 21 CFR 50 (informed consent), 21 CFR 56 (IRBs), 21 CFR 312 (investigational drugs), and 21 CFR 812 (investigational devices). FDA regulations permit exemptions for emergency use and food quality evaluation only. Investigators and the IRB of record are directly accountable to the FDA, rather than the institution itself. The FDA requires reporting of many study events directly to the FDA. The FDA also performs investigations, and the negative results are reported in "warning letters," which can be found on the FDA website. In some instances, the FDA may keep data from being used in research findings. A separate chapter of this book addresses the IND and IDE processes and provides more information regarding FDA procedures related to the testing of new drugs and devices.

The FDA rules apply to studies involving a drug, biologic, or device that is being studied, and its use is dictated by the protocol. Drugs may include vitamins, dietary supplements, and over-the-counter products as well as products available only with a prescription. A drug is defined by section 201(g) of the Federal Food Drug & Cosmetic Act (21 USC 321(g)) as:

> (A) articles recognized in the official United States Pharmacopoeia, official Homoeopathic Pharmacopoeia of the United States, or official National Formulary, or any supplement to any of them; and (B) articles intended for use in the diagnosis, cure, mitigation, treatment, or prevention of disease in man or other animals; and (C) articles (other than food) intended to affect the structure or any function of the body of man or other animals; and (D) articles intended for use as a component of any articles specified in clause (A), (B), or (C).

A device is defined as an instrument, apparatus, implement, machine, contrivance, implant, in vitro reagent, or other similar or related article, including a component part, or accessory which is:

- recognized in the official National Formulary, or the United States Pharmacopoeia, or any supplement to them,
- intended for use in the diagnosis of disease or other conditions, or in the cure, mitigation, treatment, or prevention of disease, in man or other animals, or
- intended to affect the structure or any function of the body of man or other animals, and which does not achieve its primary intended purposes through chemical action within or on the body of man or other animals and which is not dependent upon being metabolized for the achievement of any of its primary intended purposes.

Examples of devices may include wheelchairs, pacemakers, contact lenses, and diagnostic products such as pathology test kits and pregnancy tests. Devices may qualify for an IDE under some circumstances. This may be determined by the FDA within 60 days of inquiry. If the device poses a significant risk, however, it will require an IDE and is subject to IDE regulations dictating the manufacturing, marketing, and distribution. If the device is determined to pose nonsignificant risks, it does not require an IDE, but is subject to IDE regulations for manufacturing, marketing, and distribution [15].

### 3.2.3 Federal Wide Assurances

FWAs are administered by OHRP and apply to the institution pursuant to the common rule. They are signed by a signatory or institutional official and designate a human protections administrator for the institution. FWAs must also list one or more IRBs (including all internal IRBs) either registered to, or commonly used by, that institution. By signing the FWA, the institution agrees to comply with federal regulations for all federally funded research. The FWA covers the employees and agents of institution, collaborating independent researchers with written agreements with that institution, and collaborating institutional researchers with written agreements.

### 3.2.4 *Health Insurance Portability and Accountability Act of 1996*

The Health Insurance Portability and Accountability Act (HIPAA) provides federal protections for the confidentiality of protected health information from anything other than stated authorized use, access, or disclosure [16]. Under this regulation, protected health information refers to health information, including demographic information, collected from an individual or that which is created or received by a health care provider, health plan, employer, or health care clearinghouse and relates to the past, present, or future physical or mental health or condition of an individual or the provision of health care to an individual. The regulation applies to covered entities and their business associates. A covered entity is any health plan, health care clearinghouse, and health care providers who transmit any health information, including billing information, in electronic form. The regulation also specifies administrative, physical, and technical safeguards for covered entities to ensure the confidentiality, integrity, and availability of electronic protected health information. Covered entities may not use protected health information for research purposes without prior, written permission from the subject or a waiver of authorization provided by an authorized privacy board or IRB.

## 4. COMMON CHALLENGES

Every HRPP is unique in scope, in resources, and in expertise, and so, every HRPP is unique in the challenges that its leaders face. Supporting a children's hospital or a Veteran's Affairs medical center requires knowledge of specific regulations that other HRPPs may never apply. The resources required to run a large HRPP can be extremely hard to come by, requiring a risk management strategy that smaller HRPPs can barely comprehend. Yet, differences aside, today's research environment presents challenges that almost all HRPPs must face.

### 4.1 Education of Research Community

Whether serving 50 investigators or 5000, all HRPPs share the common challenge of training investigators in an area of increasingly complex regulation and increasingly complex research. While the tenets of human research protection seem like common sense, the day-to-day implementation of requirements for subject recruitment, consent, HIPAA authorization, and ongoing monitoring can be extremely difficult to describe, especially for complex research. The recent focus on translational research has attracted new players to human subject research who are unfamiliar with the requirements and often find the regulatory and institutional approval process mindboggling and burdensome. At the other end of the spectrum, those investigators who have been conducting research since the early days of the common rule find it difficult to embrace compliance leaders' attempts at finding flexibility within the research regulations. With such a varied audience, it can be difficult for HRPP staff to find the right balance of in-depth education and ongoing review courses. HRPPs must strive to present a comprehensive education program to their investigators. Courses should include regulatory basics for new investigators, and special topic discussions such as conducting research with vulnerable populations, adverse event reporting, and safety monitoring for more experienced investigators.

## 4.2 Identification of Research

While the common rule definition of research may appear black and white, applying it in practice is not always as simple as it seems. Clinical trials are easy enough to identify, but HRPP leaders often struggle to categorize other types of research. The line between research and quality improvement or program evaluation, for example, is often blurred [17]. This may also be true for the line separating bench research and human subject research, especially when the work involves biological specimens. FDA definitions equate biological specimens with human subjects, making it even more difficult to discern when IRB review is necessary. Projects that are preparatory to research are usually exempt from IRB review, as are quality improvement/quality assurance projects that are intended only for internal use. IRB leaders should be as clear as possible in their definitions and document decisions whenever possible to protect against future audits. Documentation is also extremely important to address compliance scandals, such as the recent inquiry into student athlete literacy at University of North Carolina–Chapel Hill that called the IRB's actions into question, in addition to the institution's (https://research.unc.edu/2014/01/22/irb-status-of-unc-research-on-student-athlete-literacy/).

## 4.3 Mission Creep

In many HRPPs, the IRB is the only office that touches each and every research study being conducted at an institution. As such, it often becomes the launch pad for tangential compliance efforts like scientific review, research billing, and ClinicalTrials.gov. Reporting responsibilities also seem to land on the IRB office as institutions, departments, and affiliates struggle to track and quantify research efforts. The IRB office is in the unique position as often being the first and only institutional repository for an institution's research, making it particularly susceptible to mission creep. This may include, for instance, using the IRB to oversee research that may be controversial or sensitive due, not to issues related to protection of subjects, but to the topic itself. Thus, controversial research may land on the HRPP's doorstep. Many institutions have expanded their research compliance programs to include more than just the IRB and have defined job descriptions based on compliance efforts that only graze the IRB's responsibility.

## 4.4 FDA Compliance

Institutions with investigators that conduct clinical trials and FDA-regulated research face additional challenges. FDA regulations, especially those dictating the need for INDs and IDEs, are complex, vague, and often inconsistent. For IRBs, on which the FDA has laid the responsibility for determining whether an IND or IDE is needed, interpreting FDA requirements is very difficult. Guidance documents are available, but are filled with words reminiscent of IRB terms of art, like "exempt" and "significant risk," which cause confusion for IRB members and investigators alike, thus creating additional training challenges. FDA representatives face resource issues as well and may not be available for consultation when needed. Even when they are available, the agency's risk aversion makes them loathe to provide detailed counsel in most situations and, in some situations, even agency representatives themselves find it difficult to apply regulations with confidence. In addition, institutions are struggling to apply and comply with the electronic system requirements found in 21 CFR part 11. The requirements have proven to be so onerous that the FDA has practiced enforcement discretion.

## 4.5 Addressing Noncompliance

One of the most important functions of the IRB is to review and address noncompliance actions. Noncompliance includes any failure to comply with federal, state, and local laws and regulations, encompassing actions from the most minor issues, like failing to obtain dates on informed consent statements, to major violations of the common rule such as failure to obtain IRB approval at all.

### 4.5.1 Identification of Noncompliance

Most IRBs rely largely on investigator self-reporting to identify noncompliance issues, underscoring the importance of a comprehensive investigator training program. If investigators are unaware of research requirements, they are more likely to engage in noncompliance. Few investigators, in fact, willfully stray from the regulatory tenets of human research protections. In many cases, noncompliance is the result of lack of knowledge or misunderstanding, and an HRPP that effectively addresses noncompliance includes training and a strong level of trust between the IRB office and investigators. Investigators who have trusting relationships with IRB staff are more willing to ask for guidance in difficult situations, allowing staff and investigators both to recognize and report noncompliance when it occurs.

In addition to self-reporting, ongoing monitoring of human subjects research is the second most effective way to identify noncompliance issues. Creation and implementation of a monitoring plan that includes for-cause and not-for-cause auditing is extremely important to a successful HRPP. In most institutions, both the IRB and HRPP leadership have the authority to request an audit for any reason; however, most for-cause audits are requested as follow-up to a self-report of noncompliance or complaint from a subject or colleague. No monitoring plan is complete without a not-for-cause arm to encourage and educate investigators. A not-for-cause audit plan should be the result of risk prioritization and might include auditing of new investigators and high-risk FDA-regulated research among others. Regardless of the reason for an audit, the auditing process should include careful review of the conduct of research: compliance with protocol requirements such as eligibility criteria, documentation of informed consent process including signatures and dates, obtaining of HIPAA authorization when required, and compliance with specific IRB requests.

### 4.5.2 Appropriate IRB Actions

Once noncompliance has been identified, it should be reported to the IRB per institutional policy. Most institutions require reporting within 5–10 days of discovery and review by the IRB soon after. The IRB should be provided with as much information about the incident as possible, such as scope of the noncompliance, number of subjects affected, any anticipated effect on data integrity, and proposed corrective and preventative actions. Most preventative action plans should include a plan for educating and re-training of the study team.

During review, the IRB is required to determine whether the incident represents serious and/or continuing noncompliance. Serious noncompliance may include incidents that place subjects at risk, or which have an adverse effect on subject's rights or welfare. Continuing noncompliance is that which continues even after discovery and initial attempts to address the issue. Regardless of the seriousness of the noncompliance, the IRB has several options for addressing noncompliance:

- Additional training: The IRB may require that investigators and study staff be provided specific training by IRB staff or via online educational modules to ensure understanding of regulations and research requirements.
- Auditing: As mentioned above, instances of noncompliance may lead the IRB to request for-cause audits to ensure reeducation has been successful and noncompliance is not continuing.
- Suspension of research: If subjects are placed at additional risk, the IRB can temporarily suspend the research until the noncompliance has been appropriately addressed. Suspensions can take almost any form, from suspension to further enrollment of subjects to full suspension of the research, at the IRB's discretion.
- Termination of research: If noncompliance reaches a level at which continuation of the research is no longer safe for subjects or the institution, the IRB can take the drastic step of permanently discontinuing the research.

Regardless of how noncompliance is identified and addressed, a review of such incidents remains one of the IRB's most important functions and a major component of a successful HRPP.

## 5. CURRENT INFLUENCES SHAPING THE FUTURE OF HUMAN RESEARCH SUBJECT PROTECTION

What comes next for human research protections will emerge from a complex set of activities: changing regulations, innovations by HRPPs within the regulations, and changes in the complexity and organization of research and the research community. Two trends that will clearly set the future of human subject protections are flexibility and collaborative IRB review.

### 5.1 Flexibility

HRPPs across the nation and world are currently addressing issues that will shape the future of human subject research protections well into the future. In July of 2011, the DHHS and OHRP published in the Federal Register an advance notice of proposed rulemaking (ANPRM) titled "Human Subjects Research Protections: Enhancing Protections for Research Subjects and Reducing Burden, Delay, and Ambiguity for Investigators." This proposed change to the common rule was both a reflection of, and stimulant for, a discussion already underway within the research community on how to enhance protections to subjects while reducing the burdens on researchers and the IRB. As of this writing, there is no reliable information as to what, if anything, will happen with the effort to revise the common rule. Research institutions, however, are not waiting for OHRP to act—they are actively rethinking their practices and introducing "flexibility" into their policies and procedures. This movement has matured enough to foster the development of a "Flexibility Coalition" composed of institutional representatives from universities, academic medical centers, hospitals, independent IRBs, and research institutes (http://oprs.usc.edu/initiatives/flex/). While what this means in practice varies from institution to institution, some common themes are identified below.

### 5.1.1 Approval Period

A common example of this flexibility is the granting of two or even three years, rather than one year, for approval to non-federally funded or regulated minimal risk studies. Most institutions that do this have also implemented a monitoring program to ensure that there are no "false positives," or projects awarded multiyear approvals, but are by regulations eligible for only one-year approvals.

### 5.1.2 Expanded Exempt Eligibility

While the common rule only identifies the seven categories of exempt research listed above, some institutions are expanding beyond this list the range of studies eligible for exemption from IRB review—as long as they are not federally funded or regulated, of course. Under this model, some studies reviewed by expedited means under the common rule can be determined to be exempt. Examples include:

* The common rule limits category four exemptions to studies using data that are in existence at the time of the IRB submission, as long as it was collected for purposes other than research and the data will be recorded in a manner that excludes any direct or indirect identifiers. Some institutions are expanding this to include data that is in existence at the time of the data extraction rather than IRB submission, as long as the other two conditions exist and the research is not federally funded or regulated.
* Subpart D of the common rule addresses special protections for the involvement of minors in research and prohibits the application of category two exemptions (see above) for studies involving minors "except for research involving observation of public behavior when the investigator(s) do not participate in the activities being observed." Institutions are permitting, again only for non-federally funded or regulated studies, the use of this exemption for a wide variety of research involving minors in online surveys, focus groups, and interviews, as long as identifiable information is not obtained or any disclosure would not result in reputational or other harm.

The impact of these and other "flexibility" practices should not be underestimated. For any university, these kinds of studies constitute a significant proportion of HRPP's portfolio, and the implementation of such flexibility practices may permit the HRPP to focus its effort on the studies with the greatest risks to subjects. A comparison with a change introduced over a decade ago may be illustrative. The National Institutes of Health (NIH) used to require grant applications involving human subject research to have IRB approval prior to review by a study section to determine merit and fundability. This meant that researcher and IRB time and resources were committed to the review of 100% of the submission, but less than 20% of the research was ever funded, resulting in a tremendous dedication of resources to protect subjects who may never be recruited because the projects were not conducted. There was an imbalance between effort and risks.

The flexibility initiatives described above as well as others emerging every day similarly seek to align effort and risk to permit less focus where there is less risk and greater focus where there is greater risk.

## 5.2 Collaborative IRB Review

The combined influence of limited resources and desire to reduce barriers has led investigators, institutions, and sponsors to seek efficiencies, and many are focusing on collaborations between IRBs to provide them. More and more, institutions involved in multisite research are being asked to use a single IRB model in which sites defer IRB review to one IRB that provides oversight for all sites. Single IRB review eliminates the need for each site to conduct their own IRB review, decreasing inconsistencies between sites and decreasing overall review time. While most IRB leaders agree that single IRB review is advantageous in theory, implementing a single review mechanism can be a lengthy, resource-intensive, and often frustrating process. The process begins with forging of relationships across institutions, as IRB leaders learn about each other's processes. Initial barriers often include concerns about quality of review, knowledge of local contexts, and questions of legal liability [18]. Once trust is established and leaders are comfortable with the idea of accepting the review of external IRBs, institutional agreements are required. OHRP guidance currently requires institutions to enter into agreements outlining the responsibility of each party when IRB review is deferred. These contracts require institutions to agree, at least in principle, on subjective process requirements such as review of adverse events, required informed consent language, communication of problems among parties, appropriate recruitment methods, and reporting responsibilities. Successful collaborations between IRBs are the result of months of planning and strong communication between parties, and the advantages they provide can far outweigh the challenges of implementation. These advantages are leading industry and federal sponsors to encourage single IRB review. In fact, many NIH grant applications now require certification from the applicants that collaborative IRB review models will be considered if the grant is awarded. Some programs are even conditioning membership on acceptance of single IRB review, like the National Cancer Institute's central IRB (https://ncicirb.org/cirb/default.action) and the newly established NeuroNEXT program (http://www.neuronext.org/), which has become the industry standard for IRB collaboration across institutions.

Other trends that will impact the future of human subject protections are less clear. There is, for instance, a newly regenerated push to harmonize the regulations, including, most prominently, those of OHRP and the FDA [19]. While there exists more than a little overlap between each of these agencies' regulations, there are also important and significant differences that have complicated the conduct and oversight of such research. That these two agencies are both a part of the same federal department, DHHS, has only made the differences more apparent and harder to justify. The conversation, however, has returned to harmonization of regulations between these two, and other, sets of regulations.

There will most certainly be changes in the years to come with respect to how researchers and institutions enroll and protect individuals who agree to participate in their research; changes that today we cannot even begin to imagine. The three principles (respect for persons, beneficence, and justice) and three guidelines (informed consent, assessment of risk and benefit, and equity subject selection) identified and articulated in the Belmont Report will, nonetheless, continue to frame their principles, policies, and procedures. While the specific form they take and the way that they are implemented may change, they will surely remain guiding principles in the conduct and oversight of human subject research.

## References

[1] Jones JH. Bad blood: the Tuskegee syphilis experiment. New York: Free Press; 1981.

[2] Jones JH. Bad blood: the Tuskegee syphilis experiment—new and expanded edition. New York: The Free Press; 1993.

[3] Reverby S. Examining Tuskegee: the infamous syphilis study and its legacy. Chapel Hill: University of North Carolina Press; 2009.

[4] Office of the Secretary of Department of Health, Education and Welfare. Ethical principles and guidelines for the protection of human subjects of research. The national commission for the protection of human subjects of biomedical and behavioral research. Washington, DC: U.S. Government Printing Press; 1979.

[5] Childress JF, Meslin EM, Shapiro HT, editors. Belmont revisited: ethical principles for research with human subjects. Washington, DC: Georgetown Universit Press; 2014.

[6] Hornblum AM. Acres of skin: human experiments at Holmsburg prison: a true story of abuse and exploitation in the name of medical science. New York: Routledge; 1998.

[7] Lederer SE. Subjected to science: human experimentation in America before the second world war. Baltimore: Johns Hopkins University Press; 1997.

[8] Shamoo AE, Resnik D. Responsible conduct of research. New York: Oxford University Press; 2009.

[9] Lifton RJ. The Nazi doctors: medical killing and the psychology of genocide. New York: Basic Books; 1986.

[10] Annas G, Grodin MA, editors. The Nazi doctors and the nuremberg code: human rights in human experimentation. New York: Oxford University Press; 1995.

[11] Shuster E. Fifty years later: the significance of the nuremberg code. N Engl J Med 1997;1997(337):1436–40.

[12] Emanuel EJ. Reconsidering the Declaration of Helsinki. Lancet 2013;381:1532–3.

[13] Association for the Accreditation of Human Research Protection Programs (AAHRPP). http://www.aahrpp.org/learn/accreditation/goals-principles-standards [accessed 05.14].

[14] Beauchamp TL, Childress J. Principles of biomedical research. 7th ed. New York: Oxford University Press; 2012.

[15] Henley, L What is an investigational device exemption? U.S. Food and Drug Administration, http://www.fda.gov/downloads/Training/CDRHLearn/UCM293098.pdf.

[16] Department of Health and Human Services (DHHS). Understanding health information privacy. http://www.hhs.gov/ocr/privacy/hipaa/understanding/ [accessed 05.14].

[17] Centers for Disease Control and Prevention (CDC). Distinguishing public health research and public health nonresearch. Atlanta, GA: CDC; 2010.

[18] Flynn KE, Hahn CL, Kramer JM, Check DK, Dombeck CB, Bang S, et al. Using central IRBs for multicenter clinical trials in the United States. PLoS One 2013;8:e54999.

[19] Evans BJ, Meslin EM. Encouraging translational research through harmonization of FDA and common rule informed consent requirements for research with banked specimens. J Legal Med 2006;27:119–66.

# Investigational New Drug and Device Exemption Process

*Dennis P. Swanson*

University of Pittsburgh, Pittsburgh, PA, USA

## 1. INTRODUCTION

The US Food and Drug Administration (FDA) oversees the clinical translation and final approval, for commercial marketing, of investigational drug (including biological) products and medical devices intended for human or animal use. As defined in the Federal Food, Drug and Cosmetic Act:

- A drug is any article intended for use in the diagnosis, cure, mitigation, prevention, or treatment of a disease in man or animals, including articles (other than food) intended to affect the structure or function of the body of man or animals.
- A device is an instrument, apparatus, implement, machine, in vitro reagent, or similar article intended for use in the diagnosis, cure, mitigation, prevention, or treatment of a disease in man or animals. A device must not achieve its principle intended purpose through chemical action within the body or by being metabolized.

The jurisdiction of the FDA also includes the oversight of food products (except meats and poultry) for human consumption, animal feeds and drugs, radiation-emitting products for consumer or occupational use, and cosmetics.

## 2. HISTORICAL PERSPECTIVES [1]

The FDA's oversight of drug products and medical devices has evolved and expanded over many years, primarily as a result of identified or reported hazards and safety concerns. The following discussion focuses on major congressional actions and events that have led to the FDA's current regulatory jurisdiction over drugs, biologics, and medical devices.

*Research Regulatory Compliance*
http://dx.doi.org/10.1016/B978-0-12-420058-6.00002-2

Prior to the early 1900s, the states predominantly assumed control over domestically produced food and drugs, with federal oversight being limited to respective imported products. As might be anticipated, such state-by-state oversight was inconsistent, and the adulteration and misbranding of foods and drugs were prevalent. In recognition of such, Congress passed the Food and Drugs Act in 1906. This act, which was initially administered by the Bureau of Chemistry, prohibited the interstate transport of adulterated or misbranded foods and drugs. For drug products, the act focused primarily on the regulation of appropriate drug standards and product labeling. Drug products were required to meet standards of identity, strength, quality, and purity as defined in the *United States Pharmacopeia* and *National Formulary*, unless variations from these standards were clearly stated on the product label. In 1912, the Food and Drugs Act was amended (Sherley Amendment) to prohibit the labeling of drug products with false therapeutic claims intended to defraud the consumer; however, federal oversight of this standard was difficult to enforce. There was no requirement, under this act, for federal approval of a drug product prior to its distribution in the commercial market. In 1927, the Bureau of Chemistry was reorganized into two separate entities, with regulatory functions being assumed by the Food, Drug and Insecticide Administration, which three years later became known as simply the Food and Drug Administration.

As a result of continuing false therapeutic claims and safety issues, Congress approved, in 1938, a new bill entitled the Food, Drug and Cosmetic Act (FD&C Act). A primary impetus for the passage of this new act was the death of more than 100 people, many of whom were children, from a marketed sulfanilamide "elixir" that contained an untested, highly toxic solvent similar to ethylene glycol (antifreeze). A key feature of this new law was a requirement for premarket approval of all new drugs by the FDA, based on data submitted by the manufacturer proving that the drug was safe. While the FD&C Act did not initially require, as a condition for premarket approval, the submission of data demonstrating effectiveness of the drug product, it did strengthen the FDA's oversight of false therapeutic claims by removing the requirement to prove "intent to defraud" in misbranding cases. The FD&C Act also required that drugs be labeled with adequate directions for safe use. In addition, it brought medical devices and cosmetics under the control of the FDA, authorized inspections of factories involved in the manufacture of drug products, and added court injunctions to the other processes (e.g., seizures, prosecutions) available for FDA's enforcement of the act.

In 1951, the FD&C Act was amended (Durham–Humphrey Amendment) to define drug products that could or could not be safely used in the absence of medical supervision, thereby creating two classes of drug products, prescription drugs and over-the-counter drugs. Following the 1962 thalidomide tragedy in Europe, during which thousands of children were born with birth defects associated with their mother's use of this new sedative, Congress amended (Kefauver–Harris Amendment) the FD&C Act to require that drug manufacturers prove both the safety and effectiveness of drug products as a condition for their approval for commercial marketing. This amendment also required the agency to assess the effectiveness of all drug products introduced into the commercial market since 1938. The amendment established good manufacturing practice standards for the drug industry and granted the FDA greater access to company production and control records to verify compliance with these standards. In addition, the amendment mandated the informed consent of individuals who participate in clinical trials of investigational drug products.

In 1972, the regulation of biologics, including serums, vaccines, and blood products, was transferred from the National Institutes of Health to the FDA. In 1976, the FD&C Act was once again amended (Medical Device Amendments) to provide assurance that medical devices introduced into the commercial market were also both safe and effective. Medical device manufacturers were now required to register with the FDA and comply with device-specific good manufacturing practice standards. Depending on the risk of the medical device, it must be either prior approved by the FDA for commercial marketing (i.e., for higher-risk devices) or must meet certain general performance standards (i.e., for lower-risk devices). In 1994, Congress passed the Dietary Supplement Health and Education Act, which defined "dietary supplements" and classified them as a "food." This act also established labeling requirements for dietary supplements and authorized the FDA to affect good manufacturing practice standards for such products.

# 3. RELEVANT REGULATORY/OVERSIGHT AGENCIES, REGULATIONS, AND GUIDANCE DOCUMENTS

The FDA oversees the clinical translation and final approval, for commercial marketing, of investigational drug (including biological) products and medical devices intended for human use. FDA regulations governing these processes are published under Title 21 of the Code of Federal Regulations (i.e., 21 CFR). These regulations and related FDA guidance documents may be accessed via the FDA's website at www.fda.gov.

## 3.1 Drugs and Biologics

### 3.1.1 Responsible Food and Drug Administration Entities

Within the FDA, the clinical investigation and the approval, for commercial marketing, of drugs and biologics are overseen by the Center for Drug Evaluation and Research (CDER) and the Center for Biologics Evaluation and Research (CBER), respectively. Each of these centers incorporates various offices (Tables 1 and 2) for the initial and ongoing review of investigational drug products involved in various stages of clinical translation and also offices that address compliance with applicable FDA regulations and IND commitments.

### 3.1.2 Requirements for the Submission of an Investigational New Drug Application

The use or the evaluation (for safety and/or effectiveness) of a non-FDA-approved drug or biologic in a clinical (human) research study generally requires the prior submission and FDA-acceptance of an investigational new drug (IND) application. FDA procedures and requirements governing the use of INDs, including procedures and requirements associated with the submission and FDA review of IND applications and the responsibilities of IND sponsors and investigators are addressed under 21 CFR part 312, *Investigational New Drug Application*.

As addressed within these FDA regulations, there are exceptions to the requirement for the submission of an IND application for human research studies involving certain types of products that meet, or would seem to meet, the definition of a "drug" product.

TABLE 1   Review Offices–Center for Drug Evaluation and Research [2]

**Office of antimicrobial drug products**

*OFFICE OF DRUG EVALUATION I*

Division of Cardiovascular and Renal Products

Division of Neurology Products

Division of Psychiatry Products

*OFFICE OF DRUG EVALUATION II*

Division of Anesthetic, Analgesic and Addiction Products

Division of Metabolism and Endocrinology Products

Division of Pulmonary, Allergy and Rheumatology Products

*OFFICE OF DRUG EVALUATION III*

Division of Dermatology and Dental Products

Division of Gastroenterology and Inborn Errors Products

Division of Bone, Reproductive and Urologic Products

*OFFICE OF DRUG EVALUATION IV*

Division of Medical Imaging Products

Office of Hematology/Oncology Drug Products


TABLE 2   Review Offices–Center for Biologics Evaluation and Research [3]

Office of Vaccines Research and Review

Office of Blood Research and Review

Office of Cellular, Tissue and Gene Therapy


- In accordance with the IND regulations at 21 CFR 312.2(b), clinical studies directed at the evaluation or use of an FDA-approved drug for an "off-label" indication (i.e., a clinical indication that is not currently specified in the FDA-approved product labeling) are exempt from the requirement for the submission of an IND application if the study meets each of the following criteria:
    - It is not intended to support FDA approval of a new indication or a significant change in the product labeling.
    - It is not intended to support a significant change in the advertising for the drug product.
    - It does not involve a route of administration or dosage level or use in a patient population or other factor that significantly increases the risks (or decreases the acceptability of the risks) associated with the use of the drug product.

- It is conducted in compliance with institutional review board (IRB) and informed consent regulations set forth in 21 CFR parts 50 and 56 (more information about the IRB approval process is provided in Chapter 1, Human Subjects).
- It is conducted in compliance with 21 CFR 312.7, which addresses promotion and charging for investigational drugs.

Other products that are listed under this section of the FDA regulations as being exempt from the submission of an IND application include in vitro diagnostic biologic products (blood grouping serum, reagent red blood cells, antihuman globulin) that are intended to be used in a diagnostic procedure that confirms the diagnosis made by another, medically established, diagnostic product or procedure; drugs intended solely for tests in vitro or in laboratory animals; and placebos.

- Subject to the provisions of the Dietary Supplement Health and Information Act of 1994, dietary supplements are regulated as "foods" and are therefore exempt from the regulations governing a "drug" product, provided that they are labeled or being investigated for intended use in affecting the structure or function of the body (i.e., a structure or function claim). However, the labeling or the evaluation, in a human research study, of a dietary supplement for the diagnosis, prevention, mitigation, treatment, or cure of a certain disease (i.e., a disease claim) causes the supplement to fall under the definition of a "drug" and requires the submission and FDA-acceptance of a corresponding IND application.
- Certain human cells, tissues, and cellular- and tissue-based products (HCT/Ps) are regulated solely under section 361 of the Public Health Service Act. As such, they are not regulated as "drug" products, and therefore their evaluation or use in a human research study does not require the submission of an IND application. To qualify for this exemption, the HCT/P must meet each of the following criteria [4]:
  - Minimal manipulation of the HCT/P is required for its clinical use or clinical research use or evaluation.
  - The HCT/P is intended for homologous use (i.e., a use that is the same as its natural use).
  - The HCT/P is not combined with another article, except water, crystalloids, or a sterilizing, storage, or preserving agent that does not, in itself, raise safety concerns.
  - Either the HCT/P (1) does not have a systemic effect and is not dependent on metabolic activity; or (2) the HCT/P is for autologous use, for allogeneic use in a first- or second-degree blood relative, or for reproductive use.

Entities involved in the clinical use or investigation of HCT/Ps are required to register with the FDA and provide a listing of the respective products.

- Clinical investigations involving nonapproved radioactive drugs for certain, basic research uses do not require the submission of an IND application provided that:
  - The research study is intended to obtain basic information regarding the metabolism or kinetics of the radioactive drug or regarding human physiology, pathophysiology, or biochemistry, but *not* intended for immediate therapeutic, diagnostic, or similar purposes or to determine the safety and/or effectiveness of the radioactive drug for such purposes.

- The radioactive drug/clinical investigation is prospectively approved by an institutional Radioactive Drug Research Committee (RDRC) that functions in accordance with the corresponding FDA regulations at 21 CFR 361.1. For an RDRC to approve a research study under these regulations, it must meet the following, fundamental requirements (and also several, additional specific requirements): (1) the mass of the radioactive drug to be administered must be known to not cause any clinically detectable pharmacological effect in humans based on data available from published literature or other valid human studies; (2) the total radiation dose that an individual will receive from participation in the study is the smallest radiation dose practical to perform the study and within the limits specified in the regulation; and (3) the study is approved by an IRB and is compliant with the requirements for informed consent. More information about the IRB approval process is provided in Chapter 1, Human Subjects. The RDRC approval process is discussed in more detail in Chapter 5, Radiological Hazards and Lasers.

Although substances labeled with "cold" (i.e., nonradioactive) isotopes are not technically covered by these regulations, the FDA has issued guidance specifying that the submission of an IND application is not required for basic research studies involving the use of such substances if they meet the same general regulatory requirements (i.e., with obviously the exception of the radiation dose limits) [5].

Sponsors of IND applications are required to wait for 30 days following the FDA's receipt of the application before commencing the incorporated clinical trial(s). Typically, the agency will respond to the sponsor within this 30-day interval; however if no FDA response is received, the sponsor may proceed to initiate the clinical trial (i.e., provided it has been approved by an acceptable IRB). Should the FDA identify significant concerns during its review of the IND application, it will issue a "clinical hold" notification, which, as the name implies, requires the sponsor to delay (or terminate) clinical trial initiation until the agency's concerns are adequately addressed.

### 3.1.3 *Components of an IND Application [6]*

The major components of an IND application include:

- Cover sheet (i.e., completed and signed Form FDA 1571, *Investigational New Drug*)
- Introductory statement and general investigational plan
  - The introductory statement should address the name of investigational drug (and, if applicable, other active drugs in the drug product) and its pharmacological class and structural formula (if known), the dosage form of the drug product, and the proposed route of administration of the drug product. The introductory statement should also summarize any prior human experience (i.e., in any country) with the investigational drug and address if it has previously been withdrawn from investigation or marketing.
  - The general investigational plan should briefly describe the rationale for the investigational drug or proposed human study, the clinical indication(s) that will be evaluated, the kinds of clinical trials that are planned for the first year, the number of research subjects that will be enrolled into these clinical trials, and anticipated risks.
- Investigator's brochure, to contain the following information:
  - A brief description of the drug substance and the formulation, including the structural formula, if known.
  - A summary of the pharmacological and toxicological effects of the drug in animals and, to the extent known, in humans.

- A summary of the pharmacokinetics and biological disposition of the drug in animals and, if known, in humans.
- A summary of information relating to the safety and efficacy of the drug in humans obtained from prior clinical studies.
- A description of possible risks and side effects to be anticipated based on prior experience with the drug under investigation or related drugs and of precautions or special monitoring to be done as part of the investigational use of the drug.
- Clinical trial protocol
  - Phase 1: Initial introduction of an investigational drug into humans. May involve patients or normal volunteers. Designed to determine the pharmacokinetics and pharmacologic actions of the drug, the side effects associated with increasing doses, and (if possible) gain early evidence on effectiveness. Also include human studies of drug metabolism, structure–activity relationships, and mechanism of action as well as studies in which unapproved drugs are used as research tools to explore biological phenomena or disease processes.
  - Phase 2: Controlled studies to evaluate the effectiveness of the drug for a particular indication or indications in patients with the respective disease or condition and to determine the common short-term side effects and risks of the drug.
  - Phase 3: Expanded controlled and uncontrolled evaluations of the drug to obtain additional information about its safety and effectiveness, so as to permit an overall evaluation of the benefit-to-risk relationship of the drug and to provide an adequate basis for product labeling.
  - Phase 4: Human studies conducted following FDA approval to market the drug commercially. May include additional surveillance studies mandated by the FDA as a condition of approval or, for example, studies involving pediatric or elderly patients or new clinical indications.
- Chemistry, manufacturing and (quality) control information
- Labeling
- Pharmacology and toxicology information
- Previous human experience with the investigational drug
- Additional information
  - To include, if applicable, information related to special topics such as drug dependence and abuse potential, radioactive drugs, and pediatric studies.
- FDA requested information
  - To include, if applicable, information requested by the FDA subsequent to a pre-IND meeting.

### 3.1.4 Manufacturing and Labeling Requirements

Investigational drugs and biologics being used or evaluated in phase 2 or 3 clinical trials are required to be manufactured and labeled in compliance with the FDA's current good manufacturing practice (cGMP) regulations at 21 CFR parts 210 and 211. For phase 1 (including phase 0) clinical trials, FDA regulations specify that the investigational drug or biologic must be manufactured in accordance with the principles of cGMP; however strict compliance with the FDA's cGMP regulations at 21 CFR part 211 is not required [7]. Rather, under this scenario, the FDA will oversee the manufacture and labeling of the investigational drug or biologic in accordance with respective procedures and statements contained within the submitted IND application [8].

### 3.1.5 Good Clinical Laboratory Practice Requirements for Supporting Nonclinical Safety Data

Nonclinical (i.e., laboratory or animal) safety studies, performed in support of the submission of an IND application, are required to be conducted in compliance with the FDA's current good laboratory practice (GLP) regulations at 21 CFR part 58. Note that nonclinical studies directed at evaluating the effectiveness of the investigational drug or biologic are *not* required to be conducted in compliance with these GLP regulations. Investigational drugs and biologics used for GLP-compliant safety studies must be well characterized with regard to their identity, strength, quality, and purity; however, they are not required to be manufactured in strict compliance with the previously discussed cGMP regulations. The FDA's cGLP regulations incorporate extensive validation requirements and laboratory controls, and as a result, nonclinical studies subject to these regulations are typically conducted at contract facilities that specialize in their performance. The costs associated with the conduct of cGLP-compliant, nonclinical safety studies typically represent the greatest expense associated with the initial submission of an IND application. It is thus recommended that, in the absence of an applicable (i.e., related to the class of drug under development) FDA guidance document, the nature and scope of the preclinical safety studies required for FDA acceptance of an IND application be prior discussed with the agency via the pre-IND process to include, if applicable, a discussion of the potential acceptability of existing nonclinical safety data that were not collected in strict compliance with the GLP regulations.

### 3.1.6 Good Clinical Practice Requirements

IND sponsors and study site investigators, who are involved in the performance of clinical trials being conducted under an FDA-accepted IND application, are required to comply with the good clinical practice (GCP) guidelines of the International Commission on Harmonization (ICH) [9]. These GCP guidelines represent an international ethical and scientific quality standard for designing, conducting, recording, and reporting investigations that involve the participation of human subjects. Compliance with these guidelines provides public assurance that the rights, safety, and well-being of research participants are protected and that the resulting clinical trial data are credible. Adherence to the GCP guidelines, which have been adopted by the FDA, is subject to audit by the agency. Prior to initiation of a clinical trial, study site investigators are also required to obtain the approval of an IRB that operates in compliance with the FDA's regulations at 21 CFR part 56. Informed consent of the study participants must be obtained in compliance with the FDA regulations at 21 CFR part 50.

### 3.1.7 Food and Drug Administration Guidance Documents

CDER and CBER have published numerous guidance documents (Table 3) related to the IND submission process, many of which are related to IND requirements associated with specific diseases or conditions or with specific classes of drug or biological products. FDA guidance documents may be readily searched and accessed via the FDA website at www.fda.gov.

### 3.1.8 Food and Drug Administration Approval for Commercial Marketing

FDA approves drug and biologic products for commercial marketing based on data, collected under an FDA-accepted IND application, which demonstrate that the drug is safe and effective at the recommended dosage and for the clinical indication(s) specified in the proposed product

TABLE 3    Pertinent Investigational Drug and Biologic Guidance Documents

- *Guidance for Clinical Investigators, Sponsors and IRBs: Investigational New Drug Applications (INDs)—Determining Whether Human Research Studies Can Be Conducted Without an IND, September, 2013.*
- *Guidance for Industry: IND Exemptions for Studies of Lawfully Marketed Drug or Biological Products for the Treatment of Cancer, January, 2004.*
- *Guidance for Industry: Content and Format of Investigational New Drug Applications (INDs) for Phase 1 Studies of Drugs, Including Well-Characterized, Therapeutic Biotechnology Derived Products, November, 1995*
- *Information Sheet Guidance for Sponsors, Clinical Investigators, and IRBs: Frequently Asked Questions—Statement of Investigator, May, 2010*
- *Guidance for Industry: Exploratory IND Studies, January, 2006*
- *Guidance for Industry: Expanded Access to Investigational Drugs for Treatment Use—Qs & As, May, 2013*
- *Guidance for Industry: CGMP for Phase 1 Investigational Drugs, July, 2008*
- *Guidance for Industry: INDs for Phase 2 and Phase 3 Studies—Chemistry, Manufacturing and Controls Information, May, 2003*
- *Guidance for Industry: M3(R2) Nonclinical Safety Studies for the Conduct of Human Clinical Trials and Marketing Authorization for Pharmaceuticals, January, 2010*
- *Guidance for Industry: Good Laboratory Practices—Questions and Answers, July, 2007*
- *Guidance for Industry: E6 Good Clinical Practice—Consolidated Guidance, April, 1996*
- *Guidance for Industry: Investigator Responsibilities—Protecting the Rights, Safety, and Welfare of Study Subjects, October, 2009*
- *Draft Guidance for Industry: Charging for Investigational Drugs Under an IND—Qs & As, May, 2013*
- *Guidance for Industry: Formal Meetings with Sponsors and Applicants for PDUFA Products, February, 2000*
- *Guidance for Industry: IND Meetings for Human Drugs and Biologics—Chemistry, Manufacturing and Controls Information, May, 2001*
- *Claims That Can Be Made for Conventional Foods and Dietary Supplements—Office Nutritional Products, Labeling, and Dietary Supplements, March, 2007.*
- *Guidance for Industry: Structure/Function Claims (dietary supplements)—Small Entity Compliance Guide, March, 2007.*
- *Guidance for Industry: Botanical Drug Products, June, 2004.*
- *Guidance for Industry and FDA Staff: Minimal Manipulation of Structural Tissue (i.e., human cells, tissues and cellular and tissue-based products)—Jurisdictional Update, August, 2008.*
- *Guidance for Industry and Researchers: The Radioactive Drug Research Committee—Human Research Without an Investigational New Drug Application, August, 2010.*
- *Guidance for Industry: Investigator Responsibilities—Protecting the Rights, Safety, and Welfare of Study Subjects, October, 2009.*

labeling. In the case of drug products, these data are submitted to the agency in the form of a new drug application (NDA). For biologic products, the data are submitted in the form of a biologic licensing application (BLA). Following the expiration of patent and/or market exclusivity rights, an abbreviated new drug application (ANDA) may be submitted to the FDA to obtain approval to commercially market a generic version of a currently marketed drug product. FDA approval of an ANDA is based primarily on the sponsor demonstrating bioequivalence to the innovator drug. An abbreviated BLA pathway has been established for the approval of generic biologic products, although there have been no generic biological products approved via this pathway to date.

## 3.2 Medical Devices

### 3.2.1 *Responsible Food and Drug Administration Entity*

The FDA entity responsible for the oversight of medical devices and their approval for commercial marketing is the Center for Devices and Radiological Health (CDRH).

TABLE 4    Review Offices—Center for Devices and Radiological Health [10]

**Office of Device Evaluation**

Division of Anesthesiology, General Hospital, Respiratory, Infection Control, and Dental Devices

Division of Cardiovascular Devices

Division of Ophthalmic and Ear, Nose, and Throat Devices

Division of Neurological and Physical Medicine Devices

Division of Orthopedic Devices

Division of Surgical Devices

Division of Reproductive, Gastro–Renal, and Urological Devices

**Office of In Vitro Diagnostics and Radiological Health**

Division of Chemistry and Toxicology Devices

Division of Immunology and Hematology Devices

Division of Microbiology Devices

Division of Radiological Health

Division of Mammography Quality Standards

CDRH incorporates two offices for the initial and ongoing review of investigational drug products (Table 4). It also has offices that oversee compliance with applicable FDA regulations and IDE commitments.

### 3.2.2 Investigational Device Exemption Applications

Notably, the FDA regulations that govern the submission of investigational device exemption (IDE) applications are not applicable to human research studies that involve only the use of a non-FDA-approved medical device [11]. However the evaluation, for safety and/ or effectiveness, of a nonapproved medical device in a clinical research study may require the submission and FDA acceptance of an IDE application if the reviewing IRB determines that the investigational device, or how it is being used in the study, constitutes a "significant risk device" study. The FDA's *Investigational Device Exemption* regulations at 21 CFR part 812 define a significant risk device as:

> an investigational device that (1) is intended as an implant and presents a potential for serious risk to the health, safety, or welfare of a subject; (2) is purported or represented to be for a use in supporting or sustaining human life and presents a potential for serious risk to the health, safety, or welfare of a subject; (3) is for a use of substantial importance in diagnosing, curing, mitigating, or treating disease, or otherwise preventing impairment of human health and presents a potential for serious risk to the health, safety, or welfare of a subject; or ($) otherwise presents a potential for serious risk to the health, safety, or welfare of a subject.

The submission and FDA-acceptance of an IDE application is not required for clinical research studies that have been determined by the reviewing IRB to be a nonsignificant risk device study (i.e., the study of a device that does not meet the definition of a significant risk device study). As per statements included in the FDA regulations at 21 CFR Sec. 812.2(b)(1), a nonsignificant risk device study is considered to already have an approved application for an IDE provided that the sponsor:

- labels the device in accordance with the IDE regulations (21 CFR Sec. 812.5);
- obtains approval of the study by an IRB that operates in compliance with the FDA's regulations at 21 CFR part 56 and that has reviewed the sponsor's justification as to why the device is not felt to be a significant risk device;
- obtains the informed consent of the study participants in compliance with the FDA regulations at 21 CFR part 50;
- monitors the research study in accordance with the FDA regulations at 21 CFR Sec. 812.46;
- maintains and ensures that study-site investigators maintain the records required at 21 CFR Sec 812.140 and Sec. 812.150;
- complies with the prohibitions against product promotion and other practices as addressed under 21 CFR Sec. 812.7.

The FDA regulations at 21 CFR 812.2(b) and (c) address certain categories of medical device studies that are exempt from the submission of an IDE application. Included in this category are clinical studies or comparisons of FDA-approved medical devices in which the devices are being studied for the indications specified in their FDA-approved product labeling. Clinical evaluations of the safety and effectiveness of an FDA-approved medical device for a new clinical indication (i.e., not specified in the current FDA-approved product labeling) are, however, subject to the IDE regulations and may require the submission of an IDE application based on the IRB's determination of their significant risk status. Clinical studies of in vitro diagnostic devices (IVDs) are exempt from the requirement for the submission of an IDE application provided that the IVD and its proposed evaluation meet all of the following criteria [12]:

- the IVD is labeled in accordance with the regulations at 21 CFR 809.10(c);
- the procedures associated with the use of IVD are noninvasive (with the exception of simple venipuncture);
- use of the IVD does not require an invasive sampling procedure (e.g., biopsy, use of general anesthesia, or placement of an arterial, femoral, subclavian, or iliac line or catheter) that presents significant risk;
- the IVD does not by design or intention introduce energy into a subject;
- the IVD is not used as a diagnostic procedure without confirmation of the diagnosis by another, medically established diagnostic product or procedure.

Other types of devices that are listed under Section 812.2(c) of the FDA regulations as being exempt from the submission of an IDE application include a device:

- undergoing commercial testing, testing of a modification, or testing of a combination or two or more devices in commercial distribution, if the testing does not put subjects at risk;
- intended solely for veterinary use or solely for research on or with laboratory animals and labeled in accordance with 21 CFR Sec 812.5(c); or

- that is a "custom device." A custom device is a device that deviates from an FDA-approved or approvable device to comply with the prescription order of an individual physician or dentist and is intended for use in an individual patient identified in this order. Custom devices are not generally available in finished form for purchase or for prescription use, and they cannot be offered for commercial distribution through labeling or advertising.

Sponsors of IDE applications are required to wait for 30 days following the FDA's receipt of the application before commencing the incorporated clinical investigation. Typically, the agency will respond to the sponsor within this 30-day interval; however, if no FDA response is received, the sponsor may proceed to initiate the clinical investigation (i.e., provided it has been approved by an acceptable IRB). Should the FDA identify significant concerns during its review of the IDE application, it will issue a "clinical hold" notification, which, as the name implies, requires the sponsor to delay (or terminate) the clinical investigation until the agency's concerns are adequately addressed.

### 3.2.3 Components of an IDE Application [13]

The major components of an IDE application include:

- Cover sheet, to include the name, address, and dated signature of the sponsor of the IDE application
- Overall clinical plan
  - The overall clinical plan should provide the descriptive title for each currently planned study of the investigational device and a summary of the study design, sample size, primary outcome measures, and expected principle results.
- Report of prior investigations of the device
  - This section of the IDE application should include reports of all prior laboratory, animal, and, if applicable, human testing of the investigational device. Each study should be summarized to include an adequate description of the study methods, outcome data, and relevant (i.e., safety and/or effectiveness) conclusions of the study.
- Investigational plan
  - Feasibility study: Directed at, or involving, an initial evaluation of the investigational device in humans, an evaluation of potential safety issues associated with the use of the device, an assessment of device design and/or certain human factors associated with the use of the device, or an evaluation of other device or device application characteristics.
  - Pilot study: Directed at obtaining preliminary data on which to base a subsequent pivotal study of the investigational device.
  - Pivotal study: The results of treatment or diagnosis with the investigational device are compared with a placebo, active treatment, or historical control in such a manner so as to permit a quantitative evaluation.
- Example: Investigator's agreement and certification of investigator agreements
  - All study site investigators are required to execute a written agreement specifying that they will comply with the investigator responsibilities incorporated under the IDE regulations (i.e., similar to a form FDA 1572 for investigators participating in IND studies). The IDE sponsor must certify that such a signed agreement will be obtained

from all investigators who are currently participating, or will participate, in clinical investigations of the device.
- Reviewing IRBs and other involved institutions
- Device charges
  - If applicable, the IDE sponsor must specify the amount that will be charged for the investigational device and provide an explanation of why such charges do not constitute commercialization of the device.
- Device labeling
- Consent materials
- Other relevant information
  - To include, if applicable, information requested by the FDA subsequent to a pre-IDE meeting.

### 3.2.4 *Manufacturing Requirements*

The manufacture and labeling of medical devices for human use must, with certain limited exceptions, be compliant with the FDA's cGMP regulations at 21 CFR part 820, titled *Quality System Regulation*. Of note, the manufacture of medical devices being evaluated under an IDE application is subject to compliance with only subpart C, Sec. 820.30 *Design Controls*, of these quality system regulations [14].

### 3.2.5 *Good Clinical Laboratory Practice Requirements for Supporting Nonclinical Data*

As with investigational drugs and biologics, nonclinical (i.e., laboratory or animal) safety studies conducted in support of an IDE application are subject to compliance with the FDA's current GLP regulations at 21 CFR part 58. Investigational devices used for GLP-compliant safety studies should be well characterized with regard to their design specifications.

### 3.2.6 *Good Clinical Practice Requirements*

There is no requirement, per se, for IDE sponsors and investigators involved in the conduct of medical device clinical trials to be compliant with the previously discussed ICH guidelines for good clinical practice. Rather, for medical device research, "good clinical practice" is interpreted as meaning compliance with the primary regulations addressed in the previous paragraphs and the FDA's conflict-of-interest regulations at 21 CFR part 54, *Financial Disclosure by Clinical Investigators* [15]. Also, as with investigational drugs, investigators involved in the conduct of medical device clinical trials are required to obtain the prospective approval of an IRB that operates in compliance with the FDA's regulations at 21 CFR part 56. Informed consent of the study participants must be obtained in compliance with the FDA regulations at 21 CFR part 50.

### 3.2.7 *Food and Drug Administration Guidance Documents*

CDRH has also published numerous guidance documents (Table 5) related to the clinical investigation and approval, for commercial marketing, of medical devices, and these guidance documents may be readily searched and accessed via the FDA website (www.fda.gov).

TABLE 5   Pertinent Investigational Medical Device Guidance Documents

- *Device Advice: Comprehensive Regulatory Assistance, http://www.fda.gov/medicaldevices/deviceregulationandguidance/default.htm*
- *Information Sheet Guidance for IRBs, Clinical Investigators and Sponsors: Significant Risk and Nonsignificant Risk Medical Device Studies, January, 2006*
- *Information Sheet Guidance for IRBs, Clinical Investigators and Sponsors: Frequently Asked Questions About Medical Devices, January, 2006*
- *Guidance for Industry, Clinical Investigators, Institutional Review Boards and Food and Drug Administration Staff: Design Considerations for Pivotal Clinical Investigations for Medical Devices, November, 2013*
- *Guidance for Industry and FDA Staff: in Vitro Diagnostic (IVD) Device Studies—Frequently Asked Questions, June, 2010*
- *Guidance for Industry and Food and Drug Administration Staff: Mobile Medical Applications, September, 2013.*
- *Guidance for Industry: Investigator Responsibilities—Protecting the Rights, Safety, and Welfare of Study Subjects, October, 2009.*
- *Guidance for Industry and Food and Drug Administration Staff: The 510k Program: Evaluating Substantial Equivalence in Premarket Notifications, July, 2014*

### 3.2.8 Food and Drug Administration Approval for Commercial Marketing [15]

The FDA approves medical devices for commercial marketing based on the sponsor's submission of a premarket notification (also known as a "510k") or a premarket approval (PMA) application. The regulatory "class" to which the medical device is assigned determines the type of application (i.e., 510k or PMA) that must be submitted to the agency. Class I medical devices have the lowest risk to the patient and/or user associated with their intended use and also with their labeled indications for use; whereas class III medical devices have the greatest, respective risks. If the medical device-of-interest (new device) is determined to be a class I or class II device, the submission and FDA acceptance of a 510k application is generally required to permit its commercial marketing (i.e., unless the medical device is also classified as being "exempt" from this submission and approval process). The submission and FDA-acceptance of a PMA is generally required to permit the commercial marketing of medical devices that are determined to fall under class III. FDA has established risk-based classifications for more than 17,000 medical devices and has grouped them into 16 medical specialties, referred to as "medical device classification panels," which are published in the FDA regulations at 21 CFR Parts 862–892. Within these panels are listings of applicable devices to include a general description of the device and its intended use, the risk classification (i.e., class I, class II, or class III) that has been assigned to device, and information about marketing requirements, including, if applicable, the conditions under which a class I or class II device may be considered exempt from the requirement to submit a 510k application. The information submitted to the FDA with a 510k application must demonstrate that the new device is "substantially equivalent" to a legally marketed device (i.e., a "predicate" device) that did not require the submission of a PMA for its approval (or that initially required the submission of a PMA, but was subsequently reclassified from class III to class II). A new device is considered to be substantially equivalent to a predicate device if it has the same intended use and technological characteristics as the predicate or if it has the same intended use as the predicate and different technological characteristics, and the information submitted to the FDA with the 510k application does not raise new questions of safety and effectiveness and demonstrates that the new device is at least as safe and effective as the predicate device. Thus, it is not necessary for the new device to be identical to the predicate device to obtain FDA approval of a 510k application; however, IRB-approved, clinical studies may be required to prove equivalent safety and effectiveness if they are not identical. Class III medical devices are those that support or sustain human life, are of substantial importance in preventing the impairment of human health, or which present a potential, unreasonable risk of illness or injury. For class III medical devices, the FDA has determined that the general controls (premarket notification, manufacturer registration and device listing) applied to class I and II medical devices are insufficient to assure their safety and effectiveness. Thus, FDA approval to commercially market a class III medical device is subject to the agency's review and acceptance of a PMA application, which must incorporate valid scientific data (typically collected under an IDE application) that demonstrate that the new device is safe and effective for its intended human use.

## 4. REGULATORY MANDATES

The FDA regulations that govern IND [16] and IDE [17] applications define the sponsor of the application as the individual or entity (e.g., company, governmental agency, academic organization, or other organization) who takes responsibility for and initiates the respective clinical investigation of the investigational drug or device. The sponsor does not actually conduct the investigation unless it is a sponsor–investigator application. An investigator is the individual who actually conducts the clinical investigation (i.e., under whose immediate direction the investigational drug or device is administered or dispensed to a subject) at a certain study site. In the event that a clinical investigation is conducted by a team of individuals, the investigator is the responsible leader of the team, with the other members being subinvestigators. A sponsor–investigator is an individual who both initiates and conducts a clinical investigation, and under whose immediate direction the investigational drug or device is administered or dispensed. Only an individual may be the sponsor–investigator of an IND or IDE application.

In addition to the previously addressed regulations that govern or are associated with submission of IND and IDE applications, sponsors and investigators are required to comply with certain, respective responsibilities that are defined within the IND [18] and IDE [19] regulations. Sponsor–investigators are required to comply with both of these sets of responsibilities.

### 4.1 Sponsor Responsibilities

Sponsors of IND or IDE applications are responsible for:

- Selecting appropriately qualified investigators and providing them with the information necessary to conduct the clinical investigation properly.
  - Before permitting an investigator to participate in a clinical investigation, the sponsor must obtain from the investigator a signed investigator's statement (form FDA 1572 for IND applications) or investigator's agreement (for IDE applications), curriculum vitae or other statement of qualifications, and financial disclosure information. Regarding the latter, the FDA regulations at 21 CFR part 54, *Financial Disclosure by Clinical Investigators*, require the IND or IDE sponsor to identify any substantially involved clinical investigator or subinvestigator who (or whose immediate family member) has, as defined within

these regulations, an equity interest, proprietary interest, or financial interest in the investigational drug or device or the company that owns the investigational drug or device being evaluated under the IND or IDE application. The sponsor is required to describe, in writing, any steps taken to minimize the potential for bias resulting from any of these disclosed financial conflicts-of-interest and to retain these documents on file subject to FDA review at the time of submission of an NDA, BLA, PMA, or 510k application to obtain approval to commercially market the drug or device.

- Before the clinical investigation commences, the IND or IDE sponsor is required to provide each study site investigator with a copy of the investigator's brochure (IND studies) or, at a minimum, the IRB-approved clinical protocol (for IND and IDE studies). An investigator's brochure is not required for single-site clinical investigations being conducted under a sponsor-investigator IND or IDE application [20].
- The IND or IDE sponsor must promptly inform investigators of serious and unexpected adverse events and/or other newly identified, significant risks felt to be related (or possibly related) to the investigational drug or device.

• Ensuring proper monitoring of the progress and conduct of the clinical investigation at each of the involved study sites.

- The sponsor is responsible for selecting an individual, qualified by training and experience, to monitor the clinical investigations being conducted under the FDA-accepted IND or IDE application.
- Sponsors are responsible for ensuring that the clinical investigation is being conducted in accordance with the clinical protocol contained within the FDA-accepted IND or IDE application. If it is discovered, through monitoring or other processes, that an investigator is not complying with the clinical protocol or applicable FDA or IRB requirements, the sponsor must promptly either secure compliance or terminate the investigator's participation in the investigation.

• Maintaining an up-to-date IND or IDE with regard to information concerning the pharmacology and safety of the investigational drug or device, the manufacture of the drug or device, and current or planned clinical investigations being conducted under the IND or IDE.

- The IND or IDE sponsor is required to review and evaluate evidence relating to the safety and effectiveness of the investigational drug or device as it is being obtained from the study site investigators. The sponsor is required to promptly report, to the FDA, serious and unexpected adverse events felt to be related to the investigational drug or device in accordance with the criteria and timelines specified in the IND and IDE regulations. Should it be determined that the investigational drug or device presents an unreasonable risk-to-benefit ratio for the clinical indication for which it is being evaluated, the sponsor must discontinue the respective clinical investigation(s), so notify the FDA, and so notify all involved IRBs and current and previously involved investigators.
- The IND or IDE sponsor is required to submit annual reports to the FDA summarizing the safety and efficacy data that have been accrued from ongoing clinical investigations of the investigational drug or device.
- The IND or IDE sponsor is required to submit clinical protocol modifications or new clinical protocols involving the investigational drug or device to the respective FDA-accepted IND or IDE application. As outlined in the IND and IDE regulations,

certain types of protocol modifications (e.g., modifications that affect the safety of the study participants) may require FDA notification (i.e., via the submission of a protocol amendment or supplemental IDE application) prior to implementing the modifications, whereas other types of modifications may be addressed in the annual report. New clinical protocols must be submitted to the IND or IDE application prior to their implementation. Sponsors must also update, in a timely manner, the FDA-accepted IND or IDE application with any new information related to the manufacture of the investigational drug or device or with pertinent safety or effectiveness information obtained from nonclinical studies.

- Ensuring accountability of the investigational drug or device.
  - The IND or IDE sponsor is required to maintain adequate records of the sponsor's receipt, shipment, or other disposition of the investigational drug or device.
  - The IND or IDE sponsor shall ensure that study site investigators have in place adequate records for investigational drug or device accountability and that supplies of the investigational drug or device are being stored in a secure manner in accordance with the sponsor's established storage conditions.
  - The IND or IDE sponsor shall ensure the return or other authorized disposition of remaining supplies of the investigational drug or device from each investigator whose participation in the respective clinical investigation has been completed or otherwise discontinued.
- Maintaining sponsor records and reports required under the regulations governing IND and IDE applications for the period specified in these regulations.
- Registering phase 2 and phase 3 clinical trials on the ClinicalTrials.gov database and submitting certification (form FDA 3671) of this registration to the FDA-accepted IND or IDE application [21].

## 4.2 Investigator Responsibilities

Investigators involved in the conduct of a clinical investigation under an FDA-accepted IND or IDE application are responsible for:

- Protecting the rights, safety, and welfare of research subjects.
  - The investigator must involve an IRB that complies with the FDA's regulations at 21 CFR Part 56 in the initial and continuing review and approval of the conduct of the clinical investigation at the investigator's study site.
  - The investigator must, in accordance with the FDA regulations at 21 CFR part 50, obtain the written informed consent of each human subject prior to his/her participation in any procedures being conducted for the purpose of the clinical investigation, unless the reviewing IRB approves a waiver or an exception from the requirement for written informed consent in accordance with the provisions of these regulations. The investigator is required to document the informed consent process (including the date and time that consent was obtained) in the case histories of the research subjects.
  - The investigator must promptly report unexpected adverse events that are related, or potentially related, to the investigational drug or device to the responsible IRB in accordance with IRB policies.

- Ensuring that the clinical investigation is being conducted in accordance with statements contained within the signed statement of investigator (form FDA 1572) or investigator's agreement.
  - Investigators are not permitted, in the absence of prior IRB approval, to deviate from the FDA-accepted and corresponding IRB-approved clinical protocol except when necessary to eliminate an apparent immediate hazard to the research subject(s).
  - Investigators are required to promptly report all changes in research activity (e.g., protocol deviations) and all unanticipated problems involving risks to human subjects or others to the responsible IRB.
- Ensuring control and accountability of the investigational drug or device.
  - The investigator must ensure that the investigational drug or device will be administered only to research subjects who are under the direct supervision of the investigator or under the supervision of a subinvestigator who is responsible to the investigator. The investigator must not supply the investigational drug or device to any person who is not authorized to receive it.
  - The investigator must maintain adequate records of investigational drug or device accountability, and must store supplies of the drug or device in a secure manner in accordance with the sponsor's established storage conditions. Upon completion or termination of the investigator's participation in the clinical investigation, unused supplies of the investigational drug or device must be returned to the sponsor or disposed of in accordance with the instructions of the sponsor.
- Submitting requested and required reports to the sponsor.
  - The investigator must prepare and maintain (i.e., for each research subject) adequate and accurate case histories that document all observations and other data pertinent to the evaluation of the investigational drug or device. Case histories include case report forms and respective supporting documents, such as signed and dated copies of source medical records.
  - The investigator must promptly report identified serious adverse events to the sponsor in accordance with the criteria specified by the sponsor.
  - The investigator must provide, in a timely manner, reports requested by the sponsor (e.g., progress reports, final report), including initial and routinely updated certifications and disclosures of the investigator's and subinvestigators' financial interest related to the drug or device under investigation.
- Maintaining investigator records and reports required under the regulations governing IND and IDE applications for the period specified in these regulations.

## 5. KEY PERSONNEL AND UNIVERSITY COMMITTEES DESIGNATED TO IMPLEMENT REGULATORY MANDATES

At most academic institutions, the entity responsible for ensuring compliance with the IND and IDE submission requirements will be the institution's responsible IRB. Some institutions have established specific offices to provide IND and IDE support to their faculty who are involved in this process. An example is the University of Pittsburgh's Office for Investigator-Sponsored IND and IDE Support (www.o3is.pitt.edu). Such support may also be provided by the institution's clinical and translational science institute or equivalent.

Depending on institutional policies, it may be a requirement that the institution be named as the sponsor of the IND or IDE application, on which the institution assumes the regulatory responsibilities of the sponsor. Alternately, the institution may require that the involved faculty member be designated as the sponsor-investigator or sponsor of the application.

## 6. COMMON COMPLIANCE CHALLENGES

Based on the author's experience, the most common compliance challenge for the sponsor of an IND or IDE application is in addressing the routine submission of the various reports and amendments (e.g., annual reports, safety reports, protocol amendments, information amendments, supplemental IDE applications) necessary to ensure an up-to-date application. The most common compliance challenge facing investigators are unauthorized deviations from the IRB-approved and FDA-accepted clinical protocol. The latter also becomes a compliance challenge for the IND or IDE sponsor, because it is a sponsor responsibility to routinely monitor the conduct of the clinical investigation at each study site and to take appropriate action when noncompliance with the clinical protocol is identified [22,23].

A protocol deviation refers to any unplanned instances of protocol noncompliance [24]. For example, situations in which the investigator failed to perform tests or examinations required by the protocol or failures on the part of the study subjects to complete scheduled visits as required by the protocol would be considered protocol deviations. In accordance with FDA [25] and IRB [26] regulations and statements contained within the investigator-signed form FDA 1572 or investigator's agreement [27], investigators are not permitted to deviate from the IRB-approved and FDA-accepted clinical protocol unless they have obtained prior authorization to do so from the reviewing IRB or the deviation is necessary to eliminate apparent immediate hazards to the human subject(s). As previously stated, investigators are required to promptly report to the responsible IRB all changes in research activity and all unanticipated problems involving risk to human subjects or others. Notably, the responsible IRB is subsequently required to submit all reports of unanticipated problems involving risks to human subjects or others to the responsible institutional official and to the FDA [28]. This would include reports of protocol deviations wherein the deviation (e.g., failure to perform a safety evaluation in accordance with approved clinical protocol) involves a risk to the study participant.

## 7. ADDRESSING NONCOMPLIANCE

Failure to submit the reports and protocol amendments required to maintain an up-to-date IND or IDE application should be corrected by the sponsor as soon as identified. For investigator noncompliance identified through investigator quality assurance efforts or sponsor monitoring, the investigator should ensure prompt reporting of such to the responsible IRB and to the sponsor (i.e., if not already involved). For sponsor or investigator noncompliance identified during an FDA audit, the involved agency inspector will issue a form FDA 483 with the identified items of noncompliance listed. The sponsor or investigator is instructed to respond to the form FDA 483 within a specific period (i.e. 15 days), and then the FDA's Office of Scientific Investigations will subsequently review the form FDA 483 observations, the sponsor's or investigator's response to these observations, and the inspector's establishment inspection report to determine whether additional action (e.g., issuance of an FDA warning letter) is warranted.

In responding to identified noncompliance, it should always be recognized that the IND or IDE sponsor or investigator is personally responsible for complying with applicable FDA regulations and responsibilities. It is not appropriate for the sponsor or investigator to place the blame for noncompliance on a subinvestigator, research coordinator, or other individual who is involved in the clinical investigation. For each identified item of noncompliance, the sponsor's or investigator's response should routinely include a summary of the sponsor's or investigator's conclusion, based on investigation, as to why the problem occurred and the steps or processes that have been subsequently put in place in an effort to prevent a recurrence of the problem.

## References

[1] http://www.fda.gov/AboutFDA/WhatWeDo/History/Origin/default.htm [accessed 20.11.13].
[2] http://www.fda.gov/AboutFDA/CentersOffices/OfficeofMedicalProductsandTobacco/CDER/ucm075128.htm [accessed 06.02.14].
[3] http://www.fda.gov/AboutFDA/CentersOffices/OrganizationCharts/ucm135943.htm [accessed 06.02.14].
[4] 21 CFR Part 1271, human cells, tissues, and cellular and tissue-based products, sec. 1271.10.
[5] Guidance for clinical investigators, sponsors and IRBs: investigational new drug applications (INDs)—determining whether human research studies can be conducted without an IND. U.S. Department of Health and Human Services, Food and Drug Administration; September 2013.
[6] 21 C.F.R. Part 312, investigational new drug application, sec. 312.23 IND content and format.
[7] 21 C.F.R. Part 210, current good manufacturing practice in manufacturing, processing, packing, or holding of drugs; general, sec. 210.2(c).
[8] Guidance for industry: CGMP for phase 1 investigational drugs. U.S. Department of Health and Human Services, Food and Drug Administration; July 2008.
[9] Guidance for industry: E6 good clinical practice—consolidated guidance. U.S. Department of Health and Human Services; April 1996.
[10] http://www.fda.gov/AboutFDA/CentersOffices/OfficeofMedicalProductsandTobacco/CDRH/CDRHoffices/ucm127854.htm [accessed 06.02.14].
[11] 21 C.F.R. Part 812, investigational device exemptions, sec. 812.2(a) general.
[12] 21 C.F.R. Part 812, investigational device exemptions, sec. 812.2(c)(3).
[13] 21 C.F.R. Part 812, investigational device exemptions, sec. 812.20(b).
[14] 21 C.F.R. Part 820, quality system regulation, sec. 820.1(a)(1).
[15] Device advice: comprehensive regulatory assistance, http://www.fda.gov/medicaldevices/deviceregulationandguidance/default.htm [accessed 07.02.14].
[16] 21 C.F.R. Part 312, investigational new drug application, sec. 312.3(b).
[17] 21 C.F.R. Part 812, investigational device exemptions, sec. 812.3.
[18] 21 C.F.R. Part 312, investigational new drug application, subpart D—responsibilities of sponsors and investigators.
[19] 21 C.F.R. Part 812, investigational device exemptions, subpart c—responsibilities of sponsors; subpart e—responsibilities of investigators.
[20] 21 C.F.R. Part 312, investigational new drug application, sec. 312.55(a).
[21] http://clinicaltrials.gov/.
[22] 21 C.F.R. Part 312, investigational new drug application, sec. 312.50.
[23] 21 C.F.R. Part 312, investigational new drug application, sec. 312.56(b); 21 CFR Part 812, investigational device exemptions, sec. 812.46(a).
[24] http://www.fda.gov/ICECI/EnforcementActions/BioresearchMonitoring/ucm133569.htm [accessed 07.02.14].
[25] 21 C.F.R. Part 312, investigational new drug application, sec. 312.66; sec. 312.50; sec. 312.60.
[26] 21 C.F.R. Part 56, institutional review boards, sec. 56.108(a).
[27] 21 C.F.R. part 812, investigational device exemptions, sec. 812.43(4).
[28] 21 C.F.R. Part 56, institutional review boards, sec. 56.108(b).

# 3

# The Institutional Animal Care and Use Committee

*Jerald Silverman*

University of Massachusetts Medical School, Worcester, MA, USA

## 1. INTRODUCTION

In 1981, at a congressional hearing, Rep. Douglas Walgren presided over a meeting of the House of Representatives' subcommittee on Science, Research and Technology [1]. He said that the question in front of the committee was important and sensitive: "What is the proper balance between freedom of inquiry in medical research and the suffering of animals used in experiments?" The hearing's transcript was more than 700 pages long and encompassed a plethora of information and viewpoints. Nevertheless, an unambiguous answer to that question still eludes us, and there are strong, often passionate feelings among those supporting or opposing the use of animals in research. For many years, opinion polls had shown that most Americans approved of the use of animals in biomedical research; however, that support has eroded over time, and now only about 56% of the general public supports research that uses live animals [2–4]. To help understand how public perceptions are born, and perhaps how legislators are influenced to pass laws concerning animal use, we must remember that research animals were not always afforded today's protections that provide for the ethical procurement, proper husbandry, and the alleviation of pain and distress in laboratory animals.

A past accounting of animal use and abuse for scientific purposes is not for the faint of heart. Experimentation on and dissection of living, unanesthetized animals (both human and nonhuman) has a sordid history that extends, at the least, from the time of the Alexandrian Greeks to outrages committed in modern times. The rationale behind vivisection of nonhuman animals and other forms of live animal experimentation, whether coming from notables such as Galen, Andreas Vesalius, Claude Bernard, or others, has long been a "greater good" argument. That is, what we learn from the suffering of a few will lead to benefits for the many. Of course, all experimentation with animals was not and is not vivisection, nor does all experimentation with animals lead to pain or suffering. Nevertheless, there are significant differences as to how experimenters view animals that are used in biomedical and behavioral research, ranging from those who characterize animals as no more than tools of their research to those who will not use animals for experimentation no matter how painless or nonconfining the study. Most of those who do use animals are concerned about the well-being of their animals. Yet, if we justify our use of animals for scientific purposes as being for the greater good, are there safeguards in place that are for the greater good of the animals? In this chapter, we will explore some of the existing safeguards, focusing on the institutional animal care and use committee (IACUC), which has an important role in applying safeguards. We will remain cognizant that "unlike human participants, animals will never be able to consent to experimental procedures. Accordingly, ethical evaluation ought to be very stringent to protect animals from unnecessary harm" [5].

In 1831, the English physician and physiologist, Marshall Hall, published *A Critical and Experimental Essay on the Circulation of the Blood* [6]. The introduction to this book laid out basic principles for humane experimentation with animals, which, in 1959, were expanded on in William Russell and Rex Burch's now celebrated book, *The Principles of Humane Experimental Technique* [7]. With the growth of the animal rights movement in the mid-1970s, the latter book took on increased importance, and today the so-called three "Rs" of Russell and Burch are often cited as being the basis for the consideration of humane methods of animal experimentation. In brief, the three Rs (as currently interpreted) are: (1) reduce the number of animals used to the minimum needed for valid scientific results; (2) replace the use of sentient animals (e.g., mammals) with nonanimal alternatives (such as computer simulations) or less sentient animals (e.g., insects); and (3) refine experimental techniques to provide proper husbandry, experimental skills, and pain alleviation. Each one of the three Rs can be thought of as the legs of a stool [8]. All three legs must be in place for the stool to stand, and likewise, all of the three Rs must be given full consideration by the IACUC and individual animal users to provide basic safeguards for animals that are used in research, testing, and education.

We use animals in scientific research because humans are usually capable of dominating other species of animals. Nevertheless, even the biblical account of humans having dominion over the animals is most often interpreted as humans having a responsibility to be the stewards of animals, not their outright masters. Fortunately, there has been significant moral and scientific progress since the early Hellenic and Dark Ages, and we are now part of a culture that no longer supports vivisection by arguing that animals have no soul or do not react to pain. Furthermore, we do not accept unjustified pain or distress in our experimental designs. Rather, the use of animals in research has become a highly regulated entity in many nations, including the United States. It is the purpose of this chapter to briefly discuss how some of these regulations came to be and then to focus on how they are implemented in this country.

## 2. REGULATORY HISTORY

In his review of the genesis of US federal laws providing protections to animals used in research, Rozmiarek noted, "Prior to the 20th century the responsibility for animals used in research in the US was placed directly in the hands of the research investigator" [9]. In fact, until the passage of the Laboratory Animal Welfare Act of 1966, there were many state laws but no national laws providing protections to research animals. In the early 1960s, the Animal Welfare Institute and the Humane Society of the United States influenced Congress to consider at least six different bills regulating the use of animals in laboratories. These bills were opposed by the National Institutes of Health (NIH), the American Veterinary Medical Association (AVMA), and the American Medical Association, and all eventually failed to gain passage [10]. The tide turned in 1966, perhaps influenced in part by a magazine article that related the account of a stolen dog that was found in a research laboratory [11] and another article concerning the plight of dogs in so-called puppy mills [12]. The Laboratory Animal Welfare Act of 1966 (Public Law 89–544) gave the secretary of agriculture the authority to regulate dealers who handled dogs, cats, hamsters, rabbits, guinea pigs, and nonhuman primates that were used in research. In addition to providing proper care for regulated research animals, it had an underlying second purpose of protecting dogs and cats from theft and sale to research laboratories.

The Act was amended in 1970 to change its name to the Animal Welfare Act (AWA) and concurrently give the secretary of agriculture the authorization to regulate additional warm-blooded animals when used in research, exhibition, or the wholesale pet trade. The 1970 amendment to the Act did not require the establishment of an animal care and use committee; however, the regulations that were passed to implement the act did require the establishment of such a committee, one member of which had to be a veterinarian [13]. In 1985, another amendment to the Act (via Public Law 101–624) mandated that "The Secretary [of Agriculture] shall require that each research facility establish at least one Committee" and the members of that committee "shall possess sufficient ability to assess animal care, treatment, and practices in experimental research. . ." This was the formal beginning of the IACUC for animals regulated under the authority of the AWA. The final regulations for the 1985 amendment to the AWA were published between 1989 and 1991 and provided for the approval and monitoring of research that used regulated animals. Since then, additional regulations and policies have been issued. The most significant, possibly, was a 2004 amendment to the regulations of the AWA, which reflected a 2002 change to the Act itself that altered the definition of an animal. The definition of an animal, under the AWA, now specifically excludes birds bred for use in research, rats of the genus *Rattus* used for research, and mice of the genus *Mus* that are used for research. Thus, the AWA currently regulates mammals used for biomedical research, other than common laboratory rats and mice. It also regulates farm animals used for biomedical research, but not farm animals used for agricultural research. On occasion, this can lead to confusion about whether the use of a particular animal is or is not regulated under the AWA. Although birds not bred for research are regulated under the AWA, at this time the US Department of Agriculture (USDA), which oversees compliance with the AWA, has not established specific regulatory standards for enforcing this part of the law.

National protections for animals used in research came from a second source, the Public Health Service (PHS), an organization within the US Department of Health and Human Services. As early as 1939, the NIH, which is a division of the PHS and a major funding source for biomedical research, issued "Rules Regarding Animals" to institutions receiving PHS monies for research [14]. In 1963, the PHS published a *Guide for Laboratory Animal Facilities and Care* to serve as a common source of reference for institutions using laboratory animals. Two years later, a second edition of that guidebook was published, with its purpose being "to assist scientific institutions in providing professionally appropriate care for laboratory animals" [15]. But the recommendations that were provided, although important and well-considered, were nonbinding on animal researchers and their institutions. That changed in 1971, when the NIH determined that institutions and organizations using warm-blooded animals in projects (or demonstrations) supported by NIH funds shall "assure the NIH that they will evaluate their animal facilities in regard to the maintenance of acceptable standards for the care, use and treatment of such animals." This assurance could be through a recognized laboratory animal accrediting body or an institutional committee established to evaluate the care of the warm-blooded animals held or used for animal-based activities funded by the NIH [16]. And, as did the 1970 amendment to the AWA, the 1971 NIH policy required that at least one member of this committee be a veterinarian. Thus, for the first time, institutions receiving NIH funding were required to follow NIH guidelines, the applicable portions of the AWA, and an additional set of broad guidelines known as the *Principles for Use of Laboratory Animals* [16]. Nevertheless, an IACUC-like committee was not required if the institution was accredited by a recognized laboratory animal accrediting body.

In 1973, the NIH policy was replaced by the first *Public Health Service Policy on the Humane Care and Use of Laboratory Animal* (PHS *Policy*) and a 1979 revision of the PHS *Policy* stated that every institution subject to its requirements had to have "a committee to maintain oversight of its animal care program," whether or not it was accredited by a recognized laboratory animal accrediting body [16]. For the NIH, this was the beginning of what has matured into the IACUC. An animal care and use committee also was formally required under the Health Research Extension Act of 1985 (Public Law 99–158). The current PHS policy [17] elaborates on the requirements of the Health Research Extension Act. It encompasses all vertebrate animals (not just warm-blooded animals) that are used for research, teaching, or testing that is supported by PHS funds.

There are then two federal departments having responsibilities for the welfare of laboratory animals, and both have a requirement for an IACUC or a similarly named committee. The USDA enforces compliance with the AWA and its regulations, including the requirement for an IACUC. Oversight of PHS-supported biomedical and behavioral research, using the 2002 PHS policy [17] as the guiding document, is implemented by the Department of Health and Human Services under authority given to it by the Health Research Extension Act of 1985. Much more will be said later in this chapter about the IACUC, but for now it is sufficient to understand that an IACUC is an intrainstitutional oversight committee that represents the institution and its program of animal care and use to the federal government. Its basic purpose is to assure compliance with federal animal care and use regulations and policies and to help ensure the well-being of the institution's animals that are used in research, teaching, or testing. Any institution (including colleges and universities, but not elementary or secondary schools) that receives funding from the federal government for research, teaching, or testing, using any of the federally regulated live animals noted above, is required to have an IACUC.

# 3. RELEVANT REGULATORY AND OVERSIGHT LAWS, REGULATIONS, AND GUIDANCE DOCUMENTS

## 3.1 The Animal Welfare Act [18] and the Animal Welfare Act Regulations [19]

The USDA has delegated the responsibility for compliance with the AWA and the AWA regulations (AWARs) to its Animal and Plant Health Inspection Service, and specifically to that service's Animal Care division (APHIS/AC). APHIS/AC administers the AWA and enforces it through a system of licensing, registration, cooperative efforts, and unannounced inspections. It is headquartered in Riverdale, MD, with regional offices in Fort Collins, Colo (western region), and Raleigh, NC (eastern region). The AWA and the AWAR, as noted earlier, regulate warm-blooded animals used for teaching, testing, and experimentation. However, they exclude common laboratory rats and mice, birds bred specifically for research, and farm animals that are used for food or fiber or for food or fiber research (AWAR §1.1, Animal).

The AWA is the law. Its impact extends beyond the scope of this chapter (e.g., it regulates certain animal dealers, exhibitors, operators of auction sales), but our focus will be limited to animals used for biomedical and behavioral research, training, teaching, or product testing. The AWA is about 15 printed pages in length, with the section on the IACUC comprising only about four of those pages. In contrast, the AWARs are more than 100 printed pages in length, yet the regulations addressing IACUCs still cover only about four pages. The AWARs provide the supportive details on how the AWA is to be used on a practical level. One can think of the AWA as the constitution that lays out broad principles for animal welfare, while the AWAR can be envisioned as the bylaws that go into more depth on how the law is to be applied. All institutions that have animals regulated under the AWA (such as many universities) must comply with the provisions of the AWARs.

## 3.2 Animal and Plant Health Inspection Service/Animal Care Policies

Although the AWAR is often the defining document for interpreting the AWA, there are times when even the AWARs require additional clarification. APHIS/AC accomplishes this through a series of written policies that are in its *Animal Care Policy Manual* [20]. The policy manual references specific sections of the AWAR and provides guidance on the intent and enforcement of the AWA and the AWARs. The APHIS/AC policies are not laws or regulations, but they often have the same impact as the AWAR because the courts have historically given federal departments wide leeway in interpreting their own regulations. Most of the policies contained in the *Animal Care Policy Manual* are more accurately termed interpretive rules, because they are statements that clarify or interpret the AWARs. It is only because of convention within APHIS/AC that all such documents are referred to as policies [21].

## 3.3 The Program of Veterinary Care

One small section of the AWARs (§2.33,a,1) states that if a research facility does not employ a full-time attending veterinarian (AV), then a part-time or consulting AV's employment arrangement must include a written program of veterinary care and regularly scheduled visits to the research facility. The frequency and time needed for these visits will depend on the overall size and complexity of the research program. Additional details about this program can be found in APHIS/AC policy #3 [22] and another APHIS/AC publication, the *Animal Care Inspection Guide* [23]. The basic purpose of the program of veterinary care is to assure the research institution and APHIS/AC that there is adequate veterinary oversight of the research facility's animals. This includes the availability of routine and emergency care for animals, proper vaccinations (if needed), appropriate diagnostic testing, zoonotic disease prevention, parasite control, pre- and post-procedure care of animals (including anesthesia and analgesia), proper euthanasia methods, etc.

## 3.4 The Public Health Service Policy on Humane Care and Use of Laboratory Animals

Just as the AWAR provides many of the operational details for implementing the AWA, the PHS policy provides many the operational details for the National Institutes of Health's Office of Laboratory Animal Welfare (NIH/OLAW) to oversee the implementation of the Health Research Extension Act of 1985. All institutions that use animals under the authority of the Health Research Extension Act must comply with the PHS policy. The PHS policy regulates the use of vertebrate animals (i.e., fish, amphibians, reptiles, birds, and mammals) used or intended for use in research, research training, biological testing, and similar purposes, such as teaching (PHS *Policy* III,A), when PHS funds are used for those purposes.

The PHS policy has three components:

1. The published PHS policy itself [17], which is about 12 pages in length and provides the basic information needed to comply with the pertinent sections of the Health Research Extension Act of 1985. It includes information on the animal welfare Assurance (described below), the IACUC and its functions, review of proposed research projects, reporting and record-keeping requirements, and similar items. Some of the wording of the PHS policy parallels the wording of the AWARs.

   Section IV, A of the PHS policy requires institutions that receive (or will be receiving) financial support from the PHS to provide NIH/OLAW with a written animal welfare Assurance. The Assurance is evaluated by NIH/OLAW "to determine the adequacy of the institution's proposed program for the care and use of animals in PHS-conducted or supported activities." Without an approved Assurance, no PHS-conducted or supported activity involving animals is permitted. The Assurance is based on the *Guide for the Care and Use of Laboratory Animals* [24], which is discussed below. Institutions having PHS funding submit a new Assurance to NIH/OLAW every 4 years.

2. The *US Government Principles for the Utilization and Care of Vertebrate Animals Used in Testing, Research, and Training* [25]. This part of the PHS policy consists of a list of nine brief, overarching concepts for the proper use of animals. They include commentaries on animal transportation and care, the relevance of a planned study to human or animal health, the species used and animal numbers, avoidance of pain and distress, use of proper anesthesia and analgesia, euthanasia, appropriate living conditions for animals, qualifications of investigators, and that any deviation from the principles are to be reviewed by a committee such as the IACUC. The concepts behind the *US Government Principles* are expanded on in the *Guide for the Care and Use of Laboratory Animals* and the published PHS policy.

3. The *Guide for the Care and Use of Laboratory Animals* (the *Guide*) [24] is the descendent of the original *Guide for Laboratory Animal Facilities and Care* mentioned earlier. Prepared by the Institute for Laboratory Animal Research of the National Research Council, the *Guide* is essentially an informational handbook about best practices that are intended to help institutions properly care for and use laboratory animals. The PHS policy (IV,A,1) requires institutions to use the *Guide* "as a basis for developing and implementing an institutional program for activities involving animals." Because the *Guide* and the PHS policy are published as separate documents, it is not unusual for people to refer to them separately (e.g., the *Guide* says . . . and the PHS *Policy* says . . .), but it should be

clearly understood that NIH/OLAW Assured institutions are expected to follow the recommendations of the *Guide* unless deviations are approved by the IACUC.

As indicated earlier, APHIS/AC has regulatory authority and published policies to help clarify some of the AWA regulations. NIH/OLAW oversees the implementation of the PHS policy and the *Guide*, but it is not a regulatory agency. Therefore, instead of formal policies, it provides responses to frequently asked questions [26] and has other useful information on its website [27] to help institutions remain in compliance with the PHS policy.

## 3.5 The Animal Welfare Assurance

The Assurance is a document required by Section IV,A of the PHS policy. No PHS funds involving animals can be used until a proper Assurance is in place (which means it has been accepted by NIH/OLAW). Part of the Assurance is comparable to the program of veterinary care required under the AWAR, but it differs in two major ways. First, it is required of all institutions receiving PHS funds, not just those employing a part-time or consulting veterinarian. Second, it requires information about the animal care and use program that goes beyond the veterinary care of animals. Details of what is expected to be written in the Assurance can be found in the PHS policy (IV,A,1). In brief, the Assurance attests that the institution will abide by the PHS policy, it describes the institution's program of animal care and use (including veterinary care), how that program will be evaluated, lines of authority, training, recordkeeping and reporting requirements, IACUC membership, protocol review, and related items. A sample Assurance is located on the NIH/OLAW website [28].

NIH/OLAW can approve or disapprove a proposed Assurance or negotiate an approvable Assurance. NIH/OLAW also can set conditions on an Assurance, restrict an Assurance, or even withdraw approval of an Assurance. Therefore, although NIH/OLAW is not a regulatory agency, its ability to review and possibly revoke an institution's Assurance gives it a certain amount of controlling authority.

## 3.6 AVMA Guidelines for the Euthanasia of Animals: 2013 Edition [29]

The PHS policy (IV,C,1,g) and APHIS/AC policy #3 [22] require that the methods of euthanasia used for animals regulated under the PHS policy and the AWARs will be those procedures recommended by the AVMA's euthanasia guidelines. The IACUC can approve an exception to the guidelines if the proposed deviation is scientifically justified by the investigator and is acceptable to the IACUC. The AVMA guidelines are periodically updated, and although they are termed guidelines, for practical purposes they have the impact of a federal regulation.

The basic requirement for properly performed euthanasia, as stated in the AVMA guidelines, is that "the technique employed should result in rapid loss of consciousness followed by cardiac or respiratory arrest and, ultimately, a loss of brain function. In addition, animal handling and the euthanasia technique should minimize distress experienced by the animal prior to loss of consciousness." For mice, the most common mammalian species used in biomedical research, the guidelines permit various methods of euthanasia, such as carbon dioxide gas, barbiturate overdose, cervical dislocation, decapitation, and overdosed inhalant anesthetics.

Unacceptable methods for any species include hypothermia and drowning. The AVMA guidelines often present stipulations about a method of euthanasia, and it is important that the IACUC is aware of any pertinent stipulations before approving a euthanasia method.

## 3.7 The Guide for the Care and Use of Agricultural Animals in Agricultural Research and Teaching [30]

Now in its third edition, *The Guide for the Care and Use of Agricultural Animals in Agricultural Research and Teaching,* or so-called ag guide, emphasizes basic principles for the care of farm animals whether those animals are used in research or for other purposes. The information in the ag guide is not mandated by any federal requirement and therefore does not supersede any federal requirement for animal care or use that is in the PHS policy or the AWARs. Nevertheless, the information contained in the ag guide is generally applicable to farm animals used in biomedical research and is very useful for helping to establish an effective animal care program. More will be said below on the role of the ag guide in the accreditation of laboratory animal facilities.

## 3.8 The Institutional Animal Care and Use Committee Protocol Form

A protocol form is not a federal regulatory document; rather, it is an institutional application form that commits an investigator or educator to performing his or her work as described in the protocol form once it is approved by the IACUC. The protocol form provides the IACUC with a written statement of what the investigator or educator will be doing with animals. As will be described later in this chapter, no animal activities can occur with federally regulated animals (i.e., animals regulated under the AWARs or PHS policy) unless the IACUC approves the use of the animals. Very often, by the way questions on the protocol form are written, guidance is provided to animal users about federal and institutional requirements for animal use. Although there is no federal requirement to have a protocol form, it borders on impossible to have an adequate program of animal care and use without clear and readily available documentation of what will be done using animals. This documentation need not be on paper; it can be totally electronic by having all the information required under existing regulations and any additional information requested by the IACUC entered into institutionally developed or commercially available computerized applications (programs). A sample protocol form is available on the NIH/OLAW website [31]. Some common topics and questions for investigators that are typically found on an IACUC protocol form are:

- Provide an easy to understand summary of your proposed work with animals, describing the importance of the study and how it potentially will benefit humans or other animals.
- How many animals (by species) do you anticipate using? Provide a science-based explanation for the need of that number of animals, using inferential statistical parameters when applicable.
- Justify why you need to use laboratory animals rather than performing an in vitro study, human clinical trial, using a computer simulation, epidemiological study, or other nonanimal research. Are less sentient animal models available (e.g., using certain invertebrate animals)?

- Provide in chronological order the details about what will happen to the animals you are requesting. This includes observations, operative procedures, behavioral testing, breeding, genotyping, etc. For surgical procedures, indicate how the animal, surgeon, and instruments will be prepared to accomplish aseptic surgery.
- List all drugs and chemicals to be given to the animals by dosage, route of administration, and frequency of administration. If any drugs are not of pharmaceutical quality, indicate why they must be used and how they will be prepared for use in live animals (e.g., consider sterility, pH, purity, etc.). Indicate which group of animals will be receiving each of the drugs listed.

The IACUC in general, but especially the veterinarian, should ensure that appropriate drugs are used to alleviate pain or other forms of distress. Pain and other forms of distress can sometimes be alleviated by using nondrug methods, such as petting or music. If pain or other forms of distress will not be alleviated because of research requirements, the IACUC form should request strong scientific justification from the researcher, and there should be an equally robust evaluation by the IACUC.

- For each person who will be working with animals, list the total years of direct, hands-on experience he or she has performing the specific procedure(s) described in this protocol with the species to be used (e.g., splenectomy, blood collection, intramuscular injections). How will untrained persons receive appropriate training prior to performing a procedure?
- How often will your animals be monitored for their well-being? What monitoring methods will be used (e.g., weighing, body condition score, ability to ambulate, listening for vocalizations)?
- What will be the experimental endpoint for each group of animals described in this study? Why was that endpoint chosen for your study?
- What will cause you to remove or euthanize an animal earlier than anticipated?
- What method(s) will be used to euthanize the animals and assure their death?

The above items are just examples. Most protocol forms go into additional detail, such as asking when analgesic drugs will be administered during an experiment, specific information about field studies, frequency of use of any one animal, a statement that the work to be performed is not unnecessarily duplicative, and so forth. Additional information on what might be included on a protocol form is available in the AWARs (§2.31,d; §2.31,e), the PHS policy (IV,C,1,a–g), and the *Guide* (pp. 25–33).

## 4. KEY REGULATORY MANDATES FOR THE INSTITUTIONAL ANIMAL CARE AND USE COMMITTEE

The IACUC is a committee that is qualified through the experience and expertise of its members to oversee its institution's animal program, animal facilities, and animal use procedures. No one IACUC member has to be knowledgeable about all aspects of animal care and use; that is the responsibility of the committee as a whole. As was noted earlier, the IACUC has two basic functions. The first and primary function is to ensure that its home institution (such as a university) remains in compliance with federal animal care and use laws, regulations, and policies. Its second function, which is closely related to the first, is to help ensure the welfare of animals used in research, teaching, and testing. The discussions that follow will hold true for any research, testing, or teaching institution having an IACUC. Elementary and secondary schools are not considered research facilities by the AWARs (§1.1) and the PHS policy (because they do not receive research funds from the PHS). Therefore, even if they use live animals for teaching purposes, they are exempt from being required to have an IACUC.

Because the IACUC is an institutionally based committee that derives much of its responsibility and authority from federal laws, it is understandable that it is considered to be representing its institution to the federal government. However, it also represents the federal government's regulations and policies to the institution. This puts the IACUC in the middle. For example, in academic institutions, the faculty often resents being told by the IACUC what it can or cannot do with animals because academicians do not like to be told what to do, and they flaunt the concept of academic freedom. On the other hand, APHIS/AC and NIH/OLAW expect the school's IACUC to uphold federal regulations.

With two federal departments having a requirement for an IACUC, it is fair to ask whether two separate IACUCs are required or whether an institution can have one IACUC that fulfills the requirements of the AWAR (from the Department of Agriculture) and the PHS policy (from the Department of Health and Human Services). The simple answer is yes. If an institution uses animals regulated under both the AWAR and the PHS policy, it can have one IACUC to meet the animal care and use program requirements of both federal departments. In fact, due to the many overlapping regulations and policies developed by APHIS/AC and NIH/OLAW, it would be a waste of time and other resources to have separate APHIS/AC and NIH/OLAW IACUCs. Nevertheless, there are differences between the regulations and policies emanating from the AWAR and PHS policy, and some of them will be noted in the following discussions.

The IACUC is appointed by the chief executive officer of the institution or by a person with written delegated authority from the chief executive officer. The committee's members serve for no fixed length of time (it is at the discretion of the institution). Some IACUCs prefer to keep the same members for a prolonged time, believing that their experience leads to consistency in IACUC activities. Other IACUCs rotate their membership, although chairs tend to remain on the job longer than most members. The person who has the authority to appoint the IACUC members also has the authority to remove IACUC members.

The key regulatory mandates for the IACUC are found in the AWAR (§2.31,c) and the PHS Policy (IV,B). They are described in the following sections.

## 4.1 Approve Animal Use for Research, Testing, and Research Training

The IACUC allows for two methods to approve a research protocol. The first is known as full committee review (FCR) and requires a quorum (>50%) of the IACUC members to be present at an IACUC meeting to approve animal-use activities. The FCR process will be familiar to most people who have served on any committee. Prior to reviewing protocols, all members of the IACUC are provided, at the minimum, with a list of proposed research projects (i.e., protocols) that will be reviewed at the meeting. Most IACUCs give their members more than a simple list; usually they receive a summary of the information on the protocols, or sometimes entire protocols are distributed. Typically, this distribution occurs at least a day before the meeting, and often more time than that is provided. It is also typical (but not required) for the chair of the IACUC to have previously designated one or two members of the committee to be the primary reviewers of the protocol. These reviewers will expedite the FCR by summarizing the protocol for the committee and often indicating to the other members their own opinions of the protocol's strengths and weaknesses. Once the primary reviewers have completed their presentations, the chair usually will ask for additional comments or questions from the other committee members. After any discussion is completed, the chairperson asks the IACUC to vote on the protocol. The members can vote to approve the protocol as written, disapprove the protocol as written (correctly termed withholding approval), or require the investigator to modify the protocol to obtain IACUC approval. In the last instance, the protocol still must receive IACUC approval of the modification before animal use can be initiated.

The second allowable method of protocol approval is commonly called designated member review (DMR). With DMR, a listing of the protocol or protocols to be reviewed is distributed, as was described above for FCR. Members of the IACUC are given a set amount of time (previously agreed to by the IACUC) to decide whether any member wants FCR for the protocol, and if any member requests FCR, it must be reviewed by FCR. However, if FCR is not requested, the chair designates one or more committee members to review the protocol. If there is more than one reviewer, the reviewers do not vote; they can unanimously approve the protocol as written or unanimously require the investigator to modify the protocol to obtain IACUC approval. They cannot withhold approval. If the reviewers cannot approve the protocol, which includes not being satisfied with any modifications made by the investigator, the protocol must be sent back to the IACUC for FCR.

Although many people believe that the DMR process is faster than FCR, there has been no controlled study to verify this belief. Therefore, it is appropriate to briefly look at the strengths and weaknesses of both systems of protocol review. The strength of FCR is that it solicits the opinions and knowledge of many people who are together at the same time. This often brings out issues that are not immediately obvious to the IACUC and can generate a full, hearty discussion in which everybody can have their opinions heard. A weakness of FCR is that the review occurs only when the IACUC meets, which is often once a month or even less often. Further, FCR requires a quorum of the IACUC to be present, and at certain times it can be difficult to get a quorum. When a quorum is present, there can be less than civil arguments about a protocol, rather than the desired erudite academic discussions. Lastly, it is often not necessary to use the FCR process for relatively simple studies (e.g., most animal breeding) or certain repetitive procedure studies (such as drug safety testing).

DMR also has strengths and weaknesses. It does not require the presence of a quorum, and therefore the review can be done at the leisure of the reviewer at his or her office or home. By its very nature of being individualized, DMR readily lends itself to computer-based reviews. And, because there is no waiting for a convened meeting of the IACUC, DMR can be used to review certain protocols that require a rapid turnaround time. However, using a limited number of DMR reviewers (as few as one person), there can be a narrow focus of expertise, there is often a lack of the robust discussion that can occur with FCR, the process may actually take longer than FCR if the designated reviewers get busy with other work (or go on vacation), and DMR may lead to strained relationships between reviewers if agreement cannot be reached on the disposition of the protocol. Another problem, not often mentioned because it depends on the details of how DMR is implemented at a particular institution, is that one reviewer may not want to perform his or her review until he or she sees the comments from another reviewer. This last problem can be resolved by having all DMR reviews sent to the IACUC office, where a composite review is prepared and sent to the investigator.

Once a protocol is approved by the IACUC, it must be reviewed again at least every three years if PHS policy-regulated animals are being used (PHS *Policy* IV,C,5) and at least annually if AWAR regulated animals are being used (AWAR §2.31,d,5). NIH/OLAW requires that the re-reviewed protocol be approved again by the IACUC before animal work can continue beyond the expiration date of the protocol. An extension of that date by the IACUC is not allowed. APHIS/AC does not require formal IACUC approval of the re-reviewed protocol, but some IACUCs have their own policy requiring that even APHIS/AC protocols be reapproved by the committee. If animals that are regulated under both the AWAR and PHS policy are in the same protocol, the IACUC will typically do a general review of the protocol once a year (to comply with the AWAR) and require a new protocol submission at the end of the third year of approval (to comply with the PHS policy).

It is important to understand that no person or group at the institution is allowed to pressure the IACUC or require the IACUC to approve a protocol that the committee has decided not to approve (PHS *Policy* IV,C,8; AWAR §2.31,d,8). However, for already-approved protocols, the institutional official (IO) or other officials of the institution can review the protocol and choose not to allow it to progress. (The IO is the person at the institution who has the authority to commit the school to compliance with the AWAR and/or the PHS policy.) Although it is unusual (but legal) for the IO to block the initiation of an IACUC-approved project, it might occur, for example, if adequate resources are not available.

The investigator need not be concerned with the details of the review process; that is knowledge needed by IACUC members and the IACUC administrative office. Rather, prior to approval, the take home message for investigators should be that no research, research training, teaching, or testing that uses live animals can be performed without prior IACUC approval. This includes breeding animals, identifying animals by marking, genotyping, or other means, or purchasing animals for future use.

## 4.2  To Approve Proposed Changes in Animal Use Activities

It is often necessary to make changes to a protocol to accommodate new experimental findings, help resolve research-induced problems experienced by animals, or for other research needs. Many of these changes significantly impact animal use and must be approved by the IACUC before the requested change can be implemented. The investigator need not be concerned with all of the details of the amendment process, other than how to submit an amendment. However, the message to investigators should be that no changes to already-approved research, testing, or teaching using animals can be made without prior IACUC approval. Some examples of significant changes include adding a new surgical procedure, a change of the principal investigator, and changing the species to be used [32]. The process of changing an approved animal use activity is generally termed amending a protocol. To amend a protocol, an investigator informs the IACUC of the requested change, and the change is then evaluated by the IACUC using either of the two methods described above for approving a protocol (FCR or DMR). As with a brand new protocol, and depending if FCR or DMR is used for review, the amendment can be approved as written, approval can be withheld, or the IACUC can require the investigator to modify the protocol amendment to obtain its approval.

How does an investigator inform the IACUC of a needed amendment? Many IACUCs have developed specific forms for amendments. These forms require information about the reason for the change, any increase or decrease in the number of animals needed, changes in the use of anesthesia or analgesia, the study endpoints, and so forth. Other IACUCs ask the investigator to make the requested changes directly on the already-approved protocol form, but to highlight the changes for the reviewer. Once approved, an amendment to a protocol does not change the date of the required re-review of that protocol. The review date remains as no more than one year from the date of the protocol's initial approval by the IACUC for AWAR-regulated animals and three years from the date of the initial approval for PHS policy-regulated animals.

NIH/OLAW and APHIS/AC also have procedures in place whereby certain significant changes can be handled administratively, in consultation with a veterinarian, as long as there are supporting IACUC-approved policies in place [32]. The approval of certain minor amendments that affect animals regulated under the PHS policy can be made by the IACUC's administrative office rather than by the committee itself [32,33]. Examples include changes in telephone numbers or office addresses, verification of approval from another university committee, or the addition of a trained and qualified technician.

## 4.3 To Periodically Inspect and Prepare Reports on the Institution's Animal Facilities and Laboratories where Animals Are Used

At least once every 6 months (i.e., semiannually), the IACUC is required by the AWAR (§2.31,c,1–3) and the PHS policy (IV,B,2–3) to inspect all of the institution's animal facilities where animals regulated under the AWAR or PHS policy are housed or used. The *Guide* (p. 25) recommends that these inspections occur at least once a year, but it goes on to say that they may be required more often, such as when they are required by federal regulation to occur semiannually. The definition of an animal facility differs slightly between the AWAR and PHS policy. The PHS policy defines an animal facility as an area where animals are kept for more than 24 h, and the AWAR considers an animal facility to be an area where animals are kept for more than 12 h. (The AWAR does not provide a specific definition of an animal facility, but it does provide definitions for a housing facility and a study area, which, when combined, provides a similar definition to that found in the PHS policy for an animal facility.) On a practical level, these differences are usually not of any great consequence, and IACUCs should cater to the welfare of the animals under their oversight by inspecting all laboratories and areas where animals are housed or used, no matter how long an animal is kept there and no matter whether an animal is or is not in the laboratory when an inspection is scheduled. These inspections should be done because the IACUC always has the responsibility to oversee animal well-being, wherever the animals are and for whatever length of time the animals are kept confined.

A potential problem with inspecting all areas used to study animals is faced by some IACUCs when the study area is at a distant site or a difficult-to-reach field location, such as a marsh. IACUCs have resolved this difficulty by numerous means, including direct inspections, having nearby institutions do the inspection for the IACUC, or evaluating videos of the procedures used at the sites.

There are other differences between the PHS policy and the AWAR that are of importance. One significant detail involves who can do the inspection. The PHS policy (IV,B,3) allows the IACUC to use its own discretion as to who can do the inspections; therefore, one person, many people, and IACUC members or nonmembers are all acceptable, although the IACUC always remains responsible for the inspection evaluation and a subsequent report. The wide discretion given to the IACUC under the PHS policy implies that the inspector(s) are appropriately trained to perform a suitable inspection. The AWARs (§2.31,c,1–3) are somewhat more restrictive than the PHS policy, requiring at least two IACUC members to conduct the inspections, although consultants may be used, if needed, to assist the IACUC inspectors.

There are no regulatory documents that specifically direct the IACUC on how to conduct these inspections. However, NIH/OLAW's website has a sample inspection document that provides a convenient check-off list of items that IACUCs should routinely evaluate during animal facility and laboratory inspections [34]. The information provided in the *Guide* and the AWARs are, respectively, the primary documents used to evaluate housing facilities and laboratories using animals regulated under the PHS policy and the AWARs. For agricultural animals, the ag guide is often a useful document to have during site inspections. A few of the items typically examined during the inspection of a laboratory or animal facility include:

- the apparent health and well-being of animals, paying particular attention to animals that appear to be experiencing pain or other forms of distress;
- general cleanliness;
- the construction and condition of floors, walls, and ceilings;
- the proper storage, dates of expiration, and sterility of drugs;
- room temperature, humidity, ventilation, and lighting;
- appropriate size and condition of cages, pens, or tanks;
- animals generally living in social groups are housed together when possible;
- adequacy of food, water, and shelter (the last item is primarily for animals on pastures);
- proper identification of animals or cages;
- appropriate storage facilities for food, bedding, and supplies;
- adequate facilities for washing and/or sterilizing supplies and equipment;
- appropriate medical and husbandry records are kept;
- safety procedures are in place for major equipment, high-noise areas, and other biohazards.

As important as the inspections are, they are no more important than the attitude and ability of the persons performing the inspections. The inspectors must be well-versed in the pertinent federal and institutional requirements for animal housing and use areas, they must be firm about pointing out items of noncompliance (such as a lack of medical records or conditions that might jeopardize animal safety), and they must be impartial, thorough, and polite. If for some reason a particular area cannot be inspected at a preferred time, the inspectors should plan on returning and completing the inspection.

After the inspections are completed, the IACUC discusses the findings,subsequently prepares a report of its evaluations, and submits the report to the IO. With the input of the IACUC's members, the report separates significant deficiencies from minor deficiencies and establishes a plan and a timeline to correct any significant deficiencies. Significant deficiencies are those that are or may be a threat to the health or safety of animals. The report must be signed by a majority of the IACUC membership and retained in the IACUC's records.

## 4.4 To Periodically Review and Prepare Reports on the Institution's Animal Care and Use Program

Another federal mandate for the IACUC is to semiannually review the institution's animal care and use program (AWAR §2.31,c,1; PHS *Policy* IV,B,1). This differs from the requirement to perform inspections in that the semiannual program review is accomplished by a discussion and analysis that usually does not require a visit to a specific site. However, there is nothing to say that the IACUC cannot visit an area if it is deemed to be important for the review process. Some of the many topics considered during the semiannual program review are:

1. Institutional policies and responsibilities
   a. Adequate resources are provided for animal care
   b. Appropriate training is provided for research, IACUC, and animal care personnel
   c. Contingency plans for a disaster are in place
   d. There is adequate oversight of animal use procedures after IACUC approval
   e. The use of nonpharmaceutical grade compounds or other deviations from the *Guide* are justified and have IACUC approval
   f. Occupational health and safety
2. Veterinary care
   a. A veterinarian provides oversight of surgery and postoperative care
   b. Veterinarians are properly trained to provide medical care for the species being housed
   c. Emergency veterinary service is always available
   d. Veterinarians have access to all animals and animal health records
   e. All animals are observed at least daily
   f. Procedures are in place for the surveillance, diagnosis, and treatment of diseases

There are no regulatory documents that tell the IACUC how to perform the semiannual review of the program of animal care and use. Some IACUCs perform an entire review at the same time of the year that the animal facilities and laboratories are inspected. The review can be accomplished by having either the full committee or one or more subcommittees of the IACUC meet, discuss, and evaluate the program. If subcommittees do the initial program review, they then report back to the full IACUC, because the IACUC as a whole, not a subcommittee, is responsible for approving the final program review report. Another option is for the IACUC to review specific aspects of the program of animal care and use at periodic (e.g., monthly) meetings of the committee. The results of the program review and any related discussions are then summarized semiannually and written up as a single report. There are other variations used by different institutions, but in the end, a semiannual report must be prepared and submitted to the IO (AWAR §2.31,c,3; PHS *Policy* IV,B,3) and have the signatures of a majority of the IACUC's members. The program review report is often part of the same report used to summarize the inspections of the animal facilities and laboratories. The report must distinguish significant from minor deficiencies, and if any significant deficiencies were found, there must be a plan and schedule to correct those deficiencies. NIH/OLAW provides a helpful checklist of the topics that should be included in the program review, although not every topic may be applicable to every institution [34].

## 4.5 Investigate Complaints about Animal Care and Use

The investigation of complaints concerning the program of animal care and use is required by the PHS policy (IV,b,4), the *Guide* (p. 23), and the AWARs (§2.31,c,4). Complaints can originate with faculty, staff, students, or the general public and may include allegations about animal care, protocol noncompliance, animal mistreatment, inappropriate IACUC procedures, and so forth. Perhaps the most important considerations for the IACUC when addressing complaints are to maintain neutrality and confidentiality and remember that a complaint is nothing more than a complaint unless an investigation proves otherwise. There may be times, of course, when an IACUC has to take immediate action before a full investigation is completed. For example, if an allegation is made that an animal has been maliciously injured by a particular person and an examination of the animal appears to confirm the injury, it is prudent to protect the animal from possible further harm before proceeding with a full investigation.

Different IACUCs use different methods of informing people how to report a concern to the IACUC. One of the most common means is to place informative signs throughout the animal facility. Other means include placing information on websites, using telephone or computer hotlines, newsletters, drop boxes, etc. If a complaint is not placed directly into an anonymous site such as a locked drop box, there should be multiple people who can be contacted to bring the complaint to the IACUC. This might include any member of the IACUC (especially the chair and the veterinarian); the IO; the IACUC director; a dean, provost, or chancellor; an animal care supervisor; or other persons having easy access to the IACUC. Any person receiving a complaint, or any instructions associated with filing a written complaint, should request the pertinent information that will expedite the IACUC's investigation. Typical questions are:

- What is the problem that you are reporting?
- Whom did it involve?
- Did you see or experience this yourself, or are you reporting something about which you were told?
- When did it happen?
- Where did it happen?
- Why do you think this is a problem (if not immediately apparent)?
- May we identify you as the complainant or do you wish to preserve your confidentiality?
- If necessary, may we contact you? If yes, what is the best way to reach you?

Institutions should have a policy in effect on how to transmit a complaint to the IACUC chair. The IACUC will usually conduct any ensuing investigation; however, it is the IO who is ultimately responsible for the school's compliance with the AWAR and the PHS policy. Therefore, the IO should routinely be kept apprised of any ongoing IACUC investigative activity.

It is left to the discretion of the IACUC about how to conduct an investigation if an initial review of the complaint (often by the IACUC chair or an IACUC subcommittee) requires additional inquiries. In some instances, the chair and the veterinarian conduct the investigation; in other instances, a subcommittee of the IACUC is formed for that purpose, and in still other cases (especially with small IACUCs), the entire committee may become involved in the investigation. Non-IACUC members can also serve on an investigative committee. Investigations may require talking with individuals, examining animals, examining research records, inspecting animal facilities, and the like, but in all instances confidentiality must be maintained. Lasting damage can be caused to a person's career if an allegation that is spread through the rumor mill is subsequently found to be untrue. In the next section and later in this chapter, we will discuss additional facets of an IACUC investigation.

## 4.6  Suspend an Animal Use Activity, if Justified

If the investigation of a complaint about an animal activity determines it to be true, the only sanction the IACUC can impose under the AWAR (§2.31,d,6) and the PHS policy (IV,C,6) is a suspension of the activity. A suspension is possible should the IACUC determine that the activity is not being conducted in accordance with the AWAR, the PHS policy (including the *Guide*), or the Assurance statement provided to NIH/OLAW. A suspension vote is taken at a convened meeting of a quorum of the IACUC, and it requires that the majority of the quorum present must vote for the suspension. The suspension is for a length of time determined by the IACUC, and all or part of an animal activity can be suspended (e.g., just the surgery portion of a study) or a person can be suspended. A suspension of a protocol means that no animal activity other than daily animal husbandry (provided by the animal facility) or clinical medical care (provided by the veterinary group) can be given to the animals. No breeding, no testing, no palpations, no "finishing up the work," etc. is allowed. Also, no NIH monies can be used to maintain animals on the suspended protocol without the express consent of the study's federal funding agency.

When AWAR-regulated animals are involved, the IACUC must report a suspension (with a full explanation) to APHIS/AC and any federal agency funding the suspended activity. If PHS policy-regulated animals are involved (e.g., typical laboratory mice), NIH/OLAW must be notified of the suspension, also with a full explanation. In either case, the IO, in consultation with the IACUC, must take appropriate corrective actions to help assure the problem will not recur.

Not all verified complaints are of such magnitude that a suspension is warranted, while others may be egregious enough to deserve penalties in addition to a suspension. There also are complaints reaching the IACUC that do not directly impact a specific animal activity, such as a person flaunting school rules on how to gain access to the vivarium. To address this need, many IACUCs are given authority from their institutions to impose a variety of nonsuspension penalties, such as letters of reprimand, financial penalties, retraining, barring entrance to the vivarium, and so forth.

Suspensions and other animal-related penalties are always unfortunate, because they indicate that a person has performed an activity of noncompliance with federal or institutional regulations. Many of these penalties can be eliminated if the IACUC continually emphasizes to research, teaching, and research training teams these three key points:

- do not perform any animal activity without IACUC approval;
- do not make changes to an animal activity without IACUC approval;
- do what you said you would do.

There are a plethora of regulations and policies involved with animal use in research, research training, teaching, and testing. Most researchers will focus on their study and often little more, but if they remember the above three basic and simple rules, the number of complaints investigated by IACUCs are likely to decrease dramatically.

## 4.7 Advise the Institutional Official on Animal Care and Use Items

As indicated earlier, the IO is the person who is authorized to legally commit on behalf of his or her institution that the requirements of the AWARs and/or the PHS policy will be met (AWAR 1.1; PHS *Policy* III,G). The IO, as the person ultimately responsible for the program of animal care and use, should be routinely kept informed and advised by the IACUC and the school's veterinarian about significant issues affecting the program, such as the need for animal care or surgical resources, suspensions of animal activities, significant adverse events such as flooding and power losses in a vivarium, and significant issues related to personnel training. Therefore, it is important that the IACUC chair (or IACUC manager) and the AV have ready access to the IO. As essential as the IO is in the overall animal care and use program, not all IOs may be fully cognizant of the importance and complexity of their role. In a survey of 768 IACUC members, a relatively low 82% of respondents (and only 75% of IACUC veterinarians) believed that their IO understood his or her role in the regulatory process [35].

## 5. KEY PERSONNEL AND COMMITTEES DESIGNATED TO IMPLEMENT REGULATORY MANDATES

### 5.1 Other Committees

The IACUC is the focus of this chapter, but the IACUC often does not have total responsibility for all aspects of animal care and use activities, particularly in larger academic institutions. For example, the PHS policy (IV,A,1,f) and the *Guide* (p. 17) require that any institution receiving PHS financial support have an occupational health and safety program as part of the overall program of animal care and use. Such a program includes many aspects of safety, such as microbiological, electrical, chemical, ergonomic, and radiation. While it is possible (and allowable) for the IACUC to develop, implement, and oversee such a program, given the complexity of animal-based research that is found at many institutions and the associated complexity of assuring occupational health and safety, other more dedicated committees or departments are usually given the responsibility for reviewing and approving occupational health and safety practices when using animals. Most of these institutions have an institutional biosafety committee (IBC) that typically approves and oversees studies with infectious organisms, recombinant and synthetic DNA, and perhaps biotoxins. Some institutions may have a separate environmental health and safety committee or division, which is primarily concerned with health and safety issues not overseen by the IBC. Other institutions may have a separate chemical safety committee, radiation safety committee, or other related committees. On infrequent occasions, the IACUC may even require that an institutional review board (the human-research analog of the IACUC) provide an approval for part of a study requiring the use of both laboratory animals and humans. It is the responsibility of the IACUC to ensure that all pertinent approvals from other committees, the responsibilities of which affect animal use, are in place before final IACUC approval is given to a study. It is important to remember that an approval from any other committee is in addition to IACUC approval, and not a substitute for IACUC approval.

An IACUC can approve, withhold approval, or require additional information to secure approval for an animal activity. It cannot give partial or conditional approvals that allow some parts of a study to begin, but not other parts. Yet, when an IACUC requires an approval from another committee before the IACUC can give its final approve to a study, a problem can arise. If the other committee's approval has not yet reached the IACUC, the IACUC cannot send a written approval letter to the investigator, which is what is needed for the investigator to being the approved animal activity. If this happens there are two options. First, the IACUC can simply delay sending the letter of approval until the other committee's approval reaches the IACUC. Second, the investigator can remove from the IACUC protocol the part of the study awaiting approval from the other committee, and once the other committee's approval arrives, the removed portion can be added back as an amendment [36]. Using the second option, the investigator may have to do some rewriting of the original protocol, and this may result in additional delays, assuming the IACUC has to approve the amendment. At the very least, and whenever possible, to save time, the IACUC review of a protocol should be simultaneous with any reviews being carried out by other institutional committees.

## 5.2 Association for Assessment and Accreditation of Laboratory Animal Care International

The Association for Assessment and Accreditation of Laboratory Animal Care International (AAALAC) is included in this discussion because many animal facilities are AAALAC accredited or are seeking AAALAC accreditation. AAALAC is a voluntary accrediting organization located in Frederick, MD. It is not an institutional committee, and it is independent of a direct affiliation with any research or teaching institution. The basic mission of AAALAC is to enhance "the quality of research, teaching, and testing by promoting humane, responsible animal care and use" [37]. AAALAC fulfills its mission by performing site visits every three years at accredited institutions or those seeking accreditation. Using the *Guide*, ag guide, and the AWARs as the primary standards of accreditation (the *Guide* requires that the AWARs be followed for AWAR-regulated species), the site visitors evaluate a previously submitted description of the institution's program of animal care and use, visit the animal facilities, review IACUC protocols, meet with researchers and IACUC members, and so forth. At a brief discussion at the end of the visit, the site visitors review their findings with representatives of the institution. The final decision about gaining or maintaining AAALAC accreditation is made by AAALAC's Council on Accreditation.

## 5.3 Key Personnel

### 5.3.1 General Comments

Every member of the IACUC is important because each person brings to the committee a unique set of skills and experiences. But is every member's importance equal, or paraphrasing George Orwell [38], are all members equal, but some are more equal than others?

As noted earlier, it is the committee as a whole, not each individual, that must have the appropriate ability to evaluate and oversee the program of animal care and use. For most IACUCs, the chair, as expected, takes the lead at committee meetings. The veterinarian is frequently asked to offer opinions on animal care or pain and distress. Still, the perception of who may be of prime importance depends on the issue under consideration, and any IACUC member may be of primary importance relative to the evaluation of a particular animal-related activity. Equally crucial to the proper functioning of an IACUC is the way the committee's membership interacts with each other, with investigators, and with its administrative support team to provide a humane and scientifically sound review of a proposed animal activity while remaining in compliance with federal regulations and policies.

The AWARs (§2.31,b,2) require that an IACUC be composed of a minimum of three people: a chair, a veterinarian, and a person not affiliated with the institution in any way, other than as a member of the IACUC. This last person is intended to represent general community interests in animal care and treatment. The Health Research Extension Act of 1985 (§495,b,2) requires no less than three members for an IACUC; however, the PHS policy (IV,A,3,b), which implements the Act, requires five or more members on an IACUC. There is no conflict between the act and the PHS policy because the act requires at least three people; the PHS policy has simply increased that minimum to five. Under the PHS policy, one of the IACUC members must be a veterinarian with training or experience in laboratory animal medicine, one a practicing scientist who is experienced using animals in research, one member whose primary concerns are in a nonscientific area (such as a lawyer), and one member who is unaffiliated with the institution. It is obvious that under the PHS policy there must be at least one more person on the IACUC to reach its minimum required composition of five people. Interestingly, the PHS policy does not specifically state that the chair must be a committee member, but it assumes that the committee will have a chair by stating, "The Assurance must include the names, position titles, and credentials of the IACUC chairperson and the members" (PHS *Policy* IV,A,3,b). There are no statistics available to say whether there are IACUCs in which the chair is not a voting member of the committee. That circumstance would be noncompliant with the AWARs (if the institution kept AWAR-regulated animals) and, it is fair to say, unusual, even if only PHS policy-regulated animals were being used.

Another important IACUC organizational difference between the PHS policy and the AWARs is that the AWARs do not require the IACUC to have a scientist who has worked with animals to be on the committee. In most biomedical research institutions, and for that matter in most any institution, it is best to have an IACUC membership that reflects the institution's research or teaching communities. In a research university, it would be unthinkable not to include investigators on the committee. In fact, most colleges and universities have more than the minimum number of people on the IACUC, not only to represent all of the school's constituencies, but also to ensure that they can have a quorum for meetings.

Not every IACUC member can be at every meeting or semiannual review or always be available to review a protocol. To address this problem, there is one group of people, called alternate members, who have an important role to play on the IACUC. Alternate members are "extras" who fill in for regular members who are unavailable. There is no regulation that requires an IACUC to have alternate members, but their use is common and is accepted by both NIH/OLAW and APHIS/AC. Like regular IACUC members, alternate members are appointed by the chief executive officer of the institution (or that person's designee). An alternate member must fill the same role as the regular member for whom he or she is substituting. That means an alternate for the veterinarian must be a veterinarian having training or experience with the animals housed at the institution. An alternate for a scientist who has used animals in research also must be a scientist who has used animals in research, and so forth. One person can be an alternate for more than one IACUC member (but fill in for only one person at a time), and that alternate must be able to fill the role of each person for whom he or she is an alternate. For example, if one person is named as the alternate for both the IACUC veterinarian and a specific IACUC scientist who has experience using laboratory animals, then that alternate must be a laboratory animal veterinarian who also has experience as a scientist using research animals. More information of alternates can be found in the frequently asked questions section of the NIH/OLAW website [39].

There are many behind-the-scenes people who also are important to the operation of an IACUC. They often are not members of the committee, but without them the activities of the committee would be far more difficult and in some cases, not possible. These people have titles such as IACUC manager, IACUC administrator, and compliance specialist. They are needed as much as the voting members of the committee.

### 5.3.2 *The Institutional Animal Care and Use Committee Chair*

Because everyone is important, it is the responsibility of the chair to make sure that everyone's importance is used in making the IACUC run efficiently and effectively. At academic institutions, most IACUC chairs have a faculty title (such as professor or associate professor) and are current or former animal users. This gives the chair a certain amount of credibility with committee members and the animal-using faculty. The responsibilities of the chair will vary somewhat at different institutions, but in general the chair:

- ensures that a quorum is present when necessary for the proper conduct of IACUC business requiring a vote;
- leads IACUC meetings by ensuring that all persons have an opportunity to speak and that no one person dominates the meeting;
- conducts meetings according to the rules of order previously agreed to by the IACUC and required by either the PHS policy or the AWARs (such as approving a protocol, withholding approval, or requiring modifications to secure approval);
- is impartial unless unique circumstances dictate the need for a specific direction to be taken;
- serves as a voting member of the IACUC (required by the AWARs);
- ensures that meeting minutes are kept and other reports are produced when needed;
- selects one or more reviewers for a protocol when designated member review is used (this responsibility is mandated by the AWARs and PHS policy);
- stays abreast of regulatory issues affecting the IACUC and keeps the IO informed of the same;
- communicates with the IO on specific matters of concern such as an IACUC suspension of an ongoing animal activity;
- tries to build positive relationships with IACUC members, animal care personnel, researchers, IACUC administrators, and the IO.

The chair is the face of the IACUC and has a difficult job. Although few receive direct monetary compensation for their efforts, some do receive a stipend that goes to supporting their laboratories or related institutional work.

### 5.3.3 *The Institutional Animal Care and Use Committee Veterinarian*

An IACUC constituted under the AWARs or PHS policy must have a veterinarian. The term attending veterinarian (AV) is defined in the AWARs (§1.1) as a veterinarian with training or experience in the care and management of the animal species being used and who has direct or delegated authority for animal activities at his or her institution. The PHS policy itself does not use the term attending veterinarian, but the definition of the IACUC veterinarian (PHS *Policy* IV,a,3,b) is similar to the AWAR definition of the AV. The *Guide* (p. 14) defines the AV as "The veterinarian responsible for the health and well-being of all laboratory animals used at the institution."

For the IACUC to function smoothly, it is important to have one veterinarian who is consistently on the IACUC (i.e., not one who rotates on and off the committee) and who has the authority to represent the institution's animal care and use program. Some large academic or other research institutions have campuses in many different locations and may have a different AV at each campus. Still, if there is only one IACUC for all of those campuses, then there should be one "senior" AV on the IACUC who has the authority to represent the entire institution's animal care and use program. The AWARs (§2.33,a,3) do allow for a veterinarian who is employed by the institution, but not as the AV, to be on the IACUC in place of the AV as long as that veterinarian has delegated program responsibility for animal activities. Although allowable, it is not a good idea to continually rotate veterinarians on the IACUC because this defeats the need for consistency. In contrast, the PHS policy does not make any provision for another veterinarian to replace the AV on the IACUC, although the alternate for the AV can substitute when the AV is unavailable.

With specific reference to the IACUC, what does the AV do? Some of the veterinarian's key responsibilities include:

- serves as a regular voting member of the committee with protocol review and semiannual inspection and program review responsibilities that are usually the same as for any other member of the committee;
- due to his or her training and experience, the AV brings a unique animal welfare perspective to the IACUC and is often considered to be the voice of the animals;
- as with the chairperson, the AV is typically well-versed in current regulations and policies affecting animal activities and serves as a resource for the committee;
- the AV offers the IACUC expertise in medical and surgical matters impacting animals used in research and teaching, particularly with the proper use of anesthetics, analgesics, and euthanasia agents;
- as the person immediately responsible for the animal care and use program, the AV must be able to assure the IACUC that the program is in compliance with all federal, state, and local laws and regulations.

The AV or another veterinarian often is one of the only people (or the only person) who performs unofficial pre-reviews of IACUC protocols. A pre-review gives the researcher or educator some preliminary feedback on the strengths or weaknesses of the protocol application before the official IACUC review process begins. There is no requirement at all for the researcher to accept any of the pre-review recommendations. In fact, there is no requirement at all to even have a pre-review or to have it done by a veterinarian. It is just a courtesy offered by many IACUCs, but a pre-review by a veterinarian has an additional benefit to the IACUC: It helps the committee comply with a regulation requiring consultation with the AV (or that person's designee) for procedures that may cause more than momentary or slight pain or distress to animals regulated under the AWARs (§2.31,d,1,iv,B). A veterinarian's feedback via a pre-review can be used as the required consultation if additional discussions are not needed.

### 5.3.4 Scientist Having Experience in Research Involving Animals

The breadth of research using animals ranges from small programs led by one or two research scientists to large multidisciplinary programs that may involve dozens of researchers. The scientist on the IACUC is a member who is required under the PHS policy, but not the AWARs. The IACUC scientist has three primary functions:

- to be a voting member of the IACUC and perform protocol reviews, inspections, and other IACUC functions that are assigned;
- to represent the animal use interests of the scientific community at his or her institution;
- to bring to the IACUC any unique knowledge gained from his or her research or teaching experience that, if imparted to the IACUC, might improve animal welfare or experimental results.

In one survey it was found that nearly half the scientists serving on their IACUC indicated that they did so, in part, to help ensure that the institution's research or teaching needs were not obstructed by their own IACUCs [35]. This does not imply that ensuring fairness to scientists is why a scientist joins the IACUC, but it does reinforce the importance of having all of an institution's animal-using constituencies represented on the committee.

The type of a scientist on the IACUC (e.g., an immunologist), the academic or other title of a scientist (e.g., associate professor), and any other attributes of a scientist who is being considered for service on the IACUC is at the discretion of the chief executive officer (or that person's designee) who appoints members to the IACUC. However, there is nothing prohibiting a person such as the IACUC chair or administrator from making a suggestion to the chief executive officer about the type of scientist that the IACUC might like to have, based on the needs of the committee. The minimal qualification needed is that the scientist to be chosen has experience using animals in a research setting. If the institution breeds and uses many genetically modified mice, then a mouse geneticist would likely be of value to the committee. If the institution has a focus on cardiovascular diseases, then it might consider recruiting a scientist with experience in that field. Some senior scientists in an academic setting might be involved with writing grants and serving on other school committees and not have the time to take on additional responsibilities with the IACUC. Other senior scientists, especially those no longer active in the laboratory, might relish the opportunity to serve.

### 5.3.5 Member with Primary Concerns in a Nonscientific Area

This member, required to be on the IACUC under the PHS policy only, brings to the committee a perspective that may be more neutral toward the use of animals in research than a person more prone to support animal-based research, such as the scientific member of the committee. It is expected, of course, that IACUC members will approach their committee work with a focus on animal welfare and regulatory compliance; however, human bias can never be fully dismissed. Indeed, two surveys have shown that approximately 93% of scientists support the use of animals in research [40,41], whereas one of those surveys reported only 52% support from the general public [40].

The nonscientist member can be from within or outside of the institution (the *Guide* p. 24). People serving as such a member can include ethicists, lawyers, accountants, and similar individuals. A person such as an institution's financial administrator also can serve as the nonscientific committee member as long as that person is not also a scientist as part of his or her job responsibilities. The functions of the nonscientific member are similar to that of other members:

- to be a voting member of the IACUC and perform protocol reviews, inspections, and other IACUC functions that are assigned;
- to represent the animal use interests of the nonscientific community;
- to bring to the IACUC any unique knowledge gained from his or her training and experience.

### 5.3.6 Member Who is Unaffiliated with the Institution Other than as a Member of the Institutional Animal Care and Use Committee

The AWARs (§2.31,b,3,ii) specifically state that the unaffiliated member (also known as the public member) should provide representation of the interests held by the general community in the proper care and treatment of animals. The *Guide* (p. 24) has similar wording. Both the AWARs and the *Guide* state that the unaffiliated member cannot be a member of the immediate family of a person who is affiliated with the institution.

Over the years, there have been many discussions about who can or cannot serve as the IACUC's unaffiliated member (or members, because there can be more than one unaffiliated member serving on the committee). Can a former employee serve? Can an animal researcher at another institution serve? In the latter case, the *Guide* (p. 24) and APHIS/AC policy #15 [42] say no. It is often more fruitful to answer these and similar questions by focusing on the intent of the regulation rather than trying to sort through innumerable unique situations. The intent is to have community values represented by a person who will not be influenced by any actual or perceived relationship to the institution that uses the laboratory animals. For example, a person who is long retired from a state university and receives a state pension can technically serve as the unaffiliated member because that person (assuming no direct relationship to a current employee of the school) is no longer affiliated with the school. However, the fact that the person used to be an employee and that a state pension might be construed by some people to be a school pension, suggests that this individual would not be the best person to serve on the IACUC. Who then, are typically asked to be the unaffiliated member of the IACUC? The list should be narrowed to people that have broad interactions within the community and get to know some the community's values, such as clergy, accountants, hair stylists, lawyers, etc.

The definition of "community" is not precise, but it is reasonable to include the location of the institution and its immediate surrounding area. Common sense has to be used. For example, the University of Massachusetts Medical School is in Worcester, MA. Close to Worcester are many towns where school employees live, such as Holden, Shrewsbury, and Spencer. They are all considered to be part of the medical school's community. Some employees live about an hour away, in Boston, which would not be considered by a reasonable person to be part of the Worcester community.

Unaffiliated members are not paid for their services, because any substantial payment might be interpreted as receiving a salary from the institution and making the person "affiliated." However, reimbursements for parking fees, lunch, tolls, and similar small expenses are acceptable. The unaffiliated member should receive the same training as any other IACUC member and should be provided the opportunity to participate in committee work like any other IACUC member. However, even with some help, the unaffiliated member (like the nonscientist member) may have trouble appreciating some of the concepts or language used in some research protocols. The chair and IACUC administrative office should be sensitive to this potential problem, assign achievable tasks to the unaffiliated member, and ensure that the unaffiliated member receives any needed help to make her or him comfortable with the IACUC and its functions. The roles of the unaffiliated member are:

- to be a voting member of the IACUC and perform protocol reviews, inspections, and other IACUC functions that are assigned;
- to represent the research animal use interests of the surrounding community;
- to bring to the IACUC any unique knowledge gained from his or her training and experience.

### 5.3.7 *Other Institutional Animal Care and Use Committee Members or Consultants*

The above descriptions of IACUC members include all those required by the AWARs and the PHS policy. There usually is only one chair on the IACUC (having co-chairs is rare, but possible) and one "senior" AV on the committee, but the IACUC can have other veterinarians and additional scientists, nonscientists, and unaffiliated members. It is not unusual for an IACUC to have 15–20 members in a large, research-focused university. From experience, there are other people who are not required to be on the IACUC, but, if available, are often helpful as members or consultants to the committee. For example, a biostatistician (or another person well-versed in statistics) can provide consultation on experimental design and the appropriate number of animals to be used on protocols. For institutions breeding large numbers of genetically modified mice, a mouse geneticist is an asset to the IACUC. An anesthesiologist with veterinary or human training can supplement the knowledge base of the vivarium veterinarians when complicated surgical procedures are planned. A bioethicist, although not commonly found on IACUCs, can provide guidance on complicated moral issues. A professional librarian can help provide a satisfactory database search strategy when seeking alternatives to animal use. Lastly, IACUCs in academic institutions should consider having a student on the committee to represent the views of the student body and as a learning experience for the student.

## 6. COMMON COMPLIANCE CHALLENGES

## 6.1 Overview

Noncompliance refers to a failure to adhere to the PHS policy, the Assurance the institution provided to NIH/OLAW, or the AWARs, as applicable. Noncompliance can be at the level of the individual (e.g., performing an unapproved surgical procedure), the IACUC (e.g., suspending an animal activity without a proper vote to suspend), or the institution (e.g., not having the chief executive officer or that person's designee appoint the IACUC). Determining the actual prevalence of noncompliance is not an easy task. NIH/OLAW is not required to provide a regular update of noncompliant items, but through various publications and meetings, the main compliance problems that come to its attention are known. For example, in one published study of 124 reports made to NIH/OLAW, it was found that 37% of departures from the PHS policy were related to animal care and management (such as lack of training, inadequate pain management, or inadequate animal monitoring), while 29% of noncompliant items were protocol related (such as lack of an approved protocol or not following an approved protocol) [43]. NIH/OLAW itself reported that about 30% of incidents reported to it involved animal protocols, and of that number, 40% involved protocol noncompliance [44]. Like NIH/OLAW, APHIS/AC also periodically comments on the main noncompliance problems that it finds during the course of its activities. In the federal fiscal year 2013, it was stated that 77% of APHIS/AC animal facility inspections had no direct noncompliant findings [45]. (A direct noncompliant finding is one that is affecting, or likely to soon affect, the health and well-being of an animal.)

Some of the most common reported problems with compliance [42,44,46–48] include:

- IACUCs lacking one or more of the required members (which makes the review and approval of animal activities potentially invalid);
- conducting IACUC business without a convened quorum when a quorum was needed;
- conducting animal activities that have not been reviewed and approved by the IACUC;
- inadequate semiannual inspections and program review;
- making significant changes to previously approved activities without IACUC approval;
- failure to report to NIH/OLAW instances of serious or continuing noncompliance with the policy, serious deviations from the *Guide* (PHS *Policy* IV,F,3), and for both NIH/OLAW and APHIS/AC, suspensions of animal-related activities;
- deficiencies in the use of appropriate means to minimize or avoid discomfort, distress, and pain in animals;
- deficiencies in the program of disease control and prevention;
- inadequate record-keeping, including the documentation of veterinary care;
- inadequate mechanisms by which employees can bring their concerns about animal care and use to the IACUC for consideration.

## 6.2 General Causes of Noncompliance

More important than a listing of common noncompliant items are the possible reasons for noncompliance and means for helping to assure a culture of compliance. The discussion that follows is often based on experience rather than the limited number of references on the subject matter and will focus on the research team that is performing activities with animals. After this general discussion, there is commentary about some factors that are unique to researchers and can lead to noncompliance.

### 6.2.1 Noncompliance Arising from Inadequate Training

Federal regulations (AWARs §2.32,a; §2.32,b; PHS *Policy* IV,A,1,g; the *Guide* pp. 15–17) require training and instruction of research teams, animal technicians, and other personnel (such as IACUC members) to help ensure that they are qualified to perform their animal-related duties. It is a responsibility of the IACUC to oversee the effectiveness of this training (*Guide* p. 15). The AWARs (§2.32,c) and the *Guide* (p. 17) provide training topics that should be included, such as provision for the basic needs of the species, proper animal handling, aseptic surgical methods, the use of anesthesia and analgesia, relevant legislation, and so forth. Interestingly, the three Rs are not mentioned directly in the *Guide*, AWARs, or PHS policy, but NIH/OLAW specifically states in online guidance that they should be considered during the protocol review process [49]. The challenge for the IACUC is to provide sufficient training for the research team to properly perform the planned animal use activities, but not to provide so much information that little is retained.

It is fair to ask, "Where does an investigator or IACUC member get training?" Most IACUCs require basic training on the above-mentioned subjects before a person begins work on their first animal use project. A training program may be basic and standardized for all users; nevertheless, it may meet the regulatory compliance requirements for training. Consequently, training programs can range from nothing more than a series of slides to thorough one-on-one training and evaluation. There even may be a brief written examination after the training.

There are multiple questions for the IACUC and trainers to consider. For example, will the person receiving the training actually retain much of the provided information? Is all or part of the training program ever going to be repeated as a "refresher course"? Does the trainee have an understanding of anesthesia and analgesia considerations that extends beyond the drug dosages approved by the IACUC? Is a person who received basic surgical training competent to perform even an uncomplicated surgical procedure if that is part of his or her approved protocol? If a surgical procedure is part of the study, have all potential surgeons demonstrated (to the satisfaction of the IACUC) that they can apply aseptic technique, that their tissue handling is appropriate, and that they can perform basic suture patterns? How will a neophyte surgeon learn to perform an actual operative procedure, such as an ovariohysterectomy? Many IACUCs will require initial practice of the procedure on dead animals, then the surgeon will practice the procedure as nonsurvival surgery, and only then move on to survival surgery.

None of the above and related training questions are easily answered, and much depends on the specific circumstances encountered. However, it is fair to say that one of the keys to satisfactory training of a researcher is to provide less information on items that have limited research relevance (e.g., the minuscule details of the protocol review process) and more information on items that are important for animal welfare, such as how humane endpoints can be developed, how to recognize pain, how to estimate the number of animals needed, what records must be kept, etc. Appropriate training and/or an evaluation of skills before a project starts will be worth its weight in gold after the project begins.

All of the above training issues are to help prevent noncompliance with IACUC or institutional policies and to prevent inadvertent mistreatment of animals. However, not all training must be provided directly by an institution's IACUC. There are many other possible training and learning opportunities including:

- books such as *The IACUC Handbook* [50] and *Institutional Animal Care and Use Committee Guidebook* [51];
- IACUC 101™, which is an educational program for IACUC members that is periodically presented at various institutions around the nation;

- meetings of Public Responsibility in Medicine and Research, some of which focus on IACUC issues;
- independent training companies;
- the AALAS Learning Library, sponsored by the American Association for Laboratory Animal Science;
- websites such as the NIH/OLAW website [27] and the APHIS/AC website [52].

Does every person who is involved with a research project require training or just those who do "hands-on" animal work? The principal investigator (PI) is the scientist who is responsible for designing and implementing a research project with animals. In large laboratories, the PI may not do any hands-on work with animals, delegating that responsibility to technicians, graduate students, or others. However, even when the PI does not directly work with animals, he or she should partake in basic training that covers the regulatory and animal care information required to effectively oversee and make any needed modifications to an ongoing study.

### 6.2.2 Noncompliance Arising from Unrealistic Expectations

It is important for IACUC members, particularly the chair and the AV, to have a thorough understanding of the existence and proper application of laws, regulations, and policies affecting the use of animals at their institution. Members of the IACUC also must be reasonably well-versed in their understanding of pertinent federal regulations and institutional policies in order to fulfill their obligations to the IACUC. In contrast, investigators and other members of a research or teaching team have no need to know the specific sections of the PHS policy or AWARs that are applicable to their animal work, but they do have to know some basic regulatory concepts and the terminology the IACUC is looking for when they fill out the various sections of a protocol form. Baucal [53], referring to research funding agencies, stated that a researcher has "to learn to 'translate' her/his project proposal into discourse and terminology preferable to a funding agency." The PI has to do the same for the IACUC.

As will be discussed further below, researchers want clear and simple rules to follow once a protocol is approved. If the rules are too many or too complicated, there is a good chance they will not be followed, not because of intentional resistance, but because the researcher has other priorities. The most basic and simple rules for investigators to follow and for the IACUC to repeatedly emphasize were stated earlier, and they are worth repeating:

- do not perform any animal activity without IACUC approval;
- do not make changes to an animal activity without IACUC approval;
- do what you said you would do.

### 6.2.3 Noncompliance Arising from Inadequate Oversight

Research using animals is an activity that incorporates the efforts of members of the research laboratory, the animal care team, and many others. Everybody has a job to do, and it is assumed that all involved people have been properly trained and are reasonably competent at their jobs. However, there is still a need for oversight of activities because all of us are capable of making errors. In most animal facilities, there are supervisors who oversee the provision of animal care and veterinary service. In a grants management office, there are individuals who double-check the financial work of others. Many institutions have a post-IACUC approval monitoring program, which is essentially an oversight program to help researchers remain in compliance with their protocols. (Post-approval monitoring is discussed in more detail later in this chapter.) In the research laboratory, it is the PI who ultimately is responsible for the conduct of research. In a very real sense then, research is a team effort, and no part of this broad-based research team is totally self-sufficient; therefore, if a laboratory technician does not read the IACUC protocol and just relies on what others have told him, if a PI assumes others in her lab will train a new graduate student, if an animal care technician tries to take shortcuts, or if a post-approval monitoring program is grossly understaffed, noncompliance may result and impact the entire research project, even in the most successful of research organizations. It is the PI, the AV, and the IO who have the day-to-day responsibility of assuring compliance with federal laws, regulations, and policies. The IACUC has an important role (as will be described below), but it is not the primary responsibility of the IACUC to monitor day-to-day research activities.

### 6.2.4 Noncompliance Resulting from Ethnic or Other Cultural Differences

In graduate and postdoctoral education in the United States, there are a large number of foreign scholars with varying degrees of fluency in spoken and written English and American customs. Language misunderstandings and ethnic traditions may lead to unintended noncompliance. Therefore, if a school has many foreign research or teaching personnel, it can prove helpful to translate selected training materials into a predominant language and place informational signs in the vivarium using more than one language. As another example, transporting animals on a school's public elevators is usually not acceptable to an IACUC in the United States, but may have been the norm at the institution from which a foreign researcher came. The IACUC, the PI, and the research institution have to be cognizant of and sensitive to such issues and provide appropriate support whenever possible.

### 6.2.5 Noncompliance Resulting from the Institutional Culture

The term institutional culture refers to how things are really done at an institution. It includes items such as "Friday's are dress-down days," "make sure you copy her on every email you send out," and "don't take more than a half-hour for lunch." Even an IACUC has a culture of its own. We sometimes hear that an IACUC is very strict or perhaps very lenient, but no IACUC and no institution will openly advocate noncompliance with federal regulations and policies. Yet, subtle words and actions may tell a different story, inferring that the real culture supports a degree of noncompliance. For example, assume that it is brought to the attention of the IACUC chair that an investigator performed a pilot study using animals but without IACUC approval. At the next IACUC meeting, the chair informs the committee that "Dr Childs used a few mice for a small pilot study that only involved some subcutaneous injections of a nontoxic chemical. I told him that in the future he has to get IACUC approval before he does any pilot study, otherwise we may have to inform NIH/OLAW that he's not in compliance with the PHS policy. He agreed to do so, and I thanked him for his cooperation." Clearly, the chair knew that IACUC approval was needed and that performing an animal activity without IACUC approval was a reportable noncompliance with the PHS policy. However, the IACUC culture was "if it doesn't seem like it's a big deal, we'll give you a break on a first infraction." IACUCs do have to exercise judgment in many instances, but not when it involves a clear and significant deviation from a federal regulation. The IACUC should work to establish a culture that includes trying to help investigators, but does not include sweeping problems under the rug [54].

There is one culture trait that should be entrenched in all institutions to help prevent noncompliance, that being open communication. Open communication generally refers to a culture "in which nonconfidential and nonproprietary information is actively and freely shared with both employees and interested stakeholders with the leadership's blessing and proactive participation" [55]. As a simple example of the importance of open communication in avoiding noncompliance, consider the *AVMA Guidelines for the Euthanasia of Animals: 2013 edition* [29]. For some species, these guidelines, which under the PHS policy (IV,C,1,g) and APHIS/AC policy #3 [22] must be adhered to, have either changed or modified the acceptable euthanasia methods for some laboratory animals when compared to earlier editions of the AVMA guidelines. Will the institution's IACUC (or veterinary service) announce this to the animal users? Will the IACUC point out important changes to the guidelines or just assume researchers will find them for themselves? Is there a designated person who will be able to answer questions from the research laboratories? In short, does the organizational culture encourage better regulatory compliance through open communications?

## 6.3 Noncompliance and the Individual Researcher

The five causes of noncompliance discussed above are generic and are applicable to IACUC members, researchers, IOs, animal care personnel, educators, and others working with laboratory animals. Yet, biomedical researchers often require additional support from the IACUC to help thwart noncompliance. The reason is that researchers are highly intelligent, individualistic, and motivated individuals whose short-term success, and sometimes careers, may depend on their ability to attract federal research dollars (e.g., researchers in academic institutions), publish scholarly manuscripts, and present their work at local, national, and international meetings. To advance their careers and intellectual curiosity, researchers need and expect recognition and support from their institution, including support from the IACUC. When support from the IACUC is lacking, noncompliance may be exacerbated. For example, taken as a group, researchers are uninterested in bureaucracy [56] (which includes the IACUC's protocol review and approval process) and want to have simple and clear rules to follow [57], not the plethora of rules and regulations that the IACUC must understand. Additionally, researchers do not like to be told what to do. DuBois [58] nicely summarized the needs of researchers when it comes to compliance, writing, "There are at least two fundamentally different ways that we can expect to get researchers to comply with regulations: under threat of penalty or because they have internalized it as a norm (i.e., they see it as a professional virtue, as something that ultimately contributes to the aim of producing generalizable knowledge that will serve humankind)." As a generalization, researchers prefer the latter method.

Federal laws, along with the associated regulations and policies that the IACUC and researchers are obligated to follow, are largely punishment centered and not the clear, representative rules favored by researchers (such as the rules governing tenure and promotion in academia) [57]. When the IACUC alone makes or enforces rules, researchers may comply with those rules, but only to the extent that it serves their needs. In contrast, representative rules and values that originate from the top of the organization (e.g., the president's office) and filter down through the provost, the dean, and department chairs to the individual researcher will likely have a greater chance of leading to compliance [57]. These representative rules should be clear, simple, and logical, and examples were previously stated in this chapter (i.e., do not perform any animal activity without IACUC approval; do not make changes to an animal activity without IACUC approval; and do what you said you would do).

Lastly, researchers, like most people, prefer to be represented and led by those who think and act as they do. Thus, it is important for those serving on an IACUC to be representative of their research community, and in a research-oriented institution, due consideration should be given to having a chair who has the intellectual and technical respect of the institution's researchers. To help internalize the ethical rules of research oversight throughout the organization, it has been suggested that individual researchers should be expected to rotate on and off a committee, such as the IACUC, as a natural part of their duties [58].

## 7. ADDRESSING NONCOMPLIANCE

### 7.1 Initial Responses

Try as we may to prevent it, noncompliance will likely occur at some time at most institutions. When items of known or suspected noncompliance are discovered, the immediate action to be taken depends on the nature of the noncompliant activity. If the noncompliance is not endangering the health or well-being of an animal, the first response of the IACUC should be to bring the activity back into compliance, such as by requiring a protocol amendment. However, if there is evidence that an animal is being abused (or is otherwise endangered), the initial step is to stop the abuse or endangerment and care for any immediate needs of the animal. Waiting for an IACUC to meet and make a decision about alleged abuse, even if a meeting can be hastily organized, may still take too long. But how can an animal activity be stopped without IACUC approval because IACUC approval is required to suspend an animal activity? The answer is the use of institutionally granted authority. Many institutions, through an individual such as the IO, give the AV or the IACUC chairperson (or both) the authority to stop an animal activity. If this happens, it is then incumbent on the IACUC to meet as soon as possible to review the incident and determine what additional actions, if any, may be required. If it is determined by the IACUC that significant noncompliance did occur, the incident must be reported to NIH/OLAW (assuming the institution has an NIH/OLAW Assurance), because a reportable incident includes an "IACUC suspension or other institutional intervention that results in the temporary or permanent interruption of an activity due to noncompliance with the [PHS] *Policy*, Animal Welfare Act, the *Guide*, or the institution's Animal Welfare Assurance" [59]. When an activity is stopped using institutional authority, this has occurred by an "other institutional intervention." Additionally, if the IACUC votes at a convened meeting of the committee, with a quorum present, to uphold the stopped activity (i.e., the IACUC formally votes to suspend the activity), then APHIS/AC and any federal agency funding the project also must be notified when AWAR-regulated species are involved (AWARs §2.31,d,7). The PHS does not allow NIH funds to be used to care for animals when an entire protocol is suspended. Similarly, if a person is suspended from working on a PHS-supported study such as a research grant, then NIH monies cannot be used to pay the portion of that person's salary that is associated with the study. When a suspension occurs, it is a responsibility of the IACUC, through the IO, to inform NIH/OLAW of the suspension. The institution (not necessarily the IACUC) informs the appropriate NIH funding center or institute of the suspension and provides assurance that NIH funds will not be used for animal maintenance, salaries, or related expenses until the suspension is ended by the IACUC [60].

## 7.2 Investigating Allegations of Noncompliance

The time to develop procedures to investigate noncompliance is not when noncompliance occurs, but well before that time. Although it is not possible to have specific plans that address every incident reaching the IACUC, it is possible (and recommended) to have general plans established on how to proceed with an investigation of possible noncompliance. As indicated earlier in this chapter, the first step is to maintain confidentiality because an allegation is just an unproven assertion unless determined to be correct. Following is a list of 10 questions for an IACUC to consider when developing a general plan to address allegations of noncompliance. Each institution should develop procedures that meet its unique needs.

1. Do we have procedures in place that enable people to readily bring allegations of noncompliance to the IACUC? This includes methods of making people aware that they can bring such allegations and the actual process of forwarding the allegation to the IACUC.
2. Can we ensure the confidentiality of the complainant if we are requested to do so? The IACUC should consider what confidentiality actually means. For example, does confidentiality mean that only the IACUC chairperson knows the identity of the complainant, or does it mean that the full IACUC is privy to that information? When during the investigative process will the IO be informed of the allegation, and will the IO be privy to the identification of the complainant? If you are part of an academic institution where a person who makes a complaint against another person must be identified under school policy, can the IACUC become the complainant to maintain confidentiality?
3. Will the complainant be told of any legal protections for whistleblowers? The AWARs (§2.32,c,4) prohibit reprisals against any employees or IACUC members for making an allegation of noncompliance with the AWAR. However, the PHS policy does not have such specific protection against whistleblowers, although the *Guide* (p. 24) states that there should be compliance with any existing whistleblower policies, nondiscrimination against the concerned or reporting party, and protection from reprisals.
4. Who will conduct an initial or full investigation? Will the chair, AV, IACUC subcommittee, or others do an initial investigation? Will a subsequent full investigation, if warranted, comprise the same or a different group of people?
5. When will the accused person be told of the complaint? Accused people almost invariably take an allegation seriously, and it can negatively impact their daily activities. The IACUC should carefully consider whether to contact an accused person as soon as an accusation is made or wait until a preliminary investigation provides credence to the accusation. If there is no credence to the accusation and the IACUC will take no action, will the accused person be informed of this?

6. How will an investigation be conducted? Will the IACUC develop a list of possible items to examine (e.g., animal use records, anesthesia and analgesia records, surgical packs) and possible people to interview? Or will the people performing the investigation make those decisions as the investigation progresses? Some questions that are often asked of complainants are listed earlier in this chapter (see Key Regulatory Mandates).

7. Will representation be allowed? Will either the IACUC or the accused person be allowed to have legal or other representation? If it is allowable, will the representative be allowed to speak "on the record," or is that person only allowed to provide private advice? If the accused is a member of a union, will he or she be allowed to have a union delegate present, even if the latter person provides no specific representation during the investigation?

8. What authority does the IACUC have to impose sanctions against a person? The only federally allowable sanction that the IACUC can impose against a person is to suspend an animal activity, in whole or in part, or to suspend the person from working with animals. However, some proven allegations of noncompliance may have had no actual or potential impact on animal welfare and may not have been a serious deviation from the *Guide*, the PHS policy, or the AWARs. When such a determination is made by the IACUC, it is not required to suspend a person or an animal activity. For example, if a study was approved to have five blood samples taken from a dog but only four were taken (because the four provided the PI with the needed information), an IACUC, using reasonable discretion, may remind the investigator to inform the IACUC before making such a change. In other instances, perhaps being slightly more consequential than the example just given, the IACUC might send a letter of reprimand to an investigator. This can be done if the IACUC has the authority to do so from its home institution; it has no such authority under the AWARs or PHS policy.

9. If any kind of a sanction is imposed by the IACUC, will an appeal be allowed? Neither the PHS policy nor the AWARs prohibit appeals, and it becomes a matter of IACUC policy to determine whether an appeal is allowed and whether the violator will be allowed to have some form of representation during the appeal process.

10. What information will be provided to the complainant after an allegation of noncompliance is made to the IACUC? Will the complainant (if known) be given no information, limited information, or full information about the progress and conclusion of an investigation?

## 7.3 Subsequent Actions

Once noncompliance is discovered, addressed, and the problem is resolved (or is in the process of being resolved) to the satisfaction of the IACUC, there are still more things to do. As described earlier, if a suspension of an animal activity (or a person) was voted by the IACUC, the IO, in consultation with the IACUC, is required to promptly report the suspension to NIH/OLAW if animals regulated under the PHS policy are involved and to APHIS/AC and any involved federal funding agency if the animals are regulated under the AWARs. This notification should include the identification of the involved IACUC protocol (the name of the PI is not required), the NIH/OLAW Assurance number (for PHS policy-regulated animals), a full description of the problem, the impact the problem had on the animal or on the federally supported research activity, what the corrective action was or will be, the time frame for correction of the noncompliance, and any other pertinent information [59].

Not all notifications to NIH/OLAW have to result from suspensions of animal activities. There are two other compliance-related circumstances for which NIH/OLAW must be notified, as indicated in PHS *Policy* IV,F,3. They are:

- any serious or continuing noncompliance with the PHS policy;
- any serious deviation from the provisions of the *Guide*.

Three examples of serious noncompliance with the PHS policy or deviations from the *Guide* are shown below. Additional examples have been published [59].

- failure to adhere to IACUC-approved protocols;
- inadequate programs of veterinary care or personnel training;
- inadequate animal health records.

The AWARs (§2.31,c,3) also have a reporting requirement that is in addition to reporting a suspension of an animal activity. Earlier in this chapter, the semiannual inspection and review processes were described. The AWARs require reporting any uncorrected significant deficiency that is found on the semiannual program review or semiannual inspection that is not corrected within the period determined by the IACUC. This report must be made to APHIS/ AC and any federal agency funding the activity within 15 business days after the period determined by the IACUC has expired. The report is made by the IACUC, through the IO.

## 7.4 Using Postapproval Monitoring to Improve Compliance

It was noted earlier in this chapter that a responsibility of the IACUC is to periodically review the program of animal care and use. This can be accomplished through the semiannual program review and facility inspections that were described earlier, protocol reviews, reviews of proposed changes to research activities, periodic spot-checks of certain studies, and other means. One additional method of reviewing animal care and use activities is a nonmandatory yet helpful program commonly called postapproval monitoring (PAM). PAM is a continuous process that reviews activities performed under IACUC-approved protocols for conformity with the approved protocol. In some institutions, PAM also reviews animal facility and IACUC activities. PAM is not a substitute for the semiannual review and inspection performed by the IACUC; it supplements those activities. At its heart, PAM is a collaborative auditing process that works with investigators to help ensure that they and their staffs are following their IACUC-approved protocols and when working with animals their skill level is appropriate for the task at hand.

The key to a successful PAM program is the manner in which it is implemented. It is best for PAM personnel to establish a relationship with researchers and laboratory personnel that is based on empathy and helpfulness. This avoids being regarded by the research laboratory as yet another regulatory hurdle to overcome. Establishing such a relationship can be promoted by PAM personnel who have prior experience using animals in research, are friendly, want to help facilitate research, and are able and willing to demonstrate proper techniques when practical, but at the same time are well-versed in current regulatory requirements.

PAM personnel often use a checklist of items to be reviewed during their site visit to a laboratory or other animal use area. The list may include, for example, the specific anesthetics, analgesics, or other drugs (with dosages) that are approved for use. With that information, the PAM reviewer is able to check anesthesia and analgesia records for compliance with the IACUC protocol. It may be found that adequate records are not being kept, and if that were to happen, the PAM reviewer can work with the laboratory to establish proper records. The audit list also may include the names of the people who will be performing specific techniques, the areas approved for experimentation, any IACUC-approved variances in lighting cycles, temperature, feeding, and watering schedules, and so forth. An effective PAM reviewer will not simply ask research personnel whether they are or are not following the items on their protocol, but will be proactive by observing people at work, looking at animals, and in general, observing the details of the ongoing research. If a problem is noticed, PAM personnel should work with the laboratory to correct the problem as soon as possible; however, this does not mean that a significant problem should not be reported to the IACUC. A thorough PAM evaluation can take many days because the PAM reviewer may have to return more than once to observe animal use activities.

PAM can be an extension of the IACUC, the institution's veterinary service, or it can be independent and report to a third party such as a vice-president for research. If PAM reports to the IACUC, a research laboratory might reasonably assume, albeit incorrectly, that PAM and the IACUC are one and the same. That might not help to foster the image of helpfulness that PAM tries to project. Also, a PAM program may have among its duties the review of IACUC operations, but if PAM reports to the IACUC, there is a conflict of interest. Another problem can arise when PAM reports to the IACUC, because by definition the IACUC is a committee, and the PAM staff should report to a person, not an entire committee [61]. Likewise, it would not be advisable for PAM to report to the AV because PAM often monitors the animal care program. The best option is for PAM to report to the vice-president for research or a similar individual having the authority and responsibility to oversee research compliance at the institution.

## 8. FINAL COMMENTS

Research regulatory compliance for IACUCs is a multifaceted topic. Compliance with the various regulations and policies of the federal government often is complicated by state, local, and institutional regulations and policies. Compliance concerns can arise not only from mistakes made by a research laboratory but also from errors made by the institution's administration, the vivarium staff, and the IACUC itself. Nevertheless, researchers and those with whom they work rarely are intentionally noncompliant; rather, noncompliance is often a result of misunderstandings, inadequate training, cultural differences, how researchers react to imposed regulations, and other factors discussed in this chapter.

It is true that the IACUC is a self-regulatory committee that bases its actions on federal laws and regulations, yet no IACUC should act in a vacuum and divorce itself from the realities that researchers and educators have to face. A basic understanding of how researchers react to regulatory authority and an understanding of the steps that the IACUC can take to enhance compliance can, as an end product, lead to a more compliant culture that protects the researcher, the institution, and of course, the animals.

# References

[1] Committee on Science and Technology. The use of animals in medical research and testing. Hearings before the subcommittee on science, research and technology. U.S. house of representatives. Oct. 13, 14 1981. No. 68. Washington, DC: U.S. Government Printing Office; 1982.

[2] Herzog H, Rowan A, Kossow D. Social attitudes and animals. In: Salem DJ, Rowan AN, editors. The state of the animals 2001. Washington, DC: Humane Society Press; 2001.

[3] Gallup Historical Trends. Moral issues. http://www.gallup.com/poll/1681/Moral-Issues.aspx#1 2013.

[4] Wilke J, Saad L. Older Americans' moral attitude changing Gallup Politics; August 16. http://www.gallup.com /poll/162881/older-americans-moral-attitudes-changing.aspx; 2013.

[5] Houde L, Dumas C, Leroux T. Animal ethical evaluation: an observational study of Canadian IACUCs. Ethics Behav 2003;13:333–50.

[6] Hall M. A critical and experimental essay on the circulation of the blood: especially as observed in the minute and capillary vessels of the batrachia and of fishes. London: R.B. Seeley and W. Burnside; 1831.

[7] Russell W, Burch R. The principles of humane experimental technique. London: Methuen; 1959.

[8] Van Sluyters RC. A guide to risk assessment to animal care and use programs: the metaphor of the 3-legged stool. ILAR J 2008;49:372–8.

[9] Rozmiarek H. Origins of the IACUC. In: Silverman J, Suckow MA, Murthy S, editors. The IACUC handbook. 2nd ed. Boca Raton: CRC Press; 2007.

[10] Curnutt J. Animals and the law: a sourcebook. Santa Barbara: ABC-CLIO; 2001. p. 439.

[11] Phinizy C. The lost pets that stray to the labs. Sports Illustrated November 1965;27:36–9.

[12] Wayman S. Concentration camps for dogs. Life 1966;60(5):22–9.

[13] Stewart WC. Regulatory perspectives of the United States Department of Agriculture on functions of animal care and use committees. Lab Anim Sci January 1987:22–3. Special Issue.

[14] Curnutt J. Animals and the law: a sourcebook. Santa Barbara: ABC-CLIO; 2001. p. 467.

[15] Committee on the Guide for Laboratory Animal Facilities and Care. Guide for laboratory animal facilities and care. Publication 1024. Washington DC: Public Health Service, U.S. Government Printing Office; 1965.

[16] Whitney Jr RA. Animal care and use committees: history and current national policies in the United States. Lab Anim Sci January 1987:18–21. Special Issue.

[17] National Institutes of Health, Office of Laboratory Animal Welfare. Public health service policy on humane care and use of laboratory animals. National Institutes of Health, Bethesda. http://grants2.nih.gov/grants/olaw/ references/PHSPolicyLabAnimals.pdf; 2002.

[18] Title 7, U.S. Code, Chapter 54, §§2131–2159. Animal Welfare Act.

[19] Title 9, Code of federal regulations, Chapter 1, Subchapter A, Parts 1–4. [Animal Welfare Regulations].

[20] U.S. Department of Agriculture, Animal and Plant Health Inspection Service. Animal care policy manual. http://www.aphis.usda.gov/animal_welfare/policy.php; 2011.

[21] DeHaven WR. Understanding USDA's Animal Welfare Act policies, particularly policy 12. http://www. nal.usda.gov/awic/newsletters/v9n3/9n3dehav.htm [accessed 26.11.13].

[22] U.S. Department of Agriculture, Animal and Plant Health Inspection Service. Policy #3. Veterinary care. http://www.aphis.usda.gov/animal_welfare/policy.php?policy=3; 2011.

[23] U.S. Department of Agriculture, Animal and Plant Health Inspection Service. Consolidated inspection guide. Section 8.3.1 http://www.aphis.usda.gov/animal_welfare/2011_Inspection_Guide//01%20Table%20of%20 Contents.pdf; 2010.

[24] Committee for the Update of the Guide for the Care and Use of Laboratory Animals. Guide for the care and use of laboratory animals 8th ed. Washington, D. C.: National Academies Press. http://grants2.nih.gov/grants/olaw/ Guide-for-the-Care-and-Use-of-Laboratory-Animals.pdf; 2011.

[25] National Institutes of Health, Office of Laboratory Animal Welfare. US government principles for the utilization and care of vertebrate animals used in testing, research, and training. http://grants2.nih.gov/grants/olaw/ references/phspol.htm#USGovPrinciples; 2002.

[26] National Institutes of Health, Office of Laboratory Animal Welfare. Frequently asked questions. http://gran ts2.nih.gov/grants/olaw/faqs.htm; 2013.

[27] National Institutes of Health, Office of Laboratory Animal Welfare. Internet website. http://grants2. nih.gov/grants/olaw/ [accessed 26.11.13].

[28] National Institutes of Health, Office of Extramural Research. Animal Welfare Assurance for domestic institutions. http://grants2.nih.gov/grants/olaw/sampledoc/assur.htm; 2012.

[29] American Veterinary Medical Association, Panel on Euthanasia. AVMA guidelines for the euthanasia of animals: 2013 edition. https://www.avma.org/KB/Policies/Documents/euthanasia.pdf; 2013.

[30] Committees to revise the Guide for the Care and Use of Agricultural Animals in Research and Teaching. Guide for the care and use of agricultural animals in research and teaching. Champaign, IL: Federation of Animal Science Societies; 2010.

[31] National Institutes of Health, Office of Extramural Research. Animal study proposal. http://grants2.nih.gov/grants/olaw/sampledoc/animal_study_prop.htm; 2011.

[32] National Institutes of Health. Notice NOT-OD-14-126. Guidance on significant changes to animal activities. http://grants.nih.gov/grants/guide/notice-files/NOT-OD-14-126.html; 2014.

[33] National Institutes of Health, Office of Laboratory Animal Welfare. Frequently asked question D.4, May the IACUC grant conditional or provisional approval?. http://grants.nih.gov/grants/olaw/faqs.htm#proto_4; 2013.

[34] National Institutes of Health, Office of Extramural Research. Semiannual program review and facility inspection checklist. http://grants2.nih.gov/grants/olaw/sampledoc/checklist_html.htm#3a; 2012.

[35] Silverman J, Baker SP, Lidz CW. A self-assessment survey of the institutional animal care and use committee, part 1: animal welfare and protocol compliance. Lab Anim (NY) 2012;41:230–5.

[36] Brown P, Gipson C. A word from OLAW and USDA. Lab Anim (NY) 2011;40:297.

[37] Association for Assessment and Accreditation of Laboratory Animal Care International. AAALAC International mission statement. http://www.aaalac.org/about/mission.cfm; 2013.

[38] Orwell G. Animal farm.. New York: Harcourt Brace; 1946.

[39] National Institutes of Health, Office of Laboratory Animal Welfare. Frequently asked questions B.2. May the IACUC have alternate members?. http://grants2.nih.gov/grants/olaw/faqs.htm; 2013.

[40] Pew Research Center for People & the Press. Public praises science; scientists fault public, media. http://www.people-press.org/2009/07/09/public-praises-science-scientists-fault-public-media/; 2009.

[41] Cressey D. Battle scars. Nature 2011;470:452–3. http://www.nature.com/news/2011/110223/pdf/470452a.pdf.

[42] U.S. Department of Agriculture, Animal and Plant Health Inspection Service. Policy #15. Institutional official and IACUC membership. http://www.aphis.usda.gov/animal_welfare/policy.php?policy=15; 2011.

[43] Gomez LM, Conlee KM, Stephens ML. Noncompliance with Public Health Service (PHS) policy on humane care and use of laboratory animals: an exploratory analysis. J Appl Anim Welf Sci 2010;13:123–36.

[44] Brown P, Gipson C. Noncompliance in survival surgery technique: a word from OLAW and USDA. Lab Anim (NY) 2010;39:234.

[45] Goldentyer E. Presentation at the national meeting of the American Association for Laboratory Animal Science. Baltimore, MD. October 28, 2013.

[46] Potkay S, Dehaven R, OLAW APHIS. Common areas of noncompliance. Lab Anim (NY) 2000;29(5):32–7.

[47] U.S. Department of Agriculture, Animal and Plant Health Inspection Service. Annual non-compliant item summary. http://www.aphis.usda.gov/animal_welfare/downloads/violations/2007violations.pdf; 2007.

[48] Bayne K, Brown P, Petervary N. Top 10 deficiencies from the perspective of USDA, OLAW, and AAALAC. In: "Proceedings of the PRIM&R 2011 IACUC conference." Chicago, IL, May 31–April 1, 2011.

[49] National Institutes of Health, Office of Laboratory Animal Welfare. Frequently asked question D.7, Should the IACUC consider the three "Rs" of alternatives when reviewing protocols? (Refinements to research, reduction of animal numbers, and replacement with non-animal models.). http://grants2.nih.gov/grants/olaw/faqs.htm#proto_7; 2013.

[50] Silverman J, Suckow MA, Murthy M. The IACUC handbook. Boca Raton: CRC Press; 2014.

[51] Applied Research Ethics National Association/Office of Laboratory Animal Welfare. Institutional animal care and use committee guidebook. National Institutes of Health, Bethesda; 2002.

[52] U.S. Department of Agriculture, Animal and Plant Health Inspection Service. Intranet website. http://www.aphis.usda.gov/animal_welfare/index.shtml [accessed 26.11.13].

[53] Baucal A. Reflective sociocultural psychology: lost and found in collaboration with funding agencies and ICT experts. Integr Psych Behav 2007;41:169–77.

[54] Silverman J. Do pressure and prejudice influence the IACUC? Lab Anim (NY) 1997;26(5):23–5.

[55] Melcrum Connecting Communications. Open communication cultures: best practice in a changing world. https://www.melcrum.com/research/create-high-impact-communication-plans/open-communication-cultures-best-practice-changing [accessed 11.10.13].

[56] Geoffe R, Jones G. Leading clever people. Harv Bus Rev 2007;85(3):72–9.
[57] Gouldner AW. Patterns of industrial bureaucracy. New York: The Free Press; 1964.
[58] DuBois J. Is compliance a professional virtue of researchers? Reflections on promoting the responsible conduct of research. Ethics Behav 2004;14:383–5.
[59] National Institutes of Health, Office of Laboratory Animal Welfare. Notice NOT-OD-05–034, guidance on prompt reporting to OLAW under the PHS Policy on Humane Care and Use of Laboratory Animals. http://grants.nih.gov/grants/guide/notice-files/NOT-OD-05-034.html; 2005.
[60] National Institutes of Health, Office of Extramural Research. NIH grants policy statement. Part II. Subpart A. Section 4.1.1.5, Reporting to OLAW. http://grants.nih.gov/grants/policy/nihgps_2012/nihgps_ch4.htm#olaw_reporting; 2012.
[61] Banks R. Postapproval monitoring. In: Silverman J, Suckow MA, Murthy S, editors. The IACUC handbook. 3rd ed. Boca Raton: CRC Press; 2014.

# Biological Hazards and Select Agents

*Molly Stitt-Fisher*

University of Pittsburgh, Pittsburgh, PA, USA

## 1. INTRODUCTION

Just as the field of research in the biological and health sciences encompasses a broad set of initiatives ranging from in vitro experiments in the laboratory setting to in vivo research in laboratory animals and human clinical trials, the set of regulations and guidance documents that apply to research with biological hazards is both far reaching and complex. The development of early guidance documents for safe work with biological hazards was driven in part by the efforts of the life sciences community itself [1] and in part by federal agencies. The discussion of regulatory requirements and guidance documents that follows is not intended to be an exhaustive listing of all sources. Rather, it is intended to focus on the main guidance documents, standards, and regulations that apply to work with biological materials. It is the opinion of the authors that the development and implementation of programs based on these biosafety guidance documents and regulations will form a solid foundation for investigator and institutional compliance in research with biological materials.

## 2. HISTORICAL PERSPECTIVES

Cases of laboratory workers developing infections after exposure to microorganisms that were being handled in their research laboratories (e.g., laboratory acquired infections; LAIs) were documented with increasing frequency in the literature in the early twentieth century [2–10]. As the frequency of LAIs increased, so did the development of new work practices and equipment designed to reduce the risk of infection to laboratory workers. Many of the work practices, pieces of equipment, and facility design principles that form the foundation of safe work with biological agents were developed at the United States Army Biological Research Laboratories, under the direction of Arnold G. Wedum, the director of industrial health and safety from 1944 to 1969 [11–14]. Safe work with biological hazards is based on the following foundations:

1. The Principle of Containment: Biological safety is based on the principle of containment, which can be defined as use of a combination of equipment, facility design, work practices, and personal protective equipment (PPE) to protect laboratory workers, the

public, and the environment from exposure to infectious microorganisms handled in the laboratory [14]. Containment is achieved through a combination of good microbiological work practices, use of appropriate safety equipment, and proper laboratory facility design and operation. The field of biosafety, including the regulations and guidelines that make up the current regulatory environment, is based on the principles of risk assessment and risk mitigation. These principles allow research to be performed with infectious microorganisms for the benefit of society and the environment, with a focus on protecting laboratory workers, the public, and the environment from the risks associated with release of infectious agents from the laboratory setting [14].

2. Development of National Guidelines: Work at the United States Army Medical Research Institute of Infectious Diseases in Fort Detrick, Maryland, laid the groundwork for future development of national biosafety guidelines [14], beginning with the publication by the Centers for Disease Control and Prevention (CDC) of the *Classification of Etiologic Agents on the Basis of Hazard* in 1974 [15].

   a. Classification of Etiologic Agents on the Basis of Hazard: This document represents one of the first uses of the concept of multiple levels of containment, each corresponding with increased work practice, engineering, and facility design controls developed to mitigate risks associated with handling specific categories of infectious microorganisms. Microorganisms with similar modes of transmission and which cause diseases with similar levels of severity in healthy, adult humans are placed in the same category in *Classification of Etiologic Agents on the Basis of Hazard* [15]. The *Classification of Etiologic Agents on the Basis of Hazard* describes four containment levels that serve as the basis for the biosafety levels in use today, biosafety levels one through 4 (BSL-1–BSL-4), as described in the CDC and National Institutes of Health (NIH) publication *Biosafety in Microbiological and Biomedical Laboratories* (BMBL) [14]. The *Classification of Etiologic Agents on the Basis of Hazard* also establishes a fifth classification of nonindigenous animal pathogens for which entry into the United States is restricted by the US Department of Agriculture (USDA) [15]. This fifth classification of infectious agents serves as a foundation for the groups of infectious agents that are currently regulated under the USDA's Animal and Plant Health Inspection Service (APHIS) veterinary services (VS) and plant protection and quarantine (PPQ) permitting processes [14].

   b. The NIH Guidelines for Research Involving Recombinant DNA (rDNA) Molecules: As a result of the emergence of recombinant methods for generating novel DNA molecules, the NIH developed the *NIH Guidelines for Research Involving Recombinant DNA Molecules* (NIH Guidelines), first published in 1976 [16]. The NIH Guidelines use the model developed by the CDC in *Classification of Etiologic Agents on the Basis of Hazard* to describe four ascending levels of work practice, equipment, and facility design safeguards corresponding to four levels of physical containment tailored to the potential hazard associated with the type of microorganism in use with emerging rDNA technology. Specific physical containment levels are described for work with rDNA materials in organisms within laboratories (biosafety levels one through four; BL1–BL4), plants (plant biosafety levels one through four; BL1P–BL4P), and animals (animal biosafety levels one through four; BL1N–BL4N) are described in NIH Guidelines Appendix G, P, and Q, respectively [16]. For clarity, readers should note that biosafety levels are abbreviated as "BSL" in the BMBL and as "BL" in the NIH Guidelines. Throughout this chapter the abbreviation associated with the appropriate document will be used in each section. In 1978, the NIH published the *NIH Laboratory Safety Monograph* (NIH Monograph) as an expansion of the original NIH Guidelines Appendix D "Supplementary Information on Physical Containment" [17]. The NIH Monograph contains detailed recommendations for good microbiological work practices, personal hygiene, personal protective equipment (PPE), disinfection and disposal of laboratory wastes, containment equipment (e.g., biological safety cabinets), and facility design, all of which are designed to ensure containment of research involving rDNA [17]. While the scope of the original version of the NIH Guidelines was limited to rDNA molecules constructed using recombinant techniques, advances in synthetic biology resulted in addition of synthetic nucleic acid molecules to the scope of the NIH Guidelines. These changes, along with the addition of "Synthetic Nucleic Acid Molecules" to the title of the document, became effective on March 5, 2013.

c. Biosafety in Microbiological and Biomedical Laboratories: The first edition of the joint CDC/NIH guidance document BMBL was published in 1984 [14] and supplemented the information contained in the *Classification of Etiologic Agents on the Basis of Hazard* and the *NIH Monograph* with summary statements containing specific guidance for work with infectious microorganisms known to have caused LAIs. The BMBL has been updated several times and is currently in its fifth edition [14]

3. Development of Federal Regulations

a. The Bloodborne Pathogen Standard: The Occupational Safety and Health Administration (OSHA) bloodborne pathogen standard (BBP) was published in 1991 and describes regulatory requirements in 29 CFR §1910.1030 to protect employees from exposure to infectious microorganisms that can be transmitted via blood, body fluids, and other potentially infectious materials (OPIM) [18]. In November of 2000, the Needlestick Safety and Prevention Act was passed, requiring revision of the OSHA BBP to include language specifying the evaluation and use of sharps with engineered sharps injury protection (SESIPs) [19].

b. Development of the Federal Select Agent Program (FSAP): Prior to the mid-1980s, aside from facility inspections and permits required by USDA APHIS for transfer of regulated agricultural infectious agents, there were no regulations requiring registration, licensing, or reporting of transfer of human and zoonotic pathogens within the United States [20]. Enacted in 1996, the Antiterrorism and Effective Death Penalty Act required the Department of Health and Human Services (HHS) to identify biological agents that have the potential to pose a severe threat to public health and safety and to regulate their transfer, resulting in the designation of certain biological agents and toxins as "select agents" [21] (Table 1). The CDC was required to develop and implement regulations to control the possession, use, and transfer of these select agents, resulting in the creation of the CDC Select Agent Program [21,22]. In 2001, the Uniting and Strengthening America by Providing Appropriate Tools Required to Intercept and Obstruct Terrorism Act (USA PATRIOT Act) established penalties for unauthorized possession and or transfer of select agents and toxins and established criteria for restricting access

TABLE 1    Select Agents and Toxins List

**HHS and USDA select agents and toxins 7 CFR Part 331, 9 CFR Part 121, and 42 CFR Part 73**

*HHS SELECT AGENTS AND TOXINS*

Abrin

Botulinum neurotoxins[a]

Botulinum neurotoxin producing species of *Clostridium*[a]

Conotoxins (short, paralytic alpha conotoxins containing the following amino acid sequence $X_1CCX_2PACGX_3X_4X_5X_6CX_7$)[b]

*Coxiella burnetii*

Crimean-Congo hemorrhagic fever virus

Diacetoxyscirpenol

Eastern equine encephalitis virus[d]

Ebola virus[a]

*Francisella tularensis*[a]

Lassa fever virus

Lujo virus

Marburg virus[a]

Monkeypox virus[d]

Reconstructed replication competent forms of the 1918 pandemic influenza virus containing any portion of the coding regions of all 8 gene segments (reconstructed 1918 influenza virus)

Ricin

*Rickettsia prowazekii*

SARS-associated coronavirus (SARS-CoV)

Saxitoxin

South American hemorrhagic fever viruses:
Chapare
Guanarito
Junin
Machupo
Sabia

Staphylococcal enterotoxins A, B, C, D, E subtypes

T-2 toxin

Tetrodotoxin

Tick-borne encephalitis complex (flavi) viruses:
Far eastern subtype
Siberian subtype

TABLE 1    Select Agents and Toxins List—cont'd

**HHS and USDA select agents and toxins 7 CFR Part 331, 9 CFR Part 121, and 42 CFR Part 73**

Kyasanur forest disease virus

Omsk hemorrhagic fever virus

Variola major virus (smallpox virus)[a]

Variola minor virus (Alastrim)[a]

*Yersinia pestis*[a]

***OVERLAP SELECT AGENTS AND TOXINS***

*Bacillus anthracis*[a]

*B. anthracis* Pasteur strain

*Brucella abortus*

*Brucella melitensis*

*Brucella suis*

*Burkholderia pseudomallei*[a]

Hendra virus

Nipah virus

Rift Valley fever virus

Venezuelan equine encephalitis virus[a]

***USDA SELECT AGENTS AND TOXINS***

African horse sickness virus

African swine fever virus

Avian influenza virus[d]

Classical swine fever virus

Foot-and-mouth disease virus[a]

Goat pox virus

Lumpy skin disease virus

*Mycoplasma capricolum*[d]

*Mycoplasma mycoides*[d]

Newcastle disease virus[c,d]

Peste de petits ruminants virus

Rinderpest virus[a]

Sheep pox virus

Swine vesicular disease virus

*Continued*

TABLE 1    Select Agents and Toxins List—cont'd

**HHS and USDA select agents and toxins 7 CFR Part 331, 9 CFR Part 121, and 42 CFR Part 73**

*USDA PLANT PROTECTION AND QUARANTINE SELECT AGENTS AND TOXINS*

*Peronosclerospora philippinensis (Peronosclerospora sacchari)*

*Phoma glycinicola (formerly Pyrenochaeta glycines)*

*Ralstonia solanacearum*

*Rathayibacter toxicus*

*Sclerophthora rayssiae*

*Synchytrium endobioticum*

*Xanthomonas oryzae*

This table is a listing of all select agents and toxins regulated by the Federal Select Agent Program as of April 3, 2013. Select agents and toxins regulated by HHS due to potential threat to human health are indicated as HHS select agents and toxins. Select agents and toxins regulated by HHS and the USDA due to potential threat to human and animal health are indicated as overlap select agents and toxins. Select agents and toxins regulated by the USDA due to potential threat to animal or plant health are listed as USDA select agents and toxins. Tier One select agents and toxins are indicated by [a] in the table and are subject to additional regulatory requirements due to their higher potential risk to the public as defined in the regulations.

[a]*Tier One select agents and toxins requiring compliance with additional, specific regulatory components for biological materials determined to pose higher risk to public.*

[b]*C = Cysteine residues are all present as disulfides, with the first and third cysteine, and the second and fourth systeine forming specific disulfide bridges; the consensus sequence includes known toxins α-MI and α-GI as well as α-GIA, Ac1.1a, α-CnIB; $X_1$ = any amino acid(s) or Des-X; $X_2$ = Asparagine or Histidine; P = Proline, A = Alanine; G = Glycine; $X_3$ = Arginine or Lysine; $X_4$ = Asparagine, Histidine, Lysine, Arginine, Tyrosine, Phenylalanine, or Tryptophan; $X_5$ = Tyrosine, Phenylalanine, or Tryptophan; $X_6$ = Serine, Threonine, Glutamate, Aspartate, Glutamine, or Asparagine; $X_7$ = Any amino acid(s) or Des X and; "Des X" = "an amino acid does not have to be present at this position;" e.g., in a peptide sequence XCCHPA, a related peptide CCHPA would be designated as Des-X.*

[c]*A virulent Newcastle disease virus (avian paramyxovirus serotype 2) has an intracerebral pathogenicity index in day-old chicks (Gallus gallus) of 0.7 or greater or has an amino acid sequence at the fusion (F) protein cleavage site that is not consistent with virulent strains of Newcastle disease virus. A failure to detect a cleavage site that is consistent with virulent strains does not confirm the absence of a virulent virus.*

[d]*Select agents that meet any of the following criteria are excluded from the requirements of this part: Any low pathogenic strains of avian influenza virus, South American genotype of eastern equine encephalitis virus, West African clade of monkeypox viruses, any strain of Newcastle disease virus which does not meet the criteria for virulent Newcastle disease virus, all subspecies M. capricolum except subspecies* capripneumoniae *(contagious caprine pleuropneumonia), all subspecies M. mycoides except subspecies mycoides small colony (Mmm SC; contagious bovine pleuropheumonia), any subtypes of Venezuelan equine encephalitis except for subtypes IAB or IC, and vesicular stomatitis virus (exotic): Indiana subtypes VSV-IN2, VSV-IN3, provided that the individual or entity can verify that the agent is within the exclusion category.*

of certain individuals to listed select agents and toxins [21,23]. In 2002, the Public Health Security and Bioterrorism Preparedness and Response Act (Bioterrorism Response Act) required promulgation of additional regulations to expand control of possession and transfer of biological agents and toxins that have the potential to pose a severe threat to public health and safety and biological agents and toxins that have the potential to pose a severe threat to animal or plant health or to animal or plant products by creating the HHS CDC Select Agent Program and the USDA APHIS Select Agent Program [21,24]. As a result, in 2002, the CDC Division of Select Agents and Toxins and USDA APHIS established the joint FSAP as an interagency program to regulate safety and security practices of individuals and institutions in possession of select agents and toxins [21].

# 3. RELEVANT REGULATORY/OVERSIGHT AGENCIES, REGULATIONS, AND GUIDANCE DOCUMENTS

## 3.1 Department of Health and Human Services

1. Biosafety in Microbiological and Biomedical Laboratories
   a. The CDC and the NIH jointly published the BMBL, which is the main guidance resource for biological safety in the United States [14]. The BMBL contains valuable guidance for researchers working with biological hazards, including information on risk assessment for biological agents, guiding principles of laboratory biosafety and biosecurity, and agent summary statements for many pathogens used in research laboratories. The BMBL describes sets of work practices, safety equipment, and facility design features that together can be used to mitigate risks associated with research involving human pathogens posing increasing levels of risk to human health on potential exposure [14]. Agent summary statements describing the routes of infection, infectious dose, recommendations for safe work in research laboratories, and any specialized occupational health or regulatory issues are provided for a variety of pathogens that may be used in biological research. While agent summaries are provided for a variety of bacterial, fungal, parasitic, rickettsial, and viral agents, it is important for investigators to realize that failure to list a particular biological agent in the BMBL does not indicate that there are no risks associated with the agent in question [14]. In particular, the fifth edition of the BMBL was revised to include additional information regarding occupational health and immunizations for personnel working with biological agents, decontamination and sterilization methods, requirements for agriculture pathogen safety (BSL-3 (Ag)), and updated information on safe work practices for biological toxins [14].

2. Guidelines for Safe Work Practices in Human and Animal Medical Diagnostic Laboratories
   a. In 2008, the CDC convened a Blue Ribbon Panel of laboratory experts to develop an additional guidance document to specifically address safety issues encountered in the daily operations of clinical diagnostic laboratories for human and animal patients. These additional recommendations were published in January of 2012 as the *Guidelines for Safe Work Practices in Human and Animal Medical Diagnostic Laboratories* [25] (Diagnostic Laboratories Guidelines) and are a valuable addition to the recommendations contained in the BMBL. The Diagnostic Laboratories Guidelines contain detailed safety recommendations for specific pieces of laboratory equipment (e.g., ultra-low temperature freezers, centrifuges and cytocentrifuges, ELISA plate washers, etc.) and procedures that are of value to personnel working in both clinical and nonclinical microbiological laboratories [25].

3. NIH Guidelines for Research Involving Recombinant or Synthetic Nucleic Acid Molecules
   a. The NIH publishes the *NIH Guidelines for Research Involving Recombinant or Synthetic Nucleic Acid Molecules* [16] (NIH Guidelines), which provide guidance for proper review, oversight, and containment for procedures involving the construction and/ or use of recombinant nucleic acid molecules, synthetic nucleic acid molecules, and cells, organisms, and viruses containing these molecules (Section I-A) [16].

4. CDC and USDA FSAP
   a. The CDC is tasked with developing regulations to apply to all entities that possess, use, transfer, or store infectious agents and toxins that "have the potential to pose a severe threat to public health and safety" [22], while USDA APHIS is tasked with regulation of infectious agents and toxin that "have the potential to pose a severe threat to plant health or plant products" [26] and those that "have the potential to pose a severe threat to animal health, or animal products" [27]. The CDC and APHIS have defined these agents as select agents [22,26,27]. Certain select agents and toxins that pose a severe threat to both human and animal health and animal products are designated as overlap select agents and are subject to regulation by both APHIS and CDC [22,26,27].

5. CDC Etiologic Agent Import Permit Program
   a. Import of etiological agents, hosts, and/or vectors of human disease into the United States requires an approved permit under the CDC Etiologic Agent Import Permit Program (IPP) (42 CFR §71.54). Under the regulation, etiologic agents include microorganisms and microbial toxins that can cause disease in humans, and the importation of bats, arthropods, snails, and nonhuman primate trophies.

6. USDA APHIS Import Permit Programs (IPPs)
   a. Import of a biological product as defined by USDA APHIS in 9 CFR §101 requires an individual to hold an approved US Veterinary Service Biological Product Permit (9 CFR §104.1). USDA APHIS also regulates the importation and/or interstate transfer of organisms that may be infectious to animals (including poultry) and animal vectors that have been intentionally infected with organisms or are known to be infected with or have been exposed to any contagious, infectious, or communicable disease of animals or poultry (9 CFR §122.1 (d) and (e)). Permits for importation of plant pathogens must be approved by the USDA APHIS PPQ division (7 CFR §330.2)

7. Regulations and Standards Applicable to the Proper Packaging and Shipment of Biological Agents: Dangerous Goods Regulations
   a. There are many guidelines and regulations, both internationally and within the United States, that impact the proper packaging, documentation, and shipment of dangerous goods (Table 2). In the United States, the most relevant regulations are the International Air Transport Association (IATA) Dangerous Goods Regulations (DGR) and the Department of Transportation (DOT) Federal Hazardous Materials Regulations (FHMR). Because the IATA DGR are the most restrictive of the regulations, they are usually the main source for compliance information, with specific sections being augmented by additional requirements under the DOT FHMR. Dangerous goods are defined in similar general terms in both the IATA DGR and DOT FHMR as substances that pose a risk to health, safety, and property when they are transported and which are specifically listed in applicable sections of each regulation (IATA DGR §1.0, 49 CFR §105.5) [28,29]. In research with biological materials, shipments that are known or reasonably suspected to contain pathogens, cultures of pathogens, patient specimens, biological products derived from living organisms, and that are known or reasonably believed to contain pathogens, genetically modified organisms, patient specimens, and/or shipments that contain dry ice are subject to regulation under the IATA DGR and/or the DOT FHMR [28,29].

TABLE 2    Dangerous Goods Shipping Regulations

| Organization | Regulation or standard | Brief description of regulation or standard |
|---|---|---|
| **INTERNATIONAL REGULATIONS** | | |
| The United Nations (UN) | UN recommendations on the transport of dangerous goods model regulations | Used as international model regulations by other organizations and associations to develop more specific regulations that apply to specific modes of transportation |
| International Civil Aviation Organization (ICAO) | Technical instructions for the safe transport of dangerous goods by air (ICAO TI) | All international flights must comply with the ICAO TI |
| International Air Transport Association (IATA) | IATA dangerous goods regulations (IATA DGR) | Membership includes most of the world's major airlines, and the IATA DGR is harmonized with the ICAO TI for compliance |
| International Maritime Organization (IMO) | International Maritime dangerous goods code (IMDG Code) | Required for all parties to the international convention for the safety of life at sea, including the United States (http://www.imo.org/About/Conventions/StatusOfConventions/Documents/status-x.xls; accessed 22.02.14) |
| Universal Postal Union (UPU) | The Letter Post Manual | Uses ICAO as the basis for provisions for safe shipments via post |
| **US REGULATIONS** | | |
| US Department of Transportation (US DOT) | Federal hazardous materials regulations (DOT FHMR; 49 CFR 100–185) | Pertains to the shipment of all dangerous goods shipped in the U.S. by any mode of transportation including air, road, rail, and sea |

International and US Regulations and Standards for Shipment of Dangerous Goods, including biological agents, are described [28,49,50].

8. Department of Labor OSHA
   a. The General Duty Clause: OSHA is responsible for promulgating general workplace safety regulations. In addition to regulations related to specific workplace hazards, all employers must comply with the OSHA general duty clause, which requires employers to provide employment and a place of employment free from recognized hazards that are likely to cause death or serious physical harm to employees (Section 5 (a)(1)) [30]. If serious workplace hazards are identified, the employer must implement mitigation measures that can include hazard assessment, exposure monitoring, medical surveillance, engineering and work practice controls, and the use of PPE.
   b. The BBP Standard: Compliance with the OSHA BBP Standard is required for "all occupational exposure to blood or other potentially infectious materials" (29 CFR §1910.1030a) [18]. Bloodborne pathogens are defined in the regulation as "pathogenic microorganisms that are present in human blood and can cause disease in humans" [18]. Bloodborne pathogens include the hepatitis viruses (hepatitis A, B, C, or D) and human immunodeficiency virus (HIV), but many entities choose to expand their interpretation of the regulatory definition to include other common microorganisms that may be used in research by interpreting these agents as falling under the category of OPIM.

According to the regulation, OPIM include human body fluids such as semen, vaginal secretions, cerebrospinal, synovial, pleural, pericardial, peritoneal, and/or amniotic fluids as well as saliva in dental procedures [18]. In addition, unfixed human tissues or organs, HIV-infected cell cultures, culture medium, or other solutions, or blood, organs, or other tissues from animals infected with HIV or hepatitis B virus (HBV) are considered to be OPIM. Other bodily fluids, such as urine or feces, are not considered to be OPIM unless they are visibly contaminated with blood. Many entities choose to include samples from research animals infected with other known human pathogens in their definition of bloodborne pathogens.

- Individual institutions may choose to interpret the BBP standard to exclude characterized, well-established human cell lines in culture. However, in an OSHA interpretation letter issued to biological safety professionals of the American Biological Safety Association, even well-characterized and tested human cell lines cannot be tested for every known human pathogen, and as such may be considered to fall under the BBP standard [31]. Many entities choose to extend the use of universal precautions (in which all human blood and body fluids as well as OPIM are treated as if they are known to be infected with HBV, HIV, or other pathogens) to all use of human cell lines in culture.

  **c.** The OSHA PPE Standard
- The OSHA PPE standard requires employers to provide and pay for PPE and ensure that it is used whenever employees may be exposed to hazards that may cause injury via absorption, inhalation, or physical contact (29 CFR §1910.132) [32].

**9.** The Environmental Protection Agency
  **a.** The Federal Insecticide, Fungicide, and Rodenticide Act [33] charges the Environmental Protection Agency (EPA) with regulation of the sale, distribution, and use of antimicrobial pesticides (e.g., sanitizers, disinfectants, and sterilants; 40 CFR §150–189) [34]. Disinfectants and chemical sterilants that are used routinely in hospitals, veterinary clinics, and research laboratories to decontaminate infectious materials and surfaces are registered with the EPA. The registration process requires a disinfectant manufacturer to provide safety and, more importantly, efficacy data for inactivation of specific microorganisms to the EPA to receive registration or a license [35]. Use of an EPA-registered disinfectant in accordance with its EPA-approved use instructions as provided on the product label ensures that a registered antimicrobial will be effective against its target microorganisms. Due to the requirement of rigorous efficacy testing as part of the EPA registration process of disinfectants and sterilants, it is the opinion of the author that investigators and institutions should use EPA-registered products in cleaning, sanitizing, disinfection, and decontamination whenever possible. While non-EPA-registered disinfectants such as 70% ethanol can effectively inactivate some microorganisms, standardized efficacy testing and product use instructions similar to those required for registered disinfectants are not available. Use of EPA-registered disinfectants in accordance with product label instructions provides an institution with assurance that the products in use are effective and increases confidence in inactivation procedures for infectious microorganisms. Ultimately, it is the opinion of the author that this will lead to a higher level of assurance that the health of the public and the environment are being ensured by preventing a release of pathogens to the environment.

10. Medical/Infectious Waste Handling
    a. Medical and infectious waste handling regulations are promulgated at the state level. State-specific information may be found on the EPA website [36]. It is important to note that under no circumstances should medical or infectious waste be disposed of in the normal refuse stream and that a common factor in all medical waste handling regulations is the requirement for decontamination by methods specified in each local or state regulation prior to final disposal of medical waste.

## 4. KEY REGULATORY MANDATES

### 4.1 The NIH Guidelines: Recombinant and Synthetic Nucleic Acid Oversight

1. The NIH Guidelines define recombinant and synthetic nucleic acids as follows (Section I-B) [16]. Recombinant nucleic acids are molecules that are constructed by joining nucleic acid molecules and that can replicate in a living cell. Synthetic nucleic acids are molecules that are synthesized or amplified by chemical or other means, including those that are chemically or otherwise modified, but can still pair with naturally occurring nucleic acids. Any molecules that result from the replication of recombinant or synthetic nucleic acids as defined above also fall under the scope of the NIH Guidelines.

2. While technically not a regulation, any research with recombinant or synthetic nucleic acids that is either performed or sponsored by an institution that receives any support from the NIH must comply with the NIH Guidelines. This includes all research with recombinant or synthetic nucleic acids performed at the institution, even if the individual investigator performing the research does not receive NIH support (Section I-C) [16]. The NIH Guidelines also apply to any clinical trials or testing of materials containing recombinant or synthetic nucleic acids in humans (Section I-C-1-a-(2)) [16]. Failure to comply with the NIH Guidelines could result in suspension, limitation, or termination of NIH funds for the individual noncompliant research project or suspension, limitation, or termination of NIH funds for all recombinant or synthetic nucleic acid research at the institution. Therefore the NIH Guidelines are discussed in this section as a key mandate. The NIH also reserves the right to require prior approval by the NIH of any or all projects involving recombinant or synthetic nucleic acids at an institution (Section I-D-1; Section I-D-2) [16]. While entities performing research involving recombinant or synthetic nucleic acids that do not receive funding from the NIH are not required to comply with the NIH Guidelines, many entities choose to voluntarily follow the best practices described in the document [37].

3. The NIH Guidelines describe six general categories of experiments with recombinant or synthetic nucleic acids that fall under the purview of the NIH.
    a. Major Actions: Major actions under the NIH Guidelines involve the deliberate transfer of a drug resistance trait that could compromise the control or treatment of disease in humans, veterinary medicine, or agriculture (Section III-A-1) [16]. If the drug resistance trait proposed for use in the study would confer resistance to the primary drug available for treatment in the general population and/or in a specific subpopulation (e.g., pregnant women or children), then the experiment must be approved by the NIH director, the NIH Recombinant DNA Advisory Committee (RAC), and the local institutional biosafety committee (IBC) before initiation (Section III-A-1) [16].

  b. Use of Toxin Genes: Experiments that involve deliberate formation of recombinant or synthetic nucleic acid molecules containing genes that encode toxins that are lethal for vertebrates at an LD50 of less than 100 ng per kilogram of body weight must be approved by both the NIH Office of Biotechnology Activities (OBA) and the local IBC before initiation (Section III-B-1) [16]. NIH OBA also reserves the right to determine from an investigator's application whether a proposed experiment is equivalent to an experiment previously approved as a major action, as described above. If no significant differences are present and if no information has emerged that would change the biosafety or public health recommendations for the proposed experiments, then NIH OBA may approve the similar experiment without NIH director or RAC review (Section III-B-2) [16].

  c. Human Research: Any proposed experiments that involve deliberate transfer of recombinant or synthetic nucleic acid molecules into human research participants (defined in the NIH Guidelines as human gene transfer) [16] must be reviewed by the RAC, the local institutional review board (IRB), and the local IBC prior to enrollment of any research participant (Section III-C) [16].

  d. IBC Approval Required Prior to Beginning Work: Often, an investigator's proposed research with recombinant or synthetic nucleic acids will fall under the category of experiments that require IBC approval prior to beginning work as defined in Section III-D of the NIH Guidelines [16]. An investigator is required to submit a registration document to the IBC describing the source of the nucleic acids, the nature of the inserted nucleic acid sequences, the host and vector to be used, whether a foreign gene will be expressed, and the containment level specified by the NIH Guidelines (Section III-D) [16]. Several categories of experiments are captured under this section of the NIH Guidelines:
  - Experiments using biological agents in risk groups 2–4 or biological agents that require a USDA APHIS permit due to their regulated status as plant or animal pathogens as host-vector systems (Section III-D-1) [16].
  - Experiments in which nucleic acids from risk group 2–4 or USDA APHIS-regulated plant or animal pathogens are cloned into nonpathogenic or lower eukaryotic host–vector systems (Section III-D-2) [16].
  - Experiments that involve the use of infectious DNA or RNA viruses or replication-deficient DNA or RNA viruses in combination with helper viruses in in vitro or tissue culture systems (Section III-D-3) [16].
  - Experiments involving whole animals in which the animal's genome has been altered by stable insertion of recombinant or synthetic nucleic acid molecules into the germ-line and experiments in which microorganisms that have been modified with recombinant or synthetic nucleic acids are introduced into whole animals (Section III-D-4) [16].
  - Experiments involving genetic engineering of plants via introduction of recombinant or synthetic nucleic acid molecules, propagation of such plants, and/or use of plants with microorganisms or insects containing recombinant or synthetic nucleic acid molecules (Section III-D-5) [16].
  - Large-scale experiments, which are defined as any experiment involving more than 10 L of culture (Section III-D-6) [16].

- Experiments involving influenza viruses (Section III-D-7) [16]. It should be noted that the NIH Guidelines specifically detail additional work practice, PPE and/or facility enhancements for work with certain risk group 3 influenza viruses, including strains containing the hemagglutinin segment from human H2N2 influenza strains isolated between 1957 and 1968, certain highly pathogenic avian influenza H5N1 strains, and research with any portion of the reconstructed 1918H1N1 strain (Section III-D-7 and Appendix G-II-C-5, BL-3 enhanced for research involving risk group 3 influenza viruses) [16].

e. Notification of IBC Simultaneously with Initiation of Work: Certain categories of experiments, including those involving the formation of recombinant or synthetic nucleic acid molecules containing no more than two-thirds of the genome of any eukaryotic virus, specific types of low-risk research with whole plants, and experiments that strictly involve generation of transgenic rodents that may be handled and housed appropriately at BL-1, require that the local IBC be notified simultaneously with initiation of experiments by an investigator (Section III-E) [16].

f. NIH Exempt Research: Finally, certain types of recombinant or synthetic nucleic acid molecules are exempt from the NIH Guidelines [16]:
  - Those that cannot replicate and that cannot generate nucleic acids that can replicate in any living cell, such as oligonucleotides that do not contain an origin of replication, cannot integrate into DNA, do not result in production of a toxin that is lethal for vertebrates with an LD50 less than 100 ng/kg of body weight, and are not transferred into a human research subject (Section III-F-1) [16].
  - Recombinant or synthetic nucleic acids that are not in organisms, cells, or viruses and that have not been manipulated to facilitate penetration of cellular membranes (Section III-F-2) [16].
  - Recombinant or synthetic nucleic acids that only consist of the exact nucleic acid sequence from a single source that exists contemporaneously in nature (Section III-F-3) [16].
  - Recombinant or synthetic nucleic acids from a prokaryotic host (including any indigenous plasmids or viruses) when only propagated in that same host (or a closely related strain of the same species), or when the nucleic acids are transferred to another host by well-established physiological means (Section III-F-4) [16].
  - Recombinant or synthetic nucleic acids from a eukaryotic host (including chloroplasts, mitochondria, or plasmids, but specifically excluding viruses) when propagated only in that same host (or a closely related strain of the same species) (Section III-F-5) [16].
  - Recombinant or synthetic nucleic acids consisting entirely of DNA segments from different species that are known to exchange DNA through physiological processes (e.g., known natural exchangers as defined in appendices A-I through A-IV of the NIH Guidelines; Section III-F-6) [16].
  - Genomic DNA molecules that have acquired a transposable element as long as the transposable element does not contain any recombinant or synthetic DNA (Section III-F-7) [16].
  - Experiments described in Appendix C of the NIH Guidelines, which the NIH director, with advice from the RAC and an opportunity for public comment, has determined not to pose a significant risk to health or the environment (Section III-F-8) [16].

4. The main regulatory mandate of the NIH Guidelines is to provide a framework for the proper assessment of risk, containment, and review and approval of certain classifications of experiments with recombinant and synthetic nucleic acids as defined above [16].

   a. Risk Assessment and Containment: The process of risk assessment begins with the investigator's initial assignment of a biosafety level appropriate for the research that will be performed. The NIH Guidelines provide tools to aid the investigator in the initial risk assessment by classifying biological agents into risk groups according to their potential to cause disease in a healthy adult (Appendix B) [16]. Biological agents are assigned to risk groups 1 through 4, with agents that are not associated with disease in healthy adults assigned to risk group 1, and with each successive risk group 2–4 posing a greater risk to human health. It is important to note that the listing of biological agents in the NIH Guidelines is not comprehensive, and that an investigator should not assume that biological agents not specifically listed are properly classified as a risk group 1 agent. Once an initial risk group assignment has been made by the investigator, the NIH Guidelines describe appropriate containment levels for:

     - In vitro work in the laboratory and work in small animals that are of a size that is conducive to housing in cages that provide containment of biological agents, most often laboratory rodents (Appendix G) [16],
     - Work with large animals that are of a size at which caging to provide containment of biological agents is not available and where the room itself provides containment (Appendix N) [16],
     - Work with plants (Appendix P) [16], and
     - Work with large volumes of biological agents in production facilities (Appendix K) [16].

   b. Each containment level, defined as a BL, consists of a combination of appropriate microbiological work practices, containment equipment, and facility design features. Each BL, a combination of the above risk-mitigation strategies, is developed to ensure safe research with biological agents that pose a greater risk to human health requiring progressively more complex containment practices and facilities (e.g., BL1 through BL4, BL1N-BLN4, BL1P-BL4P, good large-scale practice (GLSP), BL1-LS-BL3-LS) [16].

5. The NIH Guidelines require each institution to establish an IBC, which is responsible for reviewing research with recombinant and synthetic nucleic acids at the institution and ensuring that all such research is performed in compliance with the NIH Guidelines (Section IV-B-2) [16]. The composition of the IBC is specified in the NIH Guidelines to ensure that the committee includes members with adequate expertise to fully evaluate all research with recombinant and synthetic nucleic acids performed at an institution. For example, institutions performing recombinant or synthetic nucleic acid work in plants, animals, or human subjects are required to have at least one plant, animal, or human subject research expert as a committee member (Sections IV-B-4, IV-B-5, and IV-B-6, respectively) [16]. Similarly, any institution performing large-scale research or research at BL3 or BL4 must appoint a biological safety officer (BSO) who must serve as a member of the committee (Section IV-B-2(a-(1)) [16]. The NIH Guidelines also require at least two members of the IBC to be unaffiliated with the institution to represent the interest of the surrounding community (Section IV-B-2(a-(1)) [16]. Other recommendations for committee membership may be found in the NIH Guidelines, Section IV-B-2-a [16]. The specific review of functions of the IBC and the BSO shall be discussed later in this chapter.

## 4.2 The Federal Select Agent and Toxin Program

**1.** The select agent regulations [22,26,27] describe a strict set of requirements that apply to all entities, public or private, that possess, use, transfer, or store select agents and toxins.

   **a.** Each entity must be registered with the CDC and/or USDA APHIS (42 CFR §73.7; 7 CFR §331.7; 9 CFR §121.7) [22,26,27], and must designate a responsible official (RO) as defined in the regulation (42 CFR §73.9; 7 CFR §331.9; 9 CFR §121.9) [22,26,27]. All personnel who will have access to select agents at an entity must undergo a security risk assessment (SRA) performed by the Department of Justice's Federal Bureau of Investigation Criminal Justice Information System to identify any persons who may fall into the category of "restricted persons" as defined by the regulation (42 CFR §73.10; 7 CFR §331.10; 9 CFR §121.10) [22,26,27].

   **b.** The regulations detail specific security requirements to prevent unauthorized access to and/or theft, loss, or release of select agents and toxins, including the requirement for development of a written security plan describing physical and information security procedures, as well as inventory control measures (42 CFR §73.11; 7 CFR §331.11; 9 CFR §121.11) [22,26,27].

   **c.** A written biosafety plan is required and must be based on the best practices described in the CDC/NIH BMBL, the OSHA Hazard Communication (29 CFR §1910.1200) [38], and Occupational Exposure to Hazardous Chemicals in the Laboratory (29 CFR §1910.1450) [39] Standards, as well as the NIH Guidelines (42 CFR §73.12; 7 CFR §331.12; 9 CFR §121.12) [22,26,27].

   **d.** The regulations prohibit conduct of research involving or possession of products of a restricted experiment with a select agent or toxin unless the select agent program's review body, the Intragovernmental Select Agents and Toxins Technical Advisory Committee, provides prior review and approval. Restricted experiments include:
   - Deliberate transfer of or selection for a drug resistance trait in a select agent that does not naturally acquire such resistance if the trait confers resistance to a drug commonly used to treat disease in humans, veterinary medicine, or agriculture, or
   - Deliberate formation of recombinant or synthetic nucleic acids encoding genes for biosynthesis of select agent toxins with an LD50 of less than 100 ng per kilogram of body weight in vertebrates (42 CFR §73.13; 7 CFR §331.13; 9 CFR §121.13) [22,26,27].

   **e.** A written incident response plan based on a site-specific risk assessment must describe "the response procedures for theft, loss, or release of a select agent or toxin; inventory discrepancies; security breaches (including information systems); severe weather and other natural disasters; workplace violence; bomb threats and suspicious packages; and emergencies such as fire, gas leak, explosion, power outage, and other natural and man-made events" (42 CFR §73.14; 7 CFR §331.14; 9 CFR §121.14) [22,26,27].

   **f.** Entities are required to provide extensive training to all individuals who are approved for access to select agents and toxins (42 CFR §73.15; 7 CFR §331.15; 9 CFR §121.15) and select agents and toxins may only be transferred to another individual or entity that is registered with the CDC or APHIS to possess, use, or transfer that specific select agent or toxin, and then, only after review and approval from the CDC or APHIS (42 CFR §73.16; 7 CFR §331.16; 9 CFR §121.16) [22,26,27].

g. Detailed records of all aspects of an entity's select agent program are required (42 CFR §73.17; 7 CFR §331.17; 9 CFR §121.17), including notification of the CDC or APHIS in the event of a theft, loss, or release of select agents and toxins (42 CFR §73.19; 7 CFR §331.19; 9 CFR §121.19), and entities are subject to both announced and unannounced inspections by the CDC and/or APHIS (42 CFR §73.18; 7 CFR §331.18; 9 CFR §121.18) [22,26,27].

h. The most recent revision of the Federal Select Agent Regulations created a subset of select agents and toxins designated as "tier one select agents and toxins" due to the "greatest risk of deliberate misuse with significant potential for mass casualties or devastating effect to the economy, critical infrastructure, or public confidence, and pose a severe threat to public health and safety" [40]. Tier One select agents and toxins are indicated in Table 1 and require adherence to specific regulatory requirements in addition to those required for non-Tier One select agents and toxins. Some of the major changes associated with Tier One select agents and toxins are summarized below, but individuals seeking more information regarding Tier One requirements are strongly urged to consult the *Resource Manual for the Responsible Official* [41], which contains guidance on compliance with the Select Agent and Toxin Regulations.

   - Enhanced Security Plan Requirements for Tier One Select Agents and Toxins: Many of the enhancements required for entities possessing Tier One select agents and toxins are related to increased physical and information security requirements 42 CFR §73.11(f); 7 CFR §331.11(f); 9 CFR §121.11(f)) [22,26,27]. The requirement for entities to develop a preaccess suitability assessment program for personnel with access to Tier One select agents and toxins has posed a particular challenge for many entities. Entities are also required to develop an ongoing suitability assessment program to ensure that all workers with access to Tier One select agents and toxins continue to meet institution-specific requirements throughout their employment. Entities are also required to develop a program to ensure self- and/or peer-reporting of incidents or conditions that could affect an individual's ability to work with or have access to Tier One select agents and toxins.

   - Enhanced Incident Response Plan Requirements for Tier One Select Agents and Toxins: Entities in possession of Tier One select agents and toxins are required to detail response procedures for failure of intrusion detection systems and a process for notification of federal, state, or local law enforcement agencies of any suspicious or suspected criminal activity at the entity in their mandated incident response plan (42 CFR §73.14(e); 7 CFR §331.14(e); 9 CFR §121.14(e)) [22,26,27].

   - Occupational Health and Training Enhancements for Tier One Select Agents and Toxins: In addition to mandated annual biosafety, security, and incident response training, entities in possession of Tier One select agents and toxins are required to develop annual insider threat awareness training for all personnel with access to Tier One select agents and toxins (42 CFR §73.15(b); 7 CFR §331.15(b); 9 CFR §121.15(b)) [22,26,27]. Finally, an occupational health program, while strongly recommended for all entities in the opinion of the authors, is required for entities in possession of Tier One select agents and toxins (42 CFR §73.12(d); 7 CFR §331.12(d); 9 CFR §121.12(d)) [22,26,27].

TABLE 3    Penalties Associated with Failure to Follow Federal Regulations for the Possession, Use, and Transfer of Select Agents and Toxins

| *ADMINISTRATIVE PENALTIES* | |
| --- | --- |
| Entity | Deny, suspend, or revoke registration |
| Individual | Deny, suspend, or revoke access to select agents and toxins |
| *CIVIL PENALTIES* | |
| Entity knowingly violates any provision of the select agent regulations | Up to $500,000 fine |
| Individual knowingly violates any provision of the select agent regulations | Up to $250,000 fine |
| *CRIMINAL PENALTIES* | |
| Restricted person possesses or transfers a select agent or toxin in interstate or foreign commerce | Criminal fine, imprisonment of up to 10 years, or both |
| Transfer of a select agent or toxin to a person who is known or reasonably believed not to be registered with the federal select agent program | Criminal fine, imprisonment of up to 5 years, or both |
| A person who knowingly possesses a select agent or toxin without registration with the federal select agent program | Criminal fine, imprisonment for up to 5 years, or both |

Failure to comply with the requirements of the Federal Select Agent Program can lead to administrative, civil, and/or criminal penalties, both for the entity and for individuals in possession of select agents and toxins.

  i. Failure to comply with the regulations will result in potential administrative, civil, and/or criminal penalties for entities and/or individuals (Table 3) [22,26,27].

## 4.3 The CDC Import Permit Program: Importation of Human Pathogens

1. The CDC promulgates regulations designed to prevent the introduction, transmission, and spread of communicable human disease resulting from importation of various animal hosts or vectors or other etiological agents from foreign countries into the United States as part of the Foreign Quarantine Program (42 CFR §71.50–71.56) [42]. The CDC IPP is responsible for enforcement of the requirements for importation of infectious biological agents, as well as animals (e.g., cats, dogs, turtles, tortoises, terrapins, and nonhuman primates), animal products, and vectors capable of causing communicable disease in humans (42 CFR §71.51–71.54) [42]. An approved import permit (IP) must be obtained by an investigator prior to importation of any materials that may be infectious to humans from a foreign country [43], and approval of an IP may be accompanied by requirements and conditions, including an inspection by the CDC IPP to ensure that:
   a. The importer has implemented proper biosafety measures, and
   b. The importer ensures that the shipper meets all legal requirements regarding packaging, labeling, and shipment of infectious substances.

In some cases, the IP requires that the CDC approve an additional IP for any subsequent transfer of permitted infectious substances within the United States.

2. The Foreign Quarantine Program was modified in April of 2013 to include the provision that an approved IP is no longer required for import of a biological select agent listed in 42 CFR Part 73 [22] if the import has been approved by the FSAP under the form two transfer process described in 42 CFR 73.16 (HHS Select Agents) or 9 CFR 121.6 (Overlap Select Agents) [22,27].

## 4.4 USDA APHIS Biological Products, Organisms and Vectors, and Plant Pathogens Permitting Program: Import and Interstate Transfer of Agricultural Pathogens

1. Import of an animal product as defined by USDA APHIS in 9 CFR §101 requires an individual to hold an approved US Veterinary Animal Product Permit (9 CFR §104.1) [44]. Animal products under this definition include "vaccines, bacterins, allergens, antibodies, antitoxins, toxoids, immunostimulants, some cytokines, antigenic or immunizing components of live organisms, and diagnostic components, that are of natural or synthetic origin, or that are derived from synthesizing or altering various substances or components of substances such as microorganisms, genes or genetic sequences, carbohydrates, proteins, antigens, allergens, or antibodies" (9 CFR §104.2) as well as cell cultures (9 CFR §104.6) and seed organisms (9 CFR §104.7) [44]. There are several types of permits available for importing animal products, but the most common type required by individual researchers is the US Veterinary Permit to Import Cell Cultures and Their Products (USDA-APHIS VS 16-7) [45]. Application for a USDA-APHIS VS 16-7 requires an individual researcher to briefly describe the product, the method of propagation including composition of the medium and the species of animals or cell cultures involved, any inactivation or attenuation of the product, and the proposed plan for evaluation (9 CFR §104.4) [46].
2. USDA APHIS also regulates the importation and/or interstate transfer of organisms that may be infectious to animals (including poultry), animal vectors that have been intentionally infected with organisms or that are known to be infected with or to have been exposed to any contagious, infectious, or communicable disease of animals or poultry, or animal products and byproducts (9 CFR §122.1 (d) and (e)) [45]. A USDA APHIS VS 16-3 permit for the import or transport of controlled material or organisms or vectors is required and must be issued prior to shipment of organisms or vectors [47]. It is important to note that unlike the CDC IP, an approved USDA APHIS VS 16-3 permit is required both for importation of biological products, organisms, or vectors from foreign countries and for transfer of regulated agents from one state, US territory, or the District of Columbia to another (9 CFR §104.4 (b) (2); 9 CFR §122.2) [47].
3. USDA APHIS also requires investigators to apply for a PPQ Permit prior to importing soil, organisms, soil samples, or plants and plant products (7 CFR §330) [48].

## 4.5 Dangerous Goods Shipping Regulations: Transport of Biological Agents

1. IATA DGR and DOT FHMR regulations apply to any package containing dangerous goods that is presented for intrastate, interstate, or international shipment [28,29]. In most situations, investigators or their designees are identified as the shipper

of packages containing dangerous goods and as such, are responsible for proper classification of shipped materials, identification (by choosing a proper shipping name), selection of proper packaging materials, compliance with the proper packaging instruction while preparing the package for shipment, proper marking and labeling of packages with appropriate hazard labels, preparation of appropriate shipping documentation, and compliance with any other additional requirements (e.g., obtaining appropriate import and/or export permits) as described elsewhere in this chapter. Any individual who either prepares packages, or who presents prepared packages to a transporter (e.g., Federal Express or the United Parcel Service) must complete proper training prior to preparing or presenting the shipment. Under the IATA DGR, this training must be repeated every 24 months to ensure knowledge of the current regulations (IATA 1.5.0.3) [28], while the DOT FHMR require training to be repeated at least once every three years (49 CFR §172.704(c)(2)) [29]. Since the IATA DGR are the more stringent regulations with regard to training frequency, most institutions and/or employers choose to require that personnel who ship dangerous goods repeat training at least once every two years (24 months).

2. Classification of Dangerous Goods: Dangerous goods are divided into classes according to the type of hazard posed by the material. The individual preparing the package for shipment is responsible for correctly classifying the dangerous goods present in the shipment. While the exact list of dangerous goods varies between specific regulations, most dangerous goods associated with biological research will fall into either division 6.2 infectious substances or division 9 miscellaneous dangerous goods.

   a. Division 6.2 Infectious Substances: Any substance known or reasonably expected to contain pathogens such as bacteria, viruses, rickettsiae, parasites, fungi, and/or other agents such as prions that may cause disease in humans or animals is classified as a division 6.2 infectious substance under the IATA DGR (IATA 3.6.2.1.1) and must be packaged and shipped in accordance with the regulations for this division [28]. Cultures of pathogens must be classified as division 6.2 infectious substances, as well as patient specimens from humans or animals that are known or reasonably expected to contain pathogens. Infectious substances are further subdivided into either category A or category B substances. Category A infectious substances include those that are capable of causing permanent disability or life-threatening or fatal disease on exposure in otherwise healthy humans or animals (IATA 3.6.2.2.2.1) [28]. Infectious substances that do not meet the criteria for inclusion in category A are classified as category B infectious substances (IATA 3.6.2.2.2.2) [28].

   b. Division 9 Miscellaneous Dangerous Goods: Often biological materials, both those that may be infectious substances and those that do not meet the criteria for classification as an infectious substance, must be shipped below ambient temperatures to preserve viability. Any package presented for shipment that contains dry ice (solidified carbon dioxide) must be classified as division 9 miscellaneous dangerous goods (IATA 3.9.2.6) [28] and must be packaged and labeled in accordance with IATA DGR and DOT FHMR for this division [28,29]. Nonpathogenic, genetically modified organisms are classified as hazardous materials by the IATA DGR and must be classified as division 9 miscellaneous dangerous goods when shipped by air within the contiguous United States or when shipped by any method internationally and must be packaged and labeled in accordance with DGR (IATA 3.9.2.5.) [28]. However, it should also be noted that nonpathogenic, genetically modified organisms that are shipped by ground within the contiguous United States are not considered to be hazardous materials by the DOT FHMR and therefore are not regulated [29].

3. Identification: Dangerous goods, once properly classified, must be assigned a proper shipping name. Each proper shipping name is associated with a specific United Nations (UN) number, which may be found in Table 4 (IATA 4) [28].

4. Packaging: The regulations provide specific requirements for proper packaging of each type of dangerous good [28]. These requirements are defined in the packing instruction associated with each category of dangerous goods and may have variable maximum net quantity limits that are dependent on the exact transportation mode (e.g., shipment via passenger versus cargo aircraft). Specific requirements for use of packaging materials tested and approved to meet UN specifications may apply to each packing instruction, and the number of primary and secondary containers and the presence and type of absorbent materials may also be specified in each packing instruction. Packing instructions may be found in the IATA DGR (IATA 5) [28].

5. Marking and Labeling: All DGR provide instructions regarding the specific type of hazard labels that are required to be attached to each package, including appropriate symbols, minimum dimensions, number of labels per package, and proper placement of markings and labels on each package [28,29].

6. Documentation: In most cases, shipment of dangerous goods requires the individual responsible for the shipment to prepare a legal document, referred to under the IATA DGR as the "Shipper's Declaration for Dangerous Goods" (IATA 8.1) [28]. The regulations contain detailed requirements for proper completion of the shipper's declaration and a requirement for retention of these records by both the shipper and the carrier for two years.

TABLE 4   IATA Proper Shipping Names

| CATEGORY A INFECTIOUS SUBSTANCES | |
| --- | --- |
| UN 2814 | Infectious substance, affecting humans |
| UN 2900 | Infectious substance, affecting animals |
| **CATEGORY B INFECTIOUS SUBSTANCES** | |
| UN 3373 | Biological substance, category B |
| **GENETICALLY MODIFIED ORGANISMS OR MICRO-ORGANISMS** | |
| UN 3245 | Genetically modified organism |
| UN 3245 | Genetically modified micro-organism |
| **DRY ICE** | |
| UN 1845 | Dry ice |
| UN 1845 | Carbon dioxide, solid |

IATA DGR require all packages containing biological agents to be labeled with the proper UN identification number and shipping name. Identification numbers for category A and B infectious substances, genetically modified organisms or micro-organisms, and dry ice are listed in Table 4.

7. Special Considerations and Penalties for Violation:
   a. Transport of live infected animals by air without express authorization from the appropriate national authorities is prohibited under IATA regulations (IATA 3.6.2.6.1) [28].
   b. A technical name is required in addition to the proper shipping name for category A infectious agents in accordance with International Civil Aviation Organization (ICAO) special provision A140 [49]. The technical name consists of the genus and species of the pathogen located in parentheses following the proper shipping name and must be shown on the transport document, or shipper's declaration only. The technical name is not required to follow the proper shipping name on the outside of the package.
   c. Shipment of category A infectious substances via the US or other international postal systems *is prohibited under any circumstances* according to the Universal Postal Union (UPU; Article 132.2) [50], ICAO [49], and IATA [28] regulations.
   d. In the United States, violation of any hazardous materials regulations may result in a civil penalty of up to $50,000 for each violation, and in some cases, a criminal penalty of up to $500,000 and/or imprisonment for up to five years may apply (49 CFR §107.329 and §107.333) [29]. In cases in which the violation results in serious injury or death, penalties may be doubled [29].

## 4.6 OSHA BBP: Protection of Employees from Exposure to Bloodborne Pathogens

1. Under the BBP standard, any entity where employee(s) may have exposure to BBP must have a written exposure control plan (CFR §1910.1030, c), and this plan must be made accessible to employees [18]. The concept of universal precautions (i.e., treating all blood, body fluids, and in some cases, cultures, as infectious) is critical to compliance with the BBP standard.
2. In addition to development of an exposure control plan and adherence to universal precautions, engineering, and work practices controls must be implemented to eliminate or minimize employee exposures (CFR §1910.1030, d, (2)) [18]. Proper handwashing facilities, enforcement of proper handwashing practices following removal of gloves or other PPE, and provision of antiseptic hand sanitizers when handwashing facilities are not immediately available are required. Use of sharps in conjunction with BBPs is a high-risk activity, and the BBP standard details proper sharps handling and disposal practices (including use of approved sharps disposal containers) and prohibition of bending, recapping, or removal of contaminated sharps (unless part of a procedure specific-requirement or if no feasible alternative is available) [18]. Basic good laboratory practices, such as prohibiting mouth pipetting, eating, drinking, smoking, applying cosmetics, or handling contact lenses in work areas, storage of food and drink outside of work areas, and performing laboratory procedures carefully to minimize splashing, spraying, or generation of aerosol droplets of pathogens are also required. Laboratories where work with BBP is performed and potentially contaminated equipment and containers are used for transport of BBP must be appropriately signed and labeled [18].
3. PPE use is mandated whenever engineering and work practice controls cannot eliminate the risk of exposure to personnel [18]. Minimum PPE requirements include gloves, gowns or laboratory coats, face shields or masks, and eye protection, as well as mouthpieces,

resuscitation bags, or pocket masks or other ventilation devices. The BBP standard also requires employers to ensure that proper PPE is used by employees [18].

## 4.7 The OSHA PPE Standard

1. The PPE standard requires employers to provide training for all employees who are required to use PPE. The training must address when PPE is needed and what type, how to wear and care for PPE properly, and the limitations of PPE [32]. Specific requirements for eye and face protection (29 CFR 1910.133) [51], respiratory protection (29 CFR 1910.134) [52], and hand protection (29 CFR 1910.138) [53] are of importance for work with biological agents. In particular, respiratory protection is required for specific work with infectious agents known to be transmitted via respiratory exposure routes (work with animals and manipulations of risk group 3 pathogens and all risk group 4 pathogens). The respiratory protection standard includes requirements for medical screening prior to use of specific types of respiratory protection and requirements for proper fit testing of employees (29 CFR §1910.134(e); 29 CFR §1910.134(f), respectively) [52].

# 5. KEY PERSONNEL AND UNIVERSITY COMMITTEES DESIGNATED TO IMPLEMENT REGULATORY MANDATES

## 5.1 Research with Recombinant and Synthetic Nucleic Acids: The IBC

1. The IBC is responsible for ensuring that all work with recombinant and synthetic nucleic acids at an institution is performed in compliance with the NIH Guidelines. To achieve this function, the IBC reviews proposed research projects and assesses a variety of aspects of the research including:
   a. assessment of the containment levels required for the research (Section IV-B-2-b-(1)) [16];
   b. assessment of the facilities, procedures, practices, and training of personnel involved in the proposed project (Section IV-B-2-b-(1)) [16];
   c. ensuring that all requirements for any human gene transfer research projects are met (Section IV-B-2-b-(1) and Appendix M) [16];
   d. ensuring that no human research subject is enrolled in a human gene transfer experiment until the NIH RAC has reviewed the research, the project has been approved by both the IBC and IRB of the clinical trial site, and any other regulatory requirements have been met (Section IV-B-2-b-(1)) [16];
   e. ensuring that approval of any human gene transfer experiments chosen for public review by the RAC take into consideration any issues raised and recommendations made as a result of the RAC review and any of the principal investigator's responses to the RAC (Section IV-B-2-b-(1)) [16];
   f. ensuring that the RAC review process has been completed before granting final approval to a project (Section IV-B-2-b-(1)) [16]; and
   g. ensuring that the institution complies with all surveillance, data reporting, and adverse event reporting requirements of the NIH Guidelines (Section IV-B-2-b-(1)) [16].

2. The IBC must notify the investigator of the results of its review (Section IV-B-2-b-(2)), is responsible for lowering containment levels for specific experiments (Section IV-B-2-b-(3)) and for setting containment levels for experiments involving animals or plants (Section IV-B-2-b-(4)) [16]. The IBC must periodically review research conducted at the institution to ensure compliance with the NIH Guidelines, and adopt emergency plans detailing the institution's response to accidental spills and contamination of personnel with recombinant or synthetic nucleic acid materials (Section IV-B-2-b-(6)) [16]. Any significant violations of the NIH Guidelines and any significant research-related accidents or illnesses must be reported by the IBC to appropriate institutional officials and NIH OBA within 30 days (Section IV-B-2-b-(7)) [16].

## 5.2 Research with Recombinant and Synthetic Nucleic Acids: The BSO

1. A BSO must be appointed by institutions that perform large-scale research or are involved in production activities that use viable organisms containing recombinant or synthetic nucleic acids, or that perform research with recombinant or synthetic nucleic acids at BL3 or BL4 (Sections IV-B-3-a and IV-B-3-b) [16]. The NIH Guidelines further define specific duties for the BSO that must include:
   a. periodic inspections of laboratories to ensure that laboratory safety standards are followed by investigators and research staff (Section IV-B-3-c-(1)) [16];
   b. reporting of any significant problems or violations of the NIH Guidelines and any significant research-related accidents or illnesses to the IBC and the appropriate institutional officials (Section IV-B-2-b-(2)) [16];
   c. development of emergency plans for appropriate response to spills and personnel contamination with recombinant or synthetic nucleic acid materials and investigation of laboratory accidents involving these materials (Section IV-B-2-b-(3)) [16];
   d. providing advice to principal investigators and the IBC on laboratory safety and security procedures (Sections IV-B-2-b-(4) and IV-B-2-b-(5)) [16].

## 5.3 Research with Recombinant and Synthetic Nucleic Acids: The Principal Investigator

1. Substantial responsibility lies with the principal investigator (PI) for compliance of his or her research with the requirements of the NIH Guidelines (Section IV-B-7) [16].
   a. General requirements include a responsibility not to initiate research with recombinant or synthetic nucleic acids until appropriate approval is granted as outlined in the NIH Guidelines and ensuring simultaneous notification of the IBC with initiation of experiments described in Section III-E of the NIH Guidelines [16].
   b. The PI is responsible for reporting of accidents, exposures or violations of the NIH Guidelines to the appropriate institutional official, in addition to being trained in good microbiological techniques, adhering to institutional emergency plans for response to accidental spills and personnel contamination, and ensuring that all shipping requirements are met in any transfers of recombinant or synthetic nucleic acid molecules. Specific details regarding information that the PI is required to submit to NIH OBA and the local IBC are detailed in Section IV-B-7-b and Section IV-B-7-c of the NIH Guidelines [16].

   c. Perhaps most importantly, the NIH Guidelines place responsibility for ensuring that all personnel have adequate access to the protocols describing potential biohazards and precautions to be taken, training in the practices and techniques necessary to ensure personnel safety and proper accident response procedures, and information regarding appropriate medical surveillance programs assigned to the protocol such as vaccinations or serum collection with the PI (Section IV-B-7-d) [16]. Under the NIH Guidelines, the PI is also primarily responsible for supervision of the safety performance of the personnel in his or her laboratory and correction of any work errors or conditions that might lead to the release of recombinant or synthetic nucleic acid materials to the environment, including maintaining the integrity of physical containment devices such as biosafety cabinets and any biological containment methods (Section IV-B-7-e) [16].

   d. The PI is also responsible for complying with all applicable reporting requirements including those pertaining to reporting of problems with implementation of containment practices and/or issues associated with human gene transfer experiments (Sections IV-B-7-e-(2) and IV-B-7-e-(5), respectively) [16].

## 5.4 Research with Select Agents and Toxins: The RO

1. Designation of a RO is required as part of an entity's registration with the Select Agent Program.

   a. The RO is required to undergo the same security risk assessment process as all other personnel with access to select agents and must be given the authority and responsibility to act on behalf of the entity regarding all aspects of the Select Agent Program [22,26,27].

   b. The RO is the primary point of contact between the entity and the CDC or APHIS and is responsible for ensuring that the entity's programs comply with all of the requirements set forth in the select agent regulations [22,26,27]. Individual investigators may not communicate with the FSAP. All communications regarding an entity's registration and program are required to be coordinated by the RO.

   c. The RO is required to be physically present at the registered entity to oversee compliance and to respond to onsite incidents involving select agents and toxins, and must ensure that annual inspections are performed of each laboratory where select agents and toxins are stored or used [22,26,27]. Institutions may also designate one or more individuals to serve as alternate responsible officials (AROs), who act for the RO in his or her absence.

   d. The entity is required to designate to the RO and the ARO the authority and control needed to ensure compliance with the Select Agent Regulations [41].

## 5.5 Environmental Compliance and Research Safety: The Department of Environmental Health and Safety

1. At most institutions, compliance with other regulatory requirements not mentioned above, in addition to local and state regulations and accepted best practices for work with biological hazards, is assigned to a specific department, such as the department of environmental health and safety. The placement of this department within the

institutional reporting structure may vary, but the department should play a key role in interactions with other institutional compliance bodies.

# 6. COMMON COMPLIANCE CHALLENGES

## 6.1 NIH Guidelines

1. It is the opinion of the authors that most compliance issues associated with the NIH Guidelines fall into a category representing failure by investigators to obtain appropriate approval from NIH OBA and/or the IBC prior to beginning work that is covered by the guidelines. This can be especially challenging, because a wide variety of products based on recombinant and synthetic nucleic acid materials and/or viral vector-based systems are available for purchase from commercial vendors. Introduction of commercial products involving viral vectors or commercially produced viral particles based on recombinant or synthetic nucleic acids into mammalian cells and/or animals represents research that must be approved by the IBC prior to commencement.

2. Transfer of drug resistance traits into microorganisms can be another challenging area of compliance with the NIH Guidelines. Use of many common antimicrobial resistance markers used in molecular cloning techniques (e.g., kanamycin, puromycin, ampicillin, etc.) do not require preapproval under the major action section of the NIH Guidelines (Section III-A-1) [16]. However, investigators must perform due diligence to ensure that a particular drug resistance trait will not confer resistance to a preferred treatment for use in medicine and/or agriculture. Investigators should pay particular attention to specific drugs that are no longer considered to be preferred treatment in most human or animal populations, but are still commonly used in the treatment of special populations (e.g., pregnant women, children, or immunocompromised patients; Section III-A-1-a) [16].

3. Incident reporting is another often-challenging area of compliance for institutions and investigators. In general, incidents that involve noncompliance with the guidelines must be reported to NIH OBA within 30 days [54]. This 30-day reporting deadline also applies to accidents or exposures involving low-risk materials (generally BL1). However, in cases of accidents or exposures to higher-risk materials, expedited reporting is required. Accidents or incidents that result in known exposure of personnel to recombinant or synthetic nucleic acids materials handled at BL2 must be reported to NIH OBA immediately [54]. The reporting requirement deadlines for work with recombinant or synthetic nucleic acid materials at BL3 or BL4 are also clearly defined. In the case of work in high or maximum containment (BL3 and BL4). Accidents, spills, or incidents that result in either a known or a potential personnel exposure must be reported to NIH OBA immediately [54].

## 6.2 The Federal Select Agent Program

1. Possession of Select Agents
   a. Clinical laboratories and research laboratories, particularly those with work that includes screening of samples to identify unknown biological agents, must be aware that the Select Agent Program requires entities that identify a select agent or toxin to notify the FSAP immediately and arrange to either transfer the agent to an entity

with a current registration for possession of the select agent or toxin identified or to document destruction of the samples within seven calendar days of identification [22,26,27].

**b.** Restricted persons
- All persons who have received Security Risk Assessment (SRA) approval for access to select agents and toxins are required to notify the RO of any change in personal status that could result in the loss of SRA approval. This includes any events that would cause an individual to fall into the category of a restricted person [55].

**c.** Security Issues
- Compliance with the inventory requirements of the Select Agent (SA) regulations can be particularly challenging. The regulations provide detailed requirements that specify the information that must be contained in an inventory record, retention of records, regular auditing of an entity's inventory, etc. [41,56]. Inventory discrepancies may result from a variety of situations, including miscounting or misplacement of regulated materials. Animals infected with select agents must be accounted for from the time of infection to final carcass destruction. Documentation of destruction of materials used in in vitro experiments is required as well. The most recent version of the regulations requires that investigators document information specifying the purpose of use, amount used, and other information each time an inventoried item is accessed [41,56].
- Access to select agents and toxins must be restricted to personnel who are SRA approved, with additional personnel screening requirements applying to individuals with access to Tier One select agents and toxins [41]. Any personnel, including both internal employees of the entity and external personnel such as contractors, manufacturer service representatives, etc., who have not received SRA approval and have not completed any additional requirements as part of an entity's registration must be treated as a visitor. Visitors must be escorted at all times by an SRA-approved individual. This can pose a significant burden on small programs, because the escort is not permitted to have any duties in addition to serving as an escort [41].
- An entity is required to have detailed procedures to detect and respond to breaches in physical and information security and to perform annual drills or exercises to ensure that these procedures are effective [41]. It is the opinion of the authors that, while most entities are in compliance with the obvious requirements for physical and information security (e.g., building security and access control measures, firewall protection of information systems, etc.), it is often challenging to deal with the more subtle implications of these security requirements. Some examples include failure to collect proximity cards, remove access levels associated with proximity cards, and terminate access to electronic inventory records and other regulated electronic information upon termination of an individual's employment with an entity.

**d.** Biosafety Issues
- The FSAP inspection process is based on compliance with best practices specified in the BMBL and the NIH Guidelines. During routine, scheduled, and unannounced inspection processes, FSAP inspectors use extensive checklists based on these

guidance documents [41]. One common challenge for entities involves the requirement in the most recent edition of the BMBL for annual reverification of ventilation controls under routine operational and failure scenarios to ensure that BSL-3 and BSL-4 facilities are capable of meeting performance standards required for containment of infectious agents.

**e.** Restricted Experiments
- It is critical that investigators understand and comply with the SA regulations pertaining to performance of restricted experiments. Investigators must be aware that introduction of or selection for drug resistance traits that could confer resistance to agents used to treat diseases caused by select agents or toxins in humans, veterinary medicine, or agriculture requires preapproval from the FSAP [41]. It is also crucial to note that possession of products of restricted experiments also requires preapproval from the FSAP [41]. If an investigator plans to obtain a strain of a select agent or toxin containing drug resistance traits from another investigator or commercial repository, the entity's RO must be notified well in advance so that the appropriate approvals can be obtained.

**f.** Release of Select Agents and Toxins
- The main regulatory mandate of the FSAP is to prevent the theft, loss, or release of select agents and toxins. It can be challenging for entities to determine whether a particular scenario constitutes a release of select agents and toxins that must be reported to the FSAP. Some scenarios that require mandatory reporting include known personnel exposures to select agents and toxins (e.g., failure of respiratory protection, percutaneous injury with contaminated sharps, etc.), a spill outside of a primary containment device, or failure of an engineering control (e.g., failure of ventilation system components resulting in a reversal of airflow in a containment facility, failure of effluent decontamination systems or autoclaves, etc.) [41].

**g.** Due Diligence Requirements for Research Involving Exempt Quantities of SA Toxins
- The most recent version of the Select Agent Regulations requires entities to develop programmatic controls to ensure that investigators working with exempt quantities of select agent toxins are in compliance with the quantity limits that allow work to proceed without registration with the FSAP [57].

## 6.3 CDC and USDA APHIS IPPs

1. The most obvious compliance issue in regard to the CDC and USDA permit programs is failure on the part of an investigator to obtain a permit prior to import of a biological agent controlled under these programs. There is a distinction between CDC IPP and the USDA APHIS IPP that is of particular importance for investigators. Unlike the CDC IPP, USDA APHIS import permits are required for both import from foreign countries into the United States and shipment of regulated biological materials between states within the United States [42,45,48].

2. It is also important for investigators to pay particular attention to any conditions that are associated with the approval of an import permit by the CDC or USDA APHIS. These conditions may consist of additional containment practices (e.g., anterooms, primary containment enclosures), specific enhancements to disinfection practices, or

facility enhancements required for possession of the biological agent. Another common condition of approval restricts transfer of the biological agent from the permitee to another individual without first requiring the receiver to obtain an approved CDC or USDA APHIS permit.

## 6.4 Dangerous Goods Shipping

1. In the opinions of the authors, one of the most common compliance challenges for institutions and investigators involved in the shipment of biological materials is failure to ensure proper training of personnel. All personnel involved in the preparation of the package and in presentation of the package to the shipper must have had adequate training in compliance with the dangerous goods shipping regulations [28,29]. In the case of shipment of biological research materials, both the laboratory or research personnel preparing the actual package and any administrative personnel who may present the package to the shipper (e.g., Federal Express, United Parcel Service, etc.) must have appropriate training, and documentation of this training must be maintained by the institution.
2. Compliance with all details of the package preparation, package labeling, and paperwork preparation must be observed [28,29]. It is common for packages to be returned to the originator or for the shipper to refuse to accept packages that are improperly labeled or presented for shipment with incomplete or improperly completed paperwork.
3. Another key area of importance for investigators involves proper classification of biological materials for shipment [28,29]. While the designation of category A infectious agents is relatively straightforward, the assignment of a particular sample to either category B or an exempt specimen classification is based on the professional opinion of the individual preparing the package for shipment. In the opinion of the authors, the key concept for investigators to consider in classification of biological materials is whether the sample is known or may be reasonably suspected to contain a pathogen. For example, it is the opinion of the authors that patient samples obtained from a population in which there is a known outbreak of an infectious disease (animal or human) would be best categorized as category A samples. Again, in the opinion of the authors, most human and or animal samples may be correctly categorized as category B or exempt, unless the investigator has a reason to suspect that the samples may be infectious.

## 6.5 Occupational Safety and Health Administration Bloodborne Pathogen Standard

1. PPE and Hygiene Challenges
   a. Specific types of PPE are addressed in the BBP standard, including use of gloves when employees may have hand contact with blood and OPIM, during phlebotomy procedures (except under certain defined situations in the regulation (CFR §1910.1030(3)(ix)(d)), and when handling contaminated items or in contact with contaminated surfaces [18]. Masks in combination with eye protection (e.g., goggles, glasses with side shields, or chin-length splash shields) must be worn whenever there is a reasonably anticipated risk of generation of splashes, spray, spatter, or droplets of

blood or OPIM (CFR §1910.1030(3)(x)), and protective clothing such as a lab gown, lab coat, or similar dedicated protective apparel is required (CFR §1910.1030(3)(xii)) [18].

    **b.** The BBP standard also requires that PPE be removed before leaving the work area (CFR §1910.1030(3)(vii)) [18]. In the opinion of the authors, proper removal and storage of PPE is a commonly observed compliance issue in research and clinical settings. In addition to proper removal of PPE, hand hygiene practices are specified in the regulation. It is the responsibility of the employer to provide readily available handwashing facilities or, in areas where this is not feasible, to provide antiseptic hand cleansers or towelettes (BBP §1910.1030, d, (2), (iii and iv)) [18] for employee use. Similarly, it is the responsibility of the employer to ensure that employees wash hands as soon as possible after removing gloves and other PPE, or in the case of an area where a sink is not readily available, to sanitize hands and follow up with handwashing with soap and water as soon as possible (BBP §1910.1030, d, (2), (iii and v) [18].

    **c.** In the opinion of the authors, failure of employers to provide a broad range of sizes and types of appropriate PPE in readily accessible areas can lead to reduced employee compliance with requirements for donning and doffing of PPE (BBP §1910.1030, d, (3), iii [18]. For example, if gloves are ill fitting, dexterity can be adversely affected. Likewise, laboratory coats or coverall suits that are too large or too small for an employee can restrict movement and lead to reduced compliance. Providing employees with opportunities to evaluate different types and sizes of PPE (e.g., different types of face shields, safety glasses, gloves, etc.) can lead to increased compliance with PPE requirements.

**2.** Training and Documentation Challenges

    **a.** The BBP standard requires annual training for all employees that incorporates a specified list of topics (BBP §1910.1030 (g)(2)) [18]. Ensuring that all employees complete training on an annual schedule can be difficult to manage and enforce.

    **b.** In the section of the OSHA BBP standard pertaining to occupational health requirements, specific documentation requirements are listed (BBP §1910.1030 (h)(1)) along with specific documentation retention requirements [18].

    **c.** The required Exposure Control Plan must be reviewed and updated annually (BBP §1910.1030(c)(1)(iv)) and must include [18]:
- review and addition of new tasks and procedures that may change occupational exposure classifications, and considerations of changes to employee positions that may change the exposure assessments defined in the plan; and
- identification and evaluation of new technology and safer medical devices designed to eliminate or minimize occupational exposures.

    **d.** SESIP Challenges
- Employers are required to provide opportunities for employees directly performing work that may result in exposure to BBP or OPIM to participate in the identification, evaluation, and selection of engineering and work practice controls, including SESIPs (BBP §1910.1030(c)(1)(iv)) [18]. It is the opinion of the authors that this evaluation process often poses a challenge for personnel involved in laboratory and animal research. Because most SESIPs are engineered specifically for use in clinical applications with human patients, SESIPs are not always available

in needle gauges or configurations that lend themselves to research applications. In these cases, close communication between safety and research personnel can often result in development of additional work practice controls that mitigate the risks associated with the use of non-safety engineered sharps. It should be noted that documentation of the evaluation SESIPs in a particular procedure and specific language providing scientific rationale should be retained for experiments in which research personnel determine that use of SESIPs interferes with the research goal. Personal preference is not an acceptable rationale for noncompliance with the SESIPs provisions of the OSHA BBP standard.

- In addition to requiring evaluation and implementation of SESIPs, the OSHA BBP standard also contains provisions for proper disposal of sharps devices (BBP §1910.1030(d)(2)(vii)) [18]. Disposable, one-time use sharps devices should be disposed of in an approved sharps disposal container immediately after use. Needles should not be recapped, bent, broken, or otherwise handled prior to disposal. In cases in which there is a procedural requirement for recapping of needles, a one-handed technique or specially designed engineering control (e.g., needle recapping tray) must be used (BBP §1910.1030(d)(2)(vii)(B)) [18].

## 7. ADDRESSING NONCOMPLIANCE

### 7.1 Institutional Resources

1. Often, the same institutional resources that are appointed to ensure compliance with guidelines and/or regulations are the most useful resource for investigators. The personnel responsible for coordination of the IBC activities at a particular institution have a unique understanding of issues that are commonly experienced by investigators. Likewise, the institutional department charged with managing the health and safety program will be most familiar with the unique situations and regulatory environment consisting of local, state, and federal mandates. Often these institutional entities have established guidelines or guidance documents to assist investigators in compliance. In an ideal institutional environment, interactions between institutional departments and investigators can lead to the recognition of the need for development of improved or targeted training initiatives and guidance tools for investigators and research personnel.

## References

[1] Berg P, Baltimore D, Brenner S, Roblink R, Singer M. Summary statement of the Asilomar conference on recombinant DNA molecules. Proc Natl Acad Sci USA 1975;72(6):1981–4.

[2] Harding L, Byers KB. Epidemiology of laboratory-associated infections. In: Fleming DO, Hunt DL, editors. Biological safety: principles and practices. 4th ed. Washington, DC: ASM Press; 2006.

[3] Pike RM. Laboratory-associated infections: summary and analysis of 3921 cases. Health Lab Sci 1976;13(2):105–14.

[4] Pike RM. Past and present hazards of working with infectious agents. Arch Pathol Lab Med 1978;102(7):333–6.

[5] Pike RM. Laboratory-associated infections: incidence, fatalities, causes, and prevention. Annu Rev Microbiol 1979;33:41–66.

[6] Pike RM, Sulkin SE. Laboratory-acquired infections in the United States. Tex Rep Biol Med 1951;9(2):346–7.

[7] Pike RM, Sulkin SE, Schulze ML. Continuing importance of laboratory-acquired infections. Am J Public Health Nations Health 1965;55:190–9.

[8] Sulkin SE, Pike RM. Laboratory-acquired infections. J Am Med Assoc 1951;147(18):1740–5.

[9] Sulkin SE, Pike RM. Laboratory infections. Science 1951;114(2950):3.

[10] Sulkin SE, Pike RM. Survey of laboratory-acquired infections. Am J Public Health Nations Health 1951; 41(7):769–81.

[11] Reitman M, Wedum AG. Microbiological safety. Public Health Rep 1956;71(7):659–65.

[12] Wedum AG. Ii. Airborne infection in the laboratory. Am J Public Health Nations Health 1964;54:1669–73.

[13] Wedum AG. Laboratory safety in research with infectious aerosols. Public Health Rep 1964;79:619–33.

[14] U.S. Department of Health and Human Services: Centers for Disease Control and Prevention and National Institutes of Health. Biosafety in microbiological and biomedical laboratories. 5th ed. US Department of Health and Human Services; 2009.

[15] Ad Hoc Committee on the Safe Shipment and Handling of Etiologic Agents. Classification of etiologic agents on the basis of hazard. 4th ed. Atlanta, GA: U.S. Department of Health, Education, and Welfare, Public Health Service, Center for Disease Control, Office of Biosafety; 1974.

[16] National Institutes of Health. NIH guidelines for research involving recombinant or synthetic nucleic acid molecules. U.S. Department of Health and Human Services; 2013.

[17] National Institutes of Health Office of Research Safety NCI. National institutes of health laboratory safety monograph: a supplement to the NIH guidelines for recombinant DNA research. U.S. Department of Health, Education, and Welfare; 1978.

[18] Occupational Safety and Health Administration. Bloodborne pathogens. http://www.osha.gov/pls/oshaweb/owadisp.show_document?p_id=10051&p_table=STANDARDS [accessed 30.05.14].

[19] Needlestick safety and prevention act. 2000. http://www.osha.gov/needlesticks/needlefaq.html [accessed 30.05.14].

[20] Trans-Federal Task Force on Optimizing Biosafety and Biocontainment Oversight. Report of the Trans-Federal Task Force on Optimizing Biosafety and Biocontainment Oversight. 2009. http://www.ars.usda.gov/is/br/bbotaskforce/biosafety-FINAL-REPORT-092009.pdf. [accessed 30.05.14].

[21] Blaine JW. Establishing a national biological laboratory safety and security monitoring program. Biosecur Bioterror 2012;10(4):396–400.

[22] U.S. Department of Health and Human Services. Select agents and toxins. http://www.ecfr.gov/cgi-bin/retrieveECFR?gp=&SID=8a4be60456973b5ec6bef5dfeaffd49a&r=PART&n=42y1.0.1.6.61 [accessed 30.05.14].

[23] U.S. Congress. Uniting and strengthening America by Providing Appropriate Tools Required to Intercept and Obstruct Terrorism (USA PATRIOT) Act 2001. http://www.selectagents.gov/resources/USApatriotAct.pdf [accessed 30.05.14].

[24] U.S. Congress. Public Health Security and Bioterrorism Preparedness and Response Act. 2002. http://www.selectagents.gov/resources/PL107-188.pdf [accessed 30.05.14].

[25] Miller JM, Astles R, Baszler T, Chapin K, Carey R, Garcia L, et al. Guidelines for safe work practices in human and animal medical diagnostic laboratories. Recommendations of a CDC-convened, Biosafety Blue Ribbon Panel. Morbidity and Mortality Weekly Report Surveillance Summaries 2012;61(Suppl):1–102.

[26] U.S. Department of Agriculture Animal and Plant Health Inspection Service Plant Protection and Quarantine Programs. Possession, use, and transfer of select agents and toxins. http://www.ecfr.gov/cgi-bin/retrieveECFR?gp=&SID=8a4be60456973b5ec6bef5dfeaffd49a&r=PART&n=42y1.0.1.6.61 [accessed 30.05.14].

[27] U.S. Department of Agriculture Animal and Plant Health Inspection Service. Possession, use, and transfer of select agents and toxins. http://www.ecfr.gov/cgi-bin/retrieveECFR?gp=1&SID=b9126e9fba23e3e7933354a1d2630d72&ty=HTML&h=L&n=9y1.0.1.5.58&r=PART [accessed 30.05.14].

[28] International Air Transport Association. Dangerous goods regulations. 55th ed. International Air Transport Association; 2014.

[29] U.S. Department of Transportation. Hazardous materials and oil transportation. http://www.ecfr.gov/cgi-bin/text-idx?SID=3d06b55e9b6dc811cab4d69a32054382&c=ecfr&tpl=/ecfrbrowse/Title49/49cfrv2_02.tpl [accessed 30.05.14].

[30] U.S. Congress. Occupational safety and health act of 1970. 1970. http://www.osha.gov/pls/oshaweb/owadisp.show_document?p_table=OSHACT&p_id=2743 [accessed 30.05.14].

[31] McCully R.E. Letter of interpretation: applicability of the Occupational Safety and Health Administration's (OSHA) standard 29 CFR 1910.1030, "occupational exposure to bloodborne pathogens" to established human cell lines. 1994. http://www.osha.gov/pls/oshaweb/owadisp.show_document?p_table=INTERPRETATIONS&p_id=21519 [accessed 30.05.14].

[32] Occupational Safety and Health Administration. Personal protective equipment. http://www.osha.gov/pls/oshaweb/owadisp.show_document?p_table=STANDARDS&p_id=10118 [accessed 30.05.14].

[33] U.S. Environmental Protection Agency. Federal Insecticide, Fungicide, and Rodenticide Act (FIFRA). http://www.epa.gov/oecaagct/lfra.html [accessed 30.05.14].

[34] U.S. Environmental Protection Agency. Pesticide programs. http://www.gpo.gov/fdsys/pkg/CFR-2003-title40-vol21/pdf/CFR-2003-title40-vol21-part152.pdf [accessed 30.05.14].

[35] U.S. Environmental Protection Agency. Selected EPA-registered disinfectants. http://www.epa.gov/oppad001/chemregindex.htm [accessed 30.05.14].

[36] U.S. Environmental Protection Agency. Wastes—where you live: state programs. http://www.epa.gov/oppad001/chemregindex.htm [accessed 30.05.14].

[37] National Institutes of Health Office of Biotechnology Activities. Frequently asked questions: NIH guidelines for research involving recombinant or synthetic nucleic acid molecules (NIH Guidelines). 2013. http://osp.od.nih.gov/sites/default/files/Synthetic_FAQs_April_2013.pdf. [accessed 24.05.14].

[38] Occupational Safety and Health Administration. Hazard communication. http://www.osha.gov/pls/oshaweb/owadisp.show_document?p_table=STANDARDS&p_id=10099 [accessed 30.05.14].

[39] Occupational Safety and Health Administration. Occupational exposure to hazardous chemicals in laboratories. http://www.osha.gov/pls/oshaweb/owadisp.show_document?p_table=STANDARDS&p_id=10106 [accessed 30.05.14].

[40] National Select Agent Registry. General FAQs about select agents and toxins. http://www.selectagents.gov/FAQ_General.html - sec1q11 [accessed 24.05.14].

[41] Federal Select Agent Program. Resource manual for the responsible official. 2013. http://www.selectagents.gov/resources/Resource_Manual_All.pdf. [accessed 03.06.14].

[42] Centers for Disease Control and Prevention. Import permit program (IPP). http://www.cdc.gov/od/eaipp/ [accessed 03.06.14].

[43] Centers for Disease Control and Prevention. Import permit program (IPP): applications. http://www.cdc.gov/od/eaipp/importApplication/ [accessed 03.06.14].

[44] U.S. Department of Agriculture Animal and Plant Health Inspection Service. Veterinary Biologics. http://www.aphis.usda.gov/wps/portal/footer/topicsofinterest/applyingforpermit?1dmy&urile=wcm%3apath%3a%2Faphis_content_library%2Fsa_our_focus%2Fsa_animal_health%2Fsa_vet_biologics%2Fct_vb_import_export_products [accessed 03.06.14].

[45] U.S. Department of Agriculture Animal and Plant Health Inspection Service. Animal health permits, http://www.aphis.usda.gov/wps/portal/footer/topicsofinterest/applyingforpermit?1dmy&urile=wcm%3apath%3a%2Faphis_content_library%2Fsa_our_focus%2Fsa_animal_health%2Fsa_import_into_us%2Fsa_apply_for_permits%2Fct_animal_health_permits_home [accessed 03.06.14].

[46] U.S. Department of Agriculture Animal and Plant Health Inspection Service. VS 16.7 permit to import cell cultures and their products. http://www.aphis.usda.gov/wps/portal/footer/topicsofinterest/applyingforpermit?1dmy&urile=wcm%3apath%3a%2Faphis_content_library%2Fsa_our_focus%2Fsa_animal_health%2Fsa_import_into_us%2Fsa_apply_for_permits%2Fct_animal_health_permits_home [accessed 03.06.14].

[47] U.S. Department of Agriculture Animal and Plant Health Inspection Service. Application for permit to import or transport controlled material or organisms or vectors. http://www.aphis.usda.gov/animal_health/permits/downloads/vs16_3.pdf [accessed 03.06.14].

[48] U.S. Department of Agriculture Animal and Plant Health Inspection Service Plant Protection and Quarantine. Plant health import information. http://www.aphis.usda.gov/wps/portal/aphis/ourfocus/planthealth?1dmy&urile=wcm%3apath%3a%2FAPHIS_Content_Library%2FSA_Our_Focus%2FSA_Plant_Health%2FSA_Import%2F [accessed 03.06.14].

[49] International Civil Aviation Organization. Technical instructions for the safe transport of dangerous goods by air: International Civil Aviation Organization. 2013.

[50] Universal Postal Union. Letter post manual. 2013. http://www.upu.int/uploads/tx_sbdownloader/actInFourVolumesLetterPostManualEn.pdf. [accessed 03.06.14].

[51] Occupational Safety and Health Administration. Eye and face protection. http://www.osha.gov/pls/oshaweb/owadisp.show_document?p_table=STANDARDS&p_id=9778 [accessed 30.05.14].

[52] Occupational Safety and Health Administration. Respiratory protection. http://www.osha.gov/pls/oshaweb/owadisp.show_document?p_table=STANDARDS&p_id=12716 [accessed 30.05.14].

[53] Occupational Safety and Health Administration. Hand protection. http://www.osha.gov/pls/oshaweb/owadisp.show_document?p_table=STANDARDS&p_id=9788 [accessed 30.05.14].

[54] National Institutes of Health Office of Biotechnology Activities. Frequently asked questions for labs conducting recombinant or synthetic nucleic acid research: reporting of incidents related to research subject to the NIH guidelines for research involving recombinant or synthetic nucleic acids to the National Institutes of Health (NIH) Office of Biotechnology Activities (OBA). 2013. http://osp.od.nih.gov/sites/default/files/FAQs_about_Incident_Reporting.pdf. [accessed 24.05.14].

[55] Federal Select Agent Program. Security risk assessment FAQs. National select agent registry [accessed 03.06.14].

[56] Federal Select Agent Program. Security guidance for select agent or toxin facilities. http://www.selectagents.gov/resources/Security_Guidance_v3-English.pdf [accessed 03.06.14].

[57] Federal Select Agent Program. Due diligence FAQs. http://www.selectagents.gov/FAQ_DueDiligence.html [accessed 03.06.14].

# Radiological Hazards and Lasers

*Michael Sheetz*

University of Pittsburgh, Graduate School of Public Health, Pittsburgh, PA, USA

## 1. INTRODUCTION

Energy emitted from a source is generally referred to as radiation. Radiation can be categorized into two types: ionizing radiation and nonionizing radiation. Ionizing radiation has enough energy that during an interaction with an atom, it can remove tightly bound electrons from their orbits, causing the atom to become charged or ionized. Examples are X-rays, gamma rays, and beta particles. Nonionizing radiation is radiation without enough energy to remove tightly bound electrons from their orbits around atoms. Examples are microwaves and visible light. Educational, medical, and research institutions that use sources of ionizing and nonionizing radiation in research must develop and implement a radiation safety program to assure compliance with the applicable regulatory requirements and to provide a safe environment for personnel and the public. The purpose of this chapter is to provide guidance on the regulatory structure and safety precautions necessary for using sources of radiation in the research setting.

### 1.1 Ionizing Radiation

Ever since the discovery of X-rays and radioactivity in the late 1800s, these sources of ionizing radiation have been extensively investigated to gain an understanding of their properties and effects, and they have also been used as research tools in a variety of disciplines. The harmful biological effects of ionizing radiation were soon recognized, which lead to a series of guidelines on acceptable levels of exposure, which later evolved into an extensive set of federal and state regulatory requirements for their safe use.

#### 1.1.1 *Types and Uses of Sources*

##### 1.1.1.1 RADIOACTIVE MATERIAL

Radioisotopes of certain chemical elements have an unstable nucleus and will emit energy in the form of particles or electromagnetic waves during nuclear transformation or decay. Radioisotopes can be either naturally occurring or manmade in a nuclear reactor or particle accelerator.

*Research Regulatory Compliance*
http://dx.doi.org/10.1016/B978-0-12-420058-6.00005-8

The primary types of ionizing radiation emitted by radioisotopes are alpha particles, beta particles, gamma rays, and X-rays, which can penetrate through matter depending on their energy. The quantity or activity of radioactive material (RAM) is measured by the average number of nuclear transformations occurring per unit time. The current unit for activity is the Becquerel (Bq), which is equivalent to one nuclear transformation per second. The traditional unit previously used was the Curie, which is equivalent to $3.7 \times 10^{10}$ Bq. All radioisotopes decay or undergo a nuclear transformation at a unique rate. The number of atoms transformed per unit time decreases exponentially. The time for half of the atoms of a given radioisotope originally present to decay is called the half-life. The half-life of a radioisotope can range from seconds to many years and is therefore important in its use, radiation protection controls, and ultimate disposal as radioactive waste.

Radioisotopes are used as tracers in many areas of research because physical, chemical, and biological systems will treat the radioactive and nonradioactive forms of an element in exactly the same way. By replacing or tagging a particular atom or atoms in a molecular structure with one that is radioactive, a substance can be traced through a complex pathway. This technique provides one of the most sensitive methods for analysis because of the ability to detect very small quantities of the radiation emissions from the tracer isotope.

The typical radioisotopes used in biomedical research are H-3, C-14, P-32, P-33, S-35, Cr-51, and I-125. Examples of in vitro experimental procedures using these radioisotopes are: southern blots, northern blots, western blots, RNA and DNA synthesis, cellular process studies, radioimmunoassay, and protein metabolism, in which the radioactive tracer is detected by autoradiography (film), liquid scintillation counter, or gamma counter. These same radioisotopes, and others, are also used in animals for biodistribution studies.

Radioisotopes are also extensively used in the field of nuclear medicine for both diagnostic and therapeutic purposes. In nuclear medicine, the radioisotope is combined with other chemical compounds to form radiopharmaceuticals. These radiopharmaceuticals, once administered to the patient, can localize to specific organs to image the extent of a disease process in the body, based on the cellular function and physiology, rather than relying on physical changes in the tissue anatomy. The most widely used diagnostic radioisotope is Tc-99m, with a half-life of 6h, which delivers a relatively low radiation dose to the patient, but is ideally suited for both planar and three-dimensional single photon emission computed tomography (SPECT) imaging with a gamma camera. Another modality within the field is positron emission tomography (PET), which uses very short-lived radioisotopes produced in a cyclotron for precise three-dimensional imaging in a PET scanner. Currently, PET's most important clinical role is in the field of oncology with F-18 Fluorodeoxyglucose (FDG) as the tracer. This sugar analog is taken up in rapidly dividing cancer cells and provides an accurate noninvasive method to image the extent of disease in the body. PET is expanding into the field known as molecular imaging, in which specific probes tagged to a radioactive tracer can be developed to allow visualization, characterization, and quantification of biologic processes at the cellular and subcellular level. New technology now combines SPECT and PET with computed X-ray tomography (CT) scans to give co-registration of the two images, thus providing accurate positioning of the radiation source within the body.

Radioisotopes are also used in radiotherapy, in which the radioactive emissions (beta or alpha) deliver a lethal dose to targeted cells. The most common is the use of I-131 as sodium iodide for the treatment of thyroid cancer and hyperthyroidism. Y-90 is tagged to a monoclonal antibody for the treatment of non-Hodgkin's lymphoma and incorporated into resin or glass microspheres for the treatment of liver cancer. Sealed radioactive sources are used in brachytherapy, such as I-125 seeds for prostate cancer, and external beam gamma stereotactic radiotherapy with Co-60 sources in a gamma knife device.

#### 1.1.1.2 RADIATION PRODUCING EQUIPMENT

There is a wide variety of devices that produce ionizing radiation in the form of X-rays, a form of electromagnetic radiation, which may be generally classified as those used for medical purposes and those that are used for analytical or research purposes. Medical uses of radiation-producing equipment include radiographic, fluoroscopic, and CT for diagnostic imaging of the body in radiology. Cabinet X-ray units are used for specimen analysis in pathology. Analytical and research uses of radiation-producing equipment include X-ray diffraction/fluorescence units for material analysis of elemental composition and crystalline structure. Transmission and scanning electron microscopes are used for analysis of sample surface structure. Another type of machine-produced radiation comes from high energy particle accelerators. These devices produce a focused beam of charged particles that can be used in a variety of applications, such as experimental physics research, manufacturing using ion implantation, external beam radiotherapy, and isotope production.

## 1.2  Radiation Quantities

Radiation exposure can be from an external source irradiating the whole body, an extremity, or other organ or tissue, resulting in an external radiation dose. Alternately, internally deposited RAM may cause an internal radiation dose to the whole body, an organ, or a tissue. The terms and units used in radiation protection for measuring ionizing radiation exposure and dose are presented here [1].

1. *Exposure*: A measure of the ionization produced in air by X-rays or gamma rays. The unit of exposure is coulomb per kilogram (C/kg). The special name for exposure is roentgen (R), in which $1\,R = 2.58 \times 10^{-4}\,C/kg$.
2. *Absorbed dose*: A measure of the total energy imparted to matter by ionizing radiation per unit mass of irradiated material. The system international (SI) unit for absorbed dose is J/kg, with the special name gray (Gy). The traditional name was the rad, in which $1\,Gy = 100\,rad$.
3. *Equivalent dose*: A calculated quantity obtained by multiplying the mean absorbed dose in an organ or tissue by a factor assigned to the type of ionizing radiation incident on the body (radiation weighting factor, $W_R$). The SI unit for equivalent dose is J/kg, with the special name sievert (Sv). The traditional name is the rem, in which $1\,Sv = 100\,rem$. For low linear energy transfer (LET) radiations (e.g., X-ray, gamma ray, beta particles), the $W_R$ is assigned a value of one, and therefore 1 Gy is equivalent to 1 Sv, and 1 rad is equivalent to 1 rem. However, if the absorbed dose is from a type of radiation that is more effective in producing biological harm (e.g., alpha particles, protons, neutrons) the radiation weighting factor is greater than one and up to a value of 20, depending on the radiation type and energy.

**4.** *Effective dose*: A calculated quantity that represents the uniform whole-body dose that would pose the same overall radiation detriment or cancer risk, from nonuniform doses to the various organs and tissues actually exposed. The term effective dose (ED; or effective dose equivalent, EDE) is the sum of the weighted mean equivalent doses of the exposed organs and tissues in the body. Tissue weighting factors ($W_T$) take into account the relative radiation detriment for the organ or tissue and represent the fraction of total detriment to the whole body. Tissue weighting factors range from 0.12 for the bone marrow, colon, stomach, and breast to 0.01 for the skin, bone surface, salivary glands, and brain [2]. The SI unit for ED is also called the sievert (Sv), and the traditional name is also the rem.

## 1.3 Sources of Ionizing Radiation Exposure to the U.S. Population

Background radiation is constantly present in the environment and is emitted from a variety of natural and manmade sources. Natural background radiation comes from three sources: cosmic radiation from the sun and outer space, terrestrial radiation from radionuclides in the ground and building material, and radionuclides in the body from ingestion and inhalation of natural RAM, including radon gas. Manmade sources of radiation exposure to the population also occur from medical exposures to patients, exposure from consumer products, exposure from industrial radiation sources, and exposure of workers resulting from their occupations. Figure 1 shows the percent contribution of the various sources of exposure

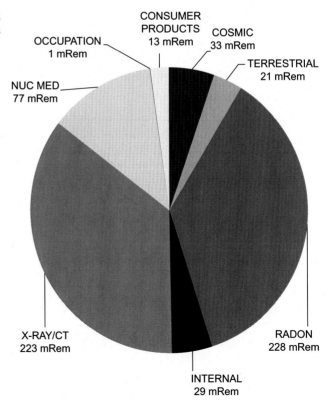

FIGURE 1   Sources of radioactive material and background radiation effective radiation dose in the United States.

to the US population as of 2006 [1]. It is of interest to note that the largest contribution from natural background sources is the inhalation of radon gas primarily in our home environment and medical exposures primarily from computed tomography, nuclear medicine, and interventional fluoroscopy. The average ED to the US population has increased by a factor of 1.7 from the early 1980s to 2006, primarily due to the increased use of these medical imaging modalities.

## 1.4 Health Effects of Ionizing Radiation Exposure

When ionizing radiation interacts with living tissue, it deposits energy at the molecular level that causes both physical and chemical changes that can result in biological damage to DNA and cells. The biological effects that may occur can be generally classified into two categories, deterministic effects and stochastic effects. Deterministic effects occur only after a relatively large threshold dose (over several Gy) is reached, and the severity of the effect will increase with increasing dose. These effects are due to cell damage and loss of tissue function and may occur early, within hours or days, or late, occurring months or years after the exposure. Examples of deterministic effects are erythema, lens opacification, and sterility or reduction in fertility. Stochastic effects are due to damage to the genetic material in cells and where the probability of the effect occurring increases with increasing dose (and not the severity). Also, for radiation protection purposes, the induction of stochastic effects is thought not to have a dose threshold, so even very low doses have a potential for causing harm. Examples are hereditary effects and cancer, and the period between the exposure and manifestation of the effect may extend from a few years to several decades. Scientific committees estimate the risk or detriment from stochastic effects to be on the order of 5% per Sv [3]. The radiation effects to the embryo-fetus from in utero exposure are dependent on the time of exposure and magnitude of dose received [4]. These range from no effect to early spontaneous abortion, malformation, mental impairment/retardation, and increased risk of childhood cancer. Other than increased risk of cancer, there is likely a threshold dose of 0.1 Gy for the deterministic effects.

## 1.5 Radiation Dose Limits

The potential harmful health effects from exposure to ionizing radiation have been and continue to be studied by both national and international expert committees. New recommendations on limits for exposure are presented by these committees as new information becomes available or revised analysis is performed on the epidemiological data. The goal of setting limits on exposure to ionizing radiation is to prevent the occurrence of any deterministic effects and to limit the potential occurrence or risk of any stochastic effects to a level considered acceptable by society. The National Council on Radiation Protection and Measurements (NCRP) report no. 116 "Limitation of Exposure to Ionizing Radiation" (1993) provides the latest US recommendations on dose limits based on the data published by the National Academy of Sciences/National Research Council Committee on the Biological Effects of Radiation (BEIR V) and the United Nations Scientific Committee on the Effects of Atomic Radiation [5]. These radiation dose limits, provided below for the applicable groups of persons involved in or affected by research activities, are for human-produced exposures, but do not include radiation doses that an individual may receive from medical care or natural background.

1. *Members of the public*: Annual ED limit of 1 mSv (100 mrem) for continuous exposures, and an annual ED limit of 5 mSv (500 mrem) for infrequent exposures. Annual equivalent dose of 15 mSv (1.5 rem) for the lens of the eyes and annual dose equivalent of 50 mSv (5 rem) for the hands, feet, and skin.

2. *Occupational worker*: Annual ED limit of 50 mSv (5 rem) and a cumulative ED limit of 10 mSv (1 rem) times the individual's age in years. Annual equivalent dose of 150 mSv (15 rem) for the lens of the eyes, and annual dose equivalent of 500 mSv (50 rem) for the hands, feet, and skin.

3. *Embryo-fetus of occupational worker*: Monthly equivalent dose limit of 0.5 mSv (50 mrem) once the pregnancy is known.

More recent recommendations from the International Commission on Radiological Protection (ICRP) publication 103 [4] provide similar recommendations on radiation exposure limits. However, as will be seen in the following sections, actual federal and state regulations on maximum permissible exposure to ionizing radiation are slow to keep up with the professional committee's recommendations.

Both the NCRP and ICRP promote three key fundamental principles of radiation protection, justification, optimization, and limitation [3,5].

a. *Justification of practice*: Any activity that involves radiation exposure must provide a net benefit that exceeds the cost or risk of harm. This means that with the introduction of a new radiation source or even the reduction of a radiation source, there should be an individual or societal benefit to offset the detriment it causes.

b. *Optimization of protection*: The number of people exposed to radiation and the magnitude of individual doses from an activity is maintained as low as reasonably achievable (the ALARA principle), taking into account economic and societal factors. This means that there is a process (establishment of dose constraint or reference levels) to keep individual and collective doses as low as reasonable to maximize the margin of benefit over harm.

c. *Application of dose limits*: The total dose to any individual from regulated sources does not exceed the applicable radiation dose limit. Regulatory dose limits are set by the applicable regulatory authority and apply to an individual's total dose from both external and internal exposures from all regulated sources.

## 1.6 Nonionizing Radiation

Nonionizing radiation refers to the portion of the electromagnetic spectrum that includes ultraviolet, visible, infrared, microwave, radiofrequency, and extremely low-frequency radiation. Unlike ionizing radiation, which interacts with atoms to remove electrons, nonionizing radiation interacts with atoms to cause excitation and production of heat. The ability for nonionizing radiation to penetrate through tissue is dependent on the particular wavelength, which will determine the type and location of biological effect. Most sources of nonionizing radiation (especially in the microwave and radiofrequency range) that are used in research have little or no known adverse health effects and do not present a significant hazard when used in accordance with the manufacturer's safety instructions [6]. However, certain classes of lasers that emit ultraviolet, visible, or infrared light are capable of causing serious harm, and these devices are also subject to certain regulatory requirements. Therefore, lasers will also be addressed in this chapter.

Laser stands for "light amplification by the stimulated emission of radiation." One basic type of laser consists of a sealed tube, containing a pair of mirrors, and a laser medium that is excited by some form of energy to produce visible light or invisible ultraviolet or infrared radiation. Unlike ordinary light, laser light has a specific wavelength, and the amplification of this specific wavelength results in a focused narrow beam of light that can be emitted in one direction. The amplification, focus, and directionality of this light concentrated in a small area can create a very high intensity light, even at large distances from the laser. Lasers have many applications in laboratories for research, measurements, and optical sources, in addition to lasers specifically designed for use in medical procedures. The risks of laser exposure must be managed to realize the benefits of their use.

## 1.7 Radiation Protection Program

Any institution that uses certain sources of ionizing or nonionizing radiation will be required by regulation to develop and implement a radiation protection pogram (RPP). The RPP will consist of a series of policies and procedures designed to assure that the sources of radiation are used safely and in accordance with regulatory requirements. The complexity of the RPP and required staff or faculty to administrate it will depend on the hazard level of the sources and corresponding regulations. The person who is responsible for overseeing the RPP is called the radiation safety officer (RSO). In small colleges and universities with limited use of radiation sources, the RSO's duties might be assigned to a part-time faculty member. Large universities with programs in medical or health sciences that have specific licenses for possession and use of RAM will have a well-defined and documented RPP with a full-time RSO who has specific training and experience for this position. The essential elements of an RPP will be discussed later in this chapter.

## 2. HISTORICAL PERSPECTIVES

### 2.1 Discovery of X-rays and Radioactivity

X-rays were discovered in 1895 by Wilhelm Roentgen, followed shortly thereafter with the discovery of natural radioactivity in certain uranium salts by Henri Becquerel in 1896. In 1898, Marie and Pierre Curie isolated and discovered the radioactive element in uranium ore that they named radium. These new discoveries marked the beginning of the study and use of radiation and radioactive substances in the fields of science, medicine, and industry. These discoveries also fascinated the public and the media, generating many magazine and newspaper articles that touted their amazing properties and cures [7]. Physicians immediately recognized that X-rays could be used as a tool to look into the interior of the body, and radium was being routinely used in self-luminous paints for watches, clocks, and instrument dials. It was also believed to have curative powers and was used in patent medicines for a number of ailments, including cancer. By the 1930s, biomedical and genetic research was being performed to study the effects of radiation on living organisms, and nuclear physics experiments increased our understanding of the mechanisms of spontaneous fission and radioactive decay.

For the first decade or so following the discovery of X-rays and radioactivity, many physicists and physicians experimented with ionizing radiation without concern for possible health effects. Soon, however, they identified effects such as skin burns, hair loss, and ulcerating sores. It quickly became apparent that the exposures to large amounts of radiation could cause serious deleterious biological effects on the human body. By 1910, many physicians, radiologists, and technicians handing radium preparations and/or X-ray equipment began to develop and report skin irritations and ulcerations, ultimately leading to premature skin cancer [7]. In 1925, an investigation conducted by a New Jersey medical examiner, Harrison Martland, suggested evidence linking the ingestion of radium by female factory workers (radium dial painters) could lead to serious illness and death [8]. This discovery concerning the dangers of internally deposited radionuclides along with the known health effects from external exposures to X-rays prompted a movement for protection against radiation hazards. Although a few early radiation pioneers called for protective measures against radiation, by the 1920s, physicians and professional organizations, primarily medical societies, acknowledged the need for control strategies and exposure limits for ionizing radiation [9].

## 2.2 Early Recommendations for Radiation Protection

In 1928, at the Second International Congress of Radiology meeting in Stockholm, Sweden, the first radiation protection commission, named the International Advisory Committee on X-ray and Radium Protection, was formed to study the problems of ionizing radiation at that time. This committee would be renamed the ICRP in 1950 to better reflect its role as a standards-setting body in all areas of radiation protection [7]. To present a unified position on various aspects of radiation safety by the United States, the American Roentgen Ray Society, the Radiological Society of North America, and the Radium Society, along with the US National Bureau of Standards, agreed in 1929 to establish a national Advisory Committee on X-ray and Radium Protection, which was renamed in 1946 the National Committee on Radiation Protection (NCRP) [10]. In 1964, the committee was congressionally chartered as the National Council on Radiation Protection and Measurements (NCRP).

To standardize the measurement of radiation exposure or the calculation of radiation dose, the International Commission on Radiation Units and Measurements (ICRU) defined the unit "roentgen" (R) as the amount of radiation that would produce a certain amount of ionization in a given volume of air at standard temperature and pressure. This unit of radiation exposure was used to quantify the levels of exposure at which observable effects occurred and to establish levels of exposure for radiation protection. In 1934, the concept of the tolerance dose was introduced as an upper limit for the exposure of workers to radiation. This concept was based on the premise of a threshold dose, that is, a level of exposure below which observable effects do not occur in an exposed person. After much study at that time, both the International and National Advisory Committees on X-ray Radium Protection concluded that they had sufficient technical basis to recommend a whole-body tolerance dose of 0.2 R per day for individuals who were occupationally exposed to X-rays. This tolerance dose was based on the assumption that a dose of one-tenth that required to produce erythema (thought to be approximately 600 R) would be acceptable for someone working with X-rays or radium over an occupational period of 250 days a year [11]. Because of uncertainties in the erythema dose, the national advisory committee reduced this dose to 0.1 R per day in 1936. This radiation exposure limit and tolerance dose model of radiation injury was maintained through World War II and was also applied to workers in the Manhattan Project [12].

In 1941, the national advisory committee also recommended a tolerance dose for hazards from internally deposited radionuclides, especially for radium. Although most of the radium in use at the time was for medical therapy applications, the US Navy also used it for several industrial applications, including watch dials and instrument panels for aircraft [7]. The recommended maximum body burden was 0.1 µCi of radium, which was based primarily on the observed radiation injuries in radium dial painters who had residual body burdens of about 10 times this limit, or 1 µCi. This limit on the radium body burden also provided the basis for control of internal exposure of workers to plutonium during the Manhattan Project. These limits for internal exposures later served as the foundation for ICRP and NCRP recommendations on maximum permissible body burdens for all bone-seeking radionuclides.

Throughout their existence, the ICRP and NCRP have worked closely together to develop radiation protection recommendations that reflect the current understanding of the risks associated with exposure to ionizing radiation. Neither organization has official status or authority to promulgate or enforce regulations. However, their recommendations often serve as the basis for the radiation protection regulations that are adopted by the regulatory authorities in the United States and most other nations.

## 2.3 Development of Radiation Protection Recommendations

After the explosions of the first atomic bombs over Hiroshima and Nagasaki in 1945 and the end of World War II, a new nuclear age was developing in the area of nuclear fission and production of new radionuclides for both medical and industrial applications. In the United States, congressional and military leaders debated on the best way to control nuclear energy for both peaceful uses and national defense. This debate culminated in the passage of the Atomic Energy Act (AEA) of 1946, which established a new federal agency, the Atomic Energy Commission (AEC), to manage the development of nuclear weapons and encourage peaceful uses of nuclear energy. The act ensured that the security and control of source (uranium and thorium), byproduct (radioisotopes produced by nuclear fission), and special nuclear (plutonium, uranium-233, or uranium enriched in the isotopes uranium-233 or uranium-235) material would remain under the federal government's jurisdiction [7].

By 1954, a broad political consensus viewed the development of nuclear energy for civilian purposes as a vital goal. In that year, Congress passed the Atomic Energy Act of 1954, as amended, which permitted for the first time the broad use of atomic energy for peaceful applications. It redefined the atomic energy program by ending the government's monopoly on technical data and making the growth of a commercial nuclear industry an important national goal. The act directed the AEC to "encourage widespread participation in the development and utilization of atomic energy for peaceful purposes." The Atomic Energy Act of 1954 also instructed the AEC to prepare regulations that would protect public health and safety from radiation hazards. Thus, it assigned the agency three major functions: (1) to continue its weapons program; (2) to promote the commercial uses of nuclear power; and (3) to protect against the hazards of those peaceful applications [13]. For the next 28 years, the AEC was responsible for programs in the development and testing of nuclear weapons, development of nuclear power for commercial use, production of radionuclides for medicine and industry, ensuring national security, and protecting the health and safety of personnel and the public from radiation hazards.

In the 1950s, new concerns about low-dose radiation from peacetime nuclear industries and from worldwide nuclear test fallout lead the ICRP and NCRP to reform their concept of "tolerance dose" to that of "permissible dose" to reflect the potential for latent effects [14]. Due to a number of new scientific concerns for the genetic hazard from radiation exposure, observed excess prevalence of leukemia among early radiologists, and the effects of radioactive fallout, the AEC in 1955 requested the National Academy of Sciences–National Research Council (NAS/NRC) to undertake a major study of the effects of low-level radiation. The NAS/NRC appointed a committee on the Biological Effects of Atomic Radiation (BEAR), which later would be renamed as the Biological Effects of Ionizing Radiation (BEIR) committee. The committee's first report was issued in 1956 and raised issues and widespread concerns about the genetic effects of ionizing radiation [15]. In 1958, the NCRP issued new recommendations for radiation exposure to workers based on a maximum permissible dose (MPD) to the most critical organs (whole body, head and trunk, active blood-forming organs, or gonads) to not exceed 3 rem in any 13 consecutive weeks or 12 rem per year. It also included a maximum lifetime dose of 5 rem multiplied by the number of years beyond age 18 years. Thus the MPD formula became equal to 5(N-18), where N was equal to the person's age, with a maximum of 12 rem per year. The NCRP also recommended limits for exposure to members of the public to 0.5 rem or one-tenth of the dose limit for workers [16]. The ICRP had issued similar recommendations two years earlier [17].

In 1959, amid the growing concerns over radioactive fallout and a recognition that at that time there was no official agency within the US government to formulate radiation protection standards or guidance for all federal agencies, the Federal Radiation Council (FRC) was created by President Eisenhower. The FRC, which comprised the secretaries of Agriculture, Health, Education and Welfare, Defense, Labor, and Commerce, and the chair of the AEC, was directed to rely on the expertise of the NAS and NCRP and propose recommendations on protection standards for all radiation activities conducted by the federal government. While the FRC was not a regulatory body, it did have the authority to act as an advisory body to establish radiation protection guidelines on occupational and population exposures for other federal agencies [7]. The FRC also issued guidance in the area of radon levels in uranium mines to protect miners from radiation-induced lung cancer and diagnostic X-ray exposures. In 1970, President Nixon issued an executive order that disbanded the FRC placing its functions in the newly created Environmental Protection Agency (EPA).

With respect to radiological protection, the EPA has issued regulatory standards for environmental radiation programs, such as underground mining, uranium fuel cycle operations (nuclear power plants), uranium mill tailings, and high-level radioactive waste disposal, along with natural sources of radioactivity such as radon. Under its authority, it has also reviewed research on the assessment of risks associated with exposures to different sources of radiation and issued standards and guidance to limit radiation exposures to workers and the general public. The EPA now encompassed two important radiation protection functions within a single agency—the promulgation of environmental standards and the development of national radiation protection guidance for federal and state agencies [7].

The US Public Health Service (PHS) had been involved in radiation-protection activities since the 1920s, and in the early years before World War II, its responsibilities included investigations of radium poisonings of watch painters, radium and X-ray hazards in hospitals, and radiation safety programs for photofluorographic technicians (X-ray technicians). In 1958, the PHS established the Division of Radiological Health to conduct research on radiation effects, provide training and technical assistance to state radiological health programs, and coordinate with other federal radiation programs. The division later expanded into environmental radiation assessment and developed recommendations for acceptable levels of radiation exposure from air, water, milk, medical procedures, and the general environment. In 1968, the division was renamed the Bureau of Radiological Health (BRH) and granted authority under the Radiation Control for Health and Safety Act (PL 90–602) to regulate performance standards for electronic product radiation and to investigate the effects and control of electronic product radiation emissions. The agency was responsible for maintaining a national program to protect the public health and safety from unnecessary exposure from machine-produced radiation. The BRH was later combined with the Bureau of Medical Devices (BMD) to form the Center for Devices and Radiological Heath (CDRH) within the Food and Drug Administration (FDA), where it exists today under the cabinet level Department of Health and Human Services (HHS).

The dual mandates of the AEC to both promote the development of nuclear technologies and regulate the protection of national security and public health and safety were viewed as contradictory functions. Those functions were in many ways inseparable and proved to be incompatible when they were carried out by a single agency. The competing responsibilities and the precedence that the AEC gave to its military and promotional duties gradually damaged its credibility on regulatory issues and undermined public confidence in its safety programs. As a result, the AEC was abolished by the Energy Reorganization Act of 1974, and two new agencies were created, the Energy Research and Development Administration (ERDA) and the Nuclear Regulatory Commission (NRC). The ERDA, which was subsequently changed to the cabinet level Department of Energy (DOE) in 1977, assumed responsibility for research and development on the various sources of energy, including nuclear power, and the military nuclear weapons program. The NRC assumed the regulatory functions for the use of byproduct, source, and special nuclear material. The mission of the NRC is to ensure adequate protection of public health and safety, the national defense and security, and the environment in the use of RAMs in the United States.

While the individual states did not have authority to regulate the use of byproduct, source, or special nuclear material, they did have responsibility for establishing their own radiation protection requirements for other sources of radiation. By the early 1960s, many states had a comprehensive radiation control program for the regulation of the use of diagnostic and therapeutic X-ray, environmental monitoring, and regulation of the use of certain RAMs, including naturally occurring and accelerator-produced radioactive material (NARM). While early state and local radiation control programs were developing, they often looked to the Federal PHS Division of Radiological Health for guidance. With many state and local radiation control programs being developed independently of each other, it became clear that unless some effort was made for uniformity, there would be inconsistencies and conflicts of rules and regulations throughout the country [18]. As a result of this identified need for uniformity of regulations, the Conference of Radiation Control Program Directors (CRCPD) was originally established in 1968 as a voluntary network of state and local governmental officials responsible for radiation regulation and enforcement. The primary purposes of the CRCPD were:

1. To serve as a forum for the many governmental radiation protection agencies to communicate with each other; and
2. To promote uniform radiation protection regulations and activities.

The CRCPD has published and periodically updates its *Suggested State Regulations for Control of Radiation* (SSRCR). Most state radiation protection programs and regulations are based on these guidelines. Despite the fact that the CRCPD is mostly composed of radiation regulators, it has no regulatory authority of its own.

The NRC has an agreement state program in which it allows states to assume NRC regulatory authority to license and regulate byproduct material, source material, and certain quantities of special nuclear material. The mechanism for the transfer of NRC's authority to a state is an agreement signed by the governor of the state and the chair of the NRC. The NRC must determine that the state's radiation control program is in accordance with and compatible to the NRC's program for regulation of such materials. Although agreement states regulate their own licensing and enforcement decisions, the NRC maintains significant authority over the states with respect to promulgation and compatibility of new regulations, and the NRC periodically reviews the adequacy of the state radiation control program. There are currently 37 states that have entered into this type of agreement with the NRC.

In 2007, under the Energy Policy Act of 2005, the NRC issued new regulations to expand the definition of byproduct material to include any discrete source of radium-226 or any material that has been made radioactive by use of a particle accelerator for use in a commercial, medical, or research activity.

## 2.4 Current Radiation Protection Recommendations

With the increasing use of sources of ionizing radiation throughout the world, the various independent scientific committees, organizations, and agencies (NCRP, ICRP, BEIR, and UNSCEAR) continued to review the large body of radiological data (primarily from the Japanese atomic bomb survivors) on the health effects from exposure to ionizing radiation to develop a more comprehensive approach to radiation protection. A risk-based system to reduce the probability of an adverse health effect was adopted to replace a system based on prevention of injury. Another concept introduced was that of ED or EDE as a way to accommodate both external exposures and intakes of RAM and variations in absorbed doses to different organs and tissues in the body in order to evaluate the overall impact and normalize the total detriment or risk to that of a uniform whole-body exposure. A new model of radiation-induced injury began to be used for the purpose of establishing guidelines for radiation protection. This model assumed that late effects of radiation exposure (late radiation injuries, namely, cancer and hereditary effects) might increase linearly with increasing dose of radiation and that a threshold dose might not exist below which late effects do not occur. This new model called the linear, no-threshold (LNT) model of radiation risk assumes that the risk of late radiation injuries at low doses can be estimated by linear extrapolation from effects at high doses. However, even today, genetic effects are only able to be observed in animal studies, and increases in cancer induction are only able to be seen in groups of people exposed to high doses (greater than approximately 0.1 Sv) of radiation. Despite this limitation, the LNT model has become widely adopted for estimating radiation risk and for quantifying the number of potentially injured persons in a population exposed to ionizing radiation. The basis for this application appears to lie largely in a conservative approach to risk assessment that has been taken to compensate for a lack of reliable data in the relevant low-dose range. With the LNT concept, the as low as reasonably achievable (ALARA) philosophy was introduced as a tenant of any radiation safety program.

Given the above assumptions, any radiation exposure must meet the following criteria [5]:

1. The need to justify any activity that involves radiation exposure on the basis that the expected benefits to society exceed the overall societal cost (*justification*);
2. The need to ensure that the total societal detriment from such justifiable activities or practices is maintained ALARA, economic and societal factors being taken into account (*optimization*); and
3. The need to apply individual dose limits to ensure that the procedures of justification and ALARA do not result in individuals or groups of individuals exceeding levels of acceptable risk (*limitation*).

Current federal and state regulations on allowable levels of radiation exposure to both workers and members of the general public are based on recommendations published by ICRP 26 in 1977. These recommendations are also consistent with the recommendations published by NCRP 91 in 1987, with an average estimated risk of fatal cancer of about $1 \times 10^{-2}$/Sv. The allowable levels of exposure are set to protect the average radiation worker to the same degree of risk from accidental death as workers in other safe industries ($1 \times 10^{-4}$) and an acceptable level of risk from radiation induced fatal cancer and serious hereditary disorders to members of the general public ($1 \times 10^{-5}$ to $1 \times 10^{-6}$). Thus the maximum recommended ED or EDE is equal to 50 mSv per year for occupational workers and 1 mSv per year to members of the public. In subsequent ICRP and NCRP reports [3,5], the risk of radiation exposure has been determined to be somewhat greater than previously thought, based on continued analysis of the latest epidemiological data, with the average estimated risk of fatal cancer now being about $5 \times 10^{-2}$/Sv. However, the current regulatory structure and occupational radiation safety standards are still considered to be adequate to protect radiation workers [19].

## 3. RELEVANT REGULATORY/OVERSIGHT AGENCIES, REGULATIONS, AND GUIDANCE DOCUMENTS

The type, quantity, and characteristics of a radiation source will determine the legal and regulatory responsibilities for its possession and use. These regulatory requirements vary greatly for different sources of radiation and its intended use. Some sources will require a license or permit, others are required to be registered, and some may be used without any regulatory oversight. The complexity and prescriptiveness of the regulations is a product of the evolution of the applicable radiation protection standards and the agency responsible for its oversight, and often does not necessarily reflect the magnitude of the health risk associated with the use of the radiation source.

## 3.1 Regulatory and Oversight Agencies

### 3.1.1 US Nuclear Regulatory Commission

The NRC is the federal agency responsible for protecting the health and safety of the public and the environment by licensing and regulating the civilian uses of the following RAMs [20]:

1. Source material (uranium and thorium);
2. Special nuclear material (enriched uranium and plutonium);
3. Byproduct material (material that is made radioactive in a reactor, residue from the milling of uranium and thorium, and any discrete source of radium-226 or any material that has been made radioactive by use of a particle accelerator for use in a commercial, medical, or research activity).

The NRC regulates the use of these RAMs through title 10, part 20, of the *Code of Federal Regulations* (10 CFR part 20), "Standards for Protection Against Radiation," which spells out the agency's requirements for the following aspects of radiation protection:

1. Dose limits for radiation workers and members of the public;
2. Exposure limits for individual radionuclides;
3. Monitoring and labeling RAMs;
4. Posting signs in and around radiation areas;
5. Reporting the theft or loss of RAM;
6. Penalties for not complying with NRC regulations.

Of more than 20,000 active source, byproduct, and special nuclear materials licenses in place in the United States, about a quarter are administered by the NRC, while the rest are administered by the 37 agreement states.

### 3.1.2 Agreement States

Under section 274 of the Atomic Energy Act of 1954, as amended, the NRC may relinquish to the states portions of its regulatory authority to license and regulate byproduct material, source material, and certain quantities of special nuclear material, as defined above [21]. The mechanism for the transfer of NRC's authority to a state is an agreement signed by the governor of the state and the chair of the commission. The state's radiation control program must be compatible and at least as stringent to the NRC's program for regulation of such materials. Some agreement states will adopt by reference the NRC regulatory requirements so that their regulations will be identical to the NRC's. Although agreement states regulate their own licensing and enforcement decisions, the NRC maintains significant authority over the states with respect to promulgation and compatibility of new regulations. The NRC also has programmatic responsibility to periodically review the actions of the agreement states to ensure that they continue to maintain adequate and compatible programs. The NRC periodically reviews each state's performance to determine whether its program is "adequate" and to ensure that its regulatory requirements do not significantly deviate from the NRC's. The NRC also provides assistance to states entering into agreements by conducting training courses and workshops, evaluating technical licensing and inspection issues, and evaluating state rule changes. The Organization of Agreement States (OAS) is a professional organization that includes the directors and staffs of agreement state programs. Initially, the OAS was established to facilitate communication between the NRC and the agreement states when most states did not have agreements with the agency. Now, the organization hosts an annual meeting to consider specific issues related to the regulation of RAMs.

### 3.1.3 Non-Agreement States

The NRC exercises regulatory authority over RAMs in states that do not have agreements. Therefore, an NRC license is required to possess RAM in these states. Prior to passage of the Energy Policy Act of 2005 redefining the definition of byproduct material, non-agreement states had regulatory authority for NARM, so a state RAMs license was required for possession and use of this material.

### 3.1.4 Conference of Radiation Control Program Directors

The CRCPD is a professional organization that was established in 1968 to promote a uniform set of radiation protection standards among the states [22]. The organization includes the directors and staffs of regulatory programs from both agreement and nonagreement states. The CRCPD maintains a standing committee to publish and periodically update a uniform set of suggested regulations. These SSRCR are used by state departments of radiological health as guidance for formulation of state law. The CRCPD also provides a forum for the states to interact with the NRC and coordinate the regulation of RAMs that are not governed by the Atomic Energy Act. The CRCPD hosts an annual meeting to consider specific issues related to the regulation of all sources of ionizing as well as nonionizing radiation.

### 3.1.5 Food and Drug Administration

The FDA has jurisdiction over the manufacturer and installation of electronic products that emit both ionizing and nonionizing radiation under the authorities of the Electronic Product Radiation Control provisions and the Medical Device Amendments of 1976 to the Food, Drug, and Cosmetic Act [23]. The FDA's CDRH regulates the performance standards for items such as tube housing leakage, beam filtration, beam collimation, accuracy and reproducibility of technique factors, and fluoroscopic exposure rates for radiation-emitting electronic products used for both medical and nonmedical applications. Manufacturers of such products must adhere to the radiation emission and safety performance standards for it to be sold or marketed in the United States. Medical X-ray imaging products, such as dental, radiographic, fluoroscopic, and CT, are regulated under 21 CFR 1020. Nonmedical products that emit ionizing radiation, such as electron microscopes, cabinet, and X-ray diffraction and fluorescence analysis equipment, must also meet certain performance standards to be sold in the United States. Medical lasers are devices that use precisely focused light sources to treat or surgically remove tissues. These laser products must also comply with the FDA medical device regulations. The CDRH also provides direction and guidance to the general public and users of radiation-emitting products to minimize unnecessary radiation exposure.

### 3.1.6 Occupational Safety and Health Administration

The Occupational Safety and Health Administration (OSHA) is part of the US Department of Labor, the mission of which is to prevent occupational-related injuries, illness, or death [24]. OSHA has standards for protection from sources of ionizing radiation that employers must follow to protect their employees from exposure hazards. OSHA covers private-sector employers and employees in all 50 states, the District of Columbia, and other US jurisdictions either directly through federal OSHA or through an OSHA-approved state program. State-run health and safety programs must be at least as effective as the federal OSHA program. There are currently 25 states that have OSHA-approved state plans and have adopted their own standards and enforcement policies. An institution in compliance with the NRC or agreement state regulations for use of RAM is considered to be in compliance with OSHA's regulations on ionizing radiation.

## 3.2 Regulation of Radioactive Materials

Because of their potentially hazardous properties, the use of certain RAMs must be closely regulated to protect the health and safety of the public and the environment. The responsibility for licensing and regulating the use and handling of certain RAMs is either the NRC or an agreement state.

### 3.2.1 Exempt Radioactive Material

Certain quantities and sources of RAM are exempt from the licensing requirements of both the NRC and the agreement states. In general, these sources are of very low activity or concentrations and have been determined not to constitute an unreasonable risk to public health and safety and the environment. A list of the exempt concentrations and quantities may be found in 10 CFR 30.70 and 10 CFR 30.71 or the equivalent agreement state regulations. Exempt quantity use includes the use of small quantities of RAM such as found in check sources and calibration standards for commercial distribution. It also includes the use and transfer of small quantities of RAM such as may occur when two labs exchange tissue samples or counting standards for intercomparison on a noncommercial basis. In addition, certain consumer products containing RAM (such as electron tubes, self-luminous watches, and smoke detectors) are exempt from licensing by the user. However, no person may incorporate the exempt RAM into products intended for commercial distribution, or combine quantities of exempt material for purposes of producing an increased radiation level.

### 3.2.2 General Licenses

Regulations provide a general license for the use of byproduct material contained in certain products. This general license allows certain persons to receive and use a device containing byproduct material if the device has been manufactured and distributed in accordance with a specific license issued by the NRC or by an agreement state. A generally licensed device usually consists of RAM contained in a sealed source within a shielded device, such as gas chromatograph units, fixed gauging devices, static eliminators, luminous exit signs, calibration or reference standards, some ice detection devices, and in vitro laboratory kits. The device is designed with inherent radiation safety features so that it can be used by persons with no radiation training or experience. In some cases, registration of the device with the applicable licensing agency is required. The owner of the device may also be required to fulfill certain regulatory obligations, such as having the sealed source leak tested, following labeling instructions, not abandoning or destroying the source, and reporting change of ownership, loss, or theft. Requirements for generally licensed sources may be found at 10 CFR 31 or the equivalent agreement state regulations.

### 3.2.3 *Specific Licenses*

Regulations require what is termed a specific license for the possession and use of RAM that is not exempt or covered under a general license as described above. An application must be submitted to the appropriate regulatory agency for review and approval to obtain the RAMs license. Information that needs to be included in the application includes:

1. Radionuclides, chemical/physical form, possession limits;
2. Purpose for which RAM will be used;
3. Locations of use;
4. Facilities and equipment to use RAM safely;
5. Individuals responsible for the radiation safety program and their training and experience;
6. RPP.

The licensee, which can be either an individual or an institution, must commit to and ensure that all uses of RAM under the issued license are in accordance with statements and representations made in the license application and the applicable regulatory requirements. There must also be a commitment from executive management to provide the oversight and resources necessary to assure safe operations. All licensees must identify a person who is designated as the RSO. This is the individual who is qualified by training and experience in radiation protection and delegated the authority to be responsible for implementing the RPP.

There are two types of specific licenses for academic, medical, research, and development applications: limited scope and broad scope. Specific licenses of limited scope are usually issued for programs that only involve a few users of RAM or for applications that are limited to specific uses that do not frequently change or involve a small number of radionuclides. The license is prescriptive in nature with respect to the policies and procedures for the use of the RAM. For such programs, one of the users (principal investigators) is often designated as the RSO. Specific licenses of broad scope are issued for programs that use a wide range of radionuclides by a large number of users for various and changing uses. The requirements for such licenses and programs are more demanding in the qualifications and experience of the RSO and the organizational structure to oversee and administer the RPP. The program often requires the establishment of a Radiation Safety Committee (RSC) to formulate institutional policy and procedures, review and approve uses and users, and monitor and audit the RPP. A specific license of broad scope allows for more flexibility on the part of the licensee to conduct research programs, in which the license authorizes the use of a large number of radionuclides with relatively high activity limits (on the order of curies) for any use approved by the RSC. The authorized user, or principal investigator, for a particular use of RAM must also meet certain training and experience requirements as required by the RPP or applicable regulations.

RAM is used for a variety of purposes in research. The following are the general categories of uses that are typically identified on academic, research and development, and other specific licenses of limited scope:

1. In vivo studies (labeling cells, studies involving animals, excluding humans);
2. In vitro studies;

3. Analytical work/studies, including gas chromatography devices (GC) and X-ray fluorescence analyzers (XRF);
4. Veterinary medicine;
5. Instrument calibration and testing;
6. Field studies.

Guidance on completing an application for this type of license may be found at: Consolidated Guidance About Materials Licenses: Program-Specific Guidance About Academic, Research and Development, and Other Licenses of Limited Scope Including Gas Chromatographs and X-ray Fluorescence Analyzers [25].

RAM may also be used for research in academic institutions and for research and development in institutions under a specific license of broad scope. Guidance on completing an application for this type of license may be found at: Consolidated Guidance About Materials Licenses: Program-Specific Guidance About Licenses of Broad Scope [26].

Sealed sources of Cs-137 are used in self-shielded irradiators in which the shielding required for operation is an integral part of the device, and the irradiation chamber is not accessible during operation. A Cs-137 source is used to irradiate a wide range of products and materials for research applications. Guidance on completing an application for this type of license may be found at: Consolidated Guidance About Materials Licenses: Program-Specific Guidance About Self-Shielded Irradiator Licenses [27].

RAM used for research involving human subjects may only be performed if the licensee has a 10 CFR part 35 medical use authorization. There are a wide variety of research uses of nuclear materials in human subjects. They include the use of nuclear materials in well-established nuclear medicine procedures to monitor a human research subject's response to a nonradioactive drug or device treatment and clinical trials to determine the safety or effectiveness of new radioactive drugs and devices. The particular medical research use must conform to the requirements in 10 CFR part 35 and the possession and medical use authorizations in the license. Guidance on completing an application for this type of license may be found at: Consolidated Guidance About Materials Licenses: Program-Specific Guidance About Medical Use Licenses [28].

### 3.3 Regulation of Ionizing Radiation-Producing Machines

While the FDA has jurisdiction over the manufacturing and marketing of electronic products that emit ionizing radiation, their use by an institution or facility is regulated by the state government. Usually, the possession and use of radiation-producing equipment is authorized by a registration process rather than licensing. The requirements for registration of radiation-producing equipment and the associated radiation safety regulations for the use of the equipment vary greatly among the different states. In some states, certain types of radiation-producing equipment, such as linear accelerators used in radiation therapy or cyclotrons used for production of PET isotopes, require a permit or license similar to that for RAM. The CRCPD has published and periodically updates its SSRCR. While most state radiation protection programs and regulations are based on these guidelines, there is no legal obligation for a state to follow the suggested regulations, and consequently, there is a significant difference in both the requirements for the use of electronic products that emit ionizing radiation and in their enforcement.

## 3.4 Regulation of Nonionizing Radiation Producing Machines

While the FDA has jurisdiction over the manufacturing and marketing of electronic products that emit nonionizing radiation, their use by an institution or facility is regulated by the state government. As with ionizing radiation-emitting products, the requirements for nonionizing radiation-producing equipment and the associated radiation safety regulations for the use of the equipment vary greatly among the different states. While the CRCPD has a section addressing radiation protection standards for certain classes of lasers in its SSRCR, currently most states do not have any requirement for registration or safety program.

## 4. KEY REGULATORY MANDATES

RAMs and radiation-producing devices are important tools in modern scientific research and in the medical diagnosis and treatment of disease. However, exposure to the various types of radiation emitted from these different sources and devices can cause certain harmful health effects. Concerns to protect workers, patients, and the public from the potential harmful effects have led to extensive federal and state regulations controlling the use of such radiation sources. The following is a description of the key regulatory mandates affecting the use of RAMs and radiation-producing devices in the research environment.

## 4.1 Radioactive Materials License

The use of RAM by an institution for research purposes will require a specific license for the use of the type and quantity of RAM unless it is "exempt" or covered under a "general license." The specific license will be issued by either the NRC or an agreement state. The license is issued to a legal entity such as a corporation, partnership, or individual. Once licensed, the entity must ensure that the radiation activities conducted are in compliance with terms and conditions of the license and applicable regulations. Accordingly, for educational, medical, and research institutions, the license is issued to the respective corporate entity and not a department or individual employee.

To obtain a RAMs license, an application must be submitted to the applicable regulatory agency for review and approval before a license document is provided to the entity. Information required to be submitted in the application include:

1. Isotope, chemical or physical form, and maximum activity;
2. Purpose for which the RAM will be used;
3. Individuals responsible for the radiation protection program and their training and experience;
4. Description of the facilities and equipment used for controlling exposures and protecting individuals;
5. Description of radiation monitoring equipment
6. Description of the RPP;
7. Radioactive waste disposal methods.

For institutions that perform a variety of research, the purpose for which RAM will be used is often listed as "research and development," which is defined in 10 CFR 30 as: (1) theoretical analysis, exploration, or experimentation; or (2) the extension of investigative findings and theories of a scientific or technical nature into practical application for experimental and demonstration purposes, including the experimental production and testing of models, devices, equipment, materials, and processes. Research and development does not include the internal or external administration of radiation or RAM to human beings. This will essentially cover the licensee for any type of research involving the use of RAM. One exception to this would be for tracer studies involving the release of RAM to the environment. This use would require specific review and approval by the regulatory agency.

The license application must also identify an individual to be named as the RSO. This individual must have the requisite training and work experience to be responsible for and manage on a day-to-day basis the RPP. Depending on the types and uses of RAM under the license, a RSC may also be required for oversight and management of the RPP. Licenses will be issued referencing applicable regulatory requirements and also include specific conditions for use of the requested RAM. Licenses are issued for periods of 5 to 10 years, after which they must be renewed by submission of an application if the licensed activities are to continue. Changes to a license, such as adding a new radioisotope or type of use or changing the RSO, are made by submitting an amendment request to the respective regulatory agency. A licensee may not transfer control to another person or entity, or dispose of the license without prior written consent from the regulatory agency. Licensing fees are associated with the application, amendment, and renewal process, along with an annual license fee assessment, the amount of which is based on the type of materials license.

The following NRC regulations are applicable to the licensing process. While these regulations will be compatible or similar to agreement state licensing regulations, the specific agreement state regulations should be addressed if under their authority:

1. 10 CFR part 2, "Rules of Practice for Domestic Licensing Proceedings and Issuance of Orders";
2. 10 CFR part 19, "Notices, Instructions and Reports to Workers: Inspection and Investigations";
3. 10 CFR part 20, "Standards for Protection Against Radiation";
4. 10 CFR part 21, "Reporting of Defects and Noncompliance";
5. 10 CFR part 30, "Rules of General Applicability to Domestic Licensing of Byproduct Material";
6. 10 CFR part 31, "General Domestic Licenses for Byproduct Material";
7. 10 CFR part 32, "Specific Domestic Licenses to Manufacture or Transfer Certain Items Containing Byproduct Material";
8. 10 CFR part 33, "Specific Domestic Licenses of Broad Scope for Byproduct Material";
9. 10 CFR part 35, "Medical Use of Byproduct Material";
10. 10 CFR part 40, "Domestic Licensing of Source Material";
11. 10 CFR part 70, "Domestic Licensing of Special Nuclear Material" (for pacemaker devices);
12. 10 CFR part 71, "Packaging and Transportation of Radioactive Material."

## 4.2 Radiation Protection Program

All RAMs licensees are required by 10 CFR 20 (or equivalent agreement state regulations) to develop, document, and implement a RPP that is commensurate with the extent and scope of licensed activities and to assure compliance with the applicable regulations. A key required component of the RPP is the ALARA program to control radiation doses to occupational workers and the public to levels as far below the regulatory limits as practicable. The content and implementation of the RPP is required to be reviewed or audited at least annually.

## 4.3 Registration of Ionizing Radiation Producing Equipment

States have the authority for the regulation of equipment that produces ionizing radiation (X-ray equipment and particle accelerators). Most states require the possession and use of this equipment to be registered, which involves the completion and submission of a standardized form. The registration process is somewhat less involved and burdensome than that required for licensing. The registration is issued to a legal entity such as a corporation, partnership, or individual. Information to be documented on the form includes:

1. Facility address;
2. Type and number of ionizing radiation-producing equipment;
3. Name of the RSO;
4. Name of administrative official, or for medical X-rays, name of licensed healing arts practitioner.

Some states will require a radiation shielding plan for any new installation, or modification of existing installation, to be submitted to the state agency for review and approval before issuing a certificate of registration. The state agency may require the applicant to use the services of a qualified health physicist or a qualified medical physicist to determine the shielding requirements.

The registrant will be responsible for maintaining and operating the radiation safety procedures for protection of patients, operators, employees, and the general public. The registrant will also be responsible for compliance with the applicable state regulatory requirements specific to the type of ionizing radiation-producing equipment. For medical X-ray equipment, a quality assurance program to assure image quality and patient protection will also be required. Registrations are typically renewed annually and associated with a fee, of which the amount is based on the facility and number and type of ionizing equipment. Some states require a license for the possession and use of particle accelerators, for which the process is similar to that for licensing RAM.

The following SSRCR from the CRCPD [29] were developed to promote consistency in addressing and resolving radiation protection issues applicable to the registration and licensing process. Because there is no requirement for a state to adopt these suggested regulations, the specific state regulations should be addressed:
SSRCR—Volume I.

1. Part A—general provisions;
2. Part B—registration (licensure) of radiation machine facilities, (services) and associated healthcare professionals;
3. Part D—standards for protection against radiation;
4. Part F—diagnostic X-rays and imaging systems in the healing arts;
5. Part H—radiation safety requirements for analytical X-ray equipment;
6. Part I—radiation safety requirements for particle accelerators;
7. Part J—notices, instructions and reports to workers; inspections.

## 4.4 Research Involving Human Subjects

The regulations addressing the use of human subjects for research that involves radiation exposure from RAM is addressed in the definition of "medical use" in the NRC regulations 10 CFR 35.2 or equivalent agreement state regulations. Medical use is defined as the intentional internal or external administration of byproduct material or the radiation from byproduct material to patients or human research subjects under the supervision of an authorized user. Furthermore, in 10 CFR 35.6 (or equivalent agreement state regulations), "Provisions for the protection of human research subjects," the protection of the rights of human subjects involved in research by medical use licensees is addressed to require that:

1. The licensee may conduct research involving human research subjects only if it uses the byproduct materials specified on its license for the uses authorized on its license.
2. The research is conducted, funded, supported, or regulated by another federal agency that has implemented the federal policy for the protection of human subjects (federal policy), the licensee shall, before conducting research—
   a. Obtain review and approval of the research from an "institutional review board," as defined and described in the federal policy; and
   b. Obtain "informed consent," as defined and described in the federal policy, from the human research subject.
3. If the research will not be conducted, funded, supported, or regulated by another federal agency that has implemented the federal policy, the licensee shall, before conducting research, apply for and receive a specific amendment to its NRC or agreement state medical use license. The amendment request must include a written commitment that the licensee will, before conducting research, adhere to the requirements in (a) and (b) above.

   Otherwise, nothing in the section above relieves the licensee from complying with the other applicable requirements in the medical use regulations. If the research use does not conform to the conditions stated above, then a licensee must apply for and receive a specific amendment request for approval to conduct the research protocol. Similarly, the CRCPD SSRCR addresses the use of research on human subjects involving machine-produced radiation to require:

   In addition to the other requirements of Part B, any research using radiation machines on humans shall be approved by an Institutional Review Board (IRB) as required by title 45, CFR, part 46 and title 21, CFR, part 56. The IRB shall include at least one practitioner of the healing arts to direct any use of radiation in accordance with part F. Detailed information about the management of IRBs is provided in Chapter 1, "Human subjects."

   Therefore, a licensee or registrant is permitted to perform research involving the internal or external administration of radiation or RAM to human subjects as long as the research is reviewed and approved by an IRB in accordance with the human subject protection requirements.

## 4.5 Authorized Users

An authorized user (AU), more commonly known as a principal investigator (PI) in the research setting, is a person who meets certain specified training and experience requirements and uses or directly supervises the use of licensed RAM. The AU is responsible for the safe use of RAM in his or her laboratory or area. Every type of RAMs use under a license must have an AU. An AU is considered to be supervising the use of RAM when it is being handled or experiments being performed by others. While the AU may delegate specific tasks to others who work with the RAM, the AU is responsible that they will use the material safely and in accordance with regulatory requirements. For in vitro studies, animal research, use of self-shielded gamma irradiators, and other uses that do not involve the exposure of humans, the training and experience requirements for an AU generally include: (1) a college degree at the bachelor level or equivalent training and experience in the physical or biological sciences or in engineering; and (2) at least 40 h of training and experience in the safe handling of RAMs, characteristics of ionizing radiation, units of radiation dose and quantities, radiation detection instrumentation, and biological hazards of exposure to radiation appropriate to the type and forms of RAM to be used. For limited scope licensees, the AU's training and experience will be reviewed by the regulatory agency, and the AU will be named on the license for the approved uses. For broad scope licensees, the AU's training and experience will be reviewed by the RSC, and an internal permit will be provided to the AU for the approved uses.

AUs for the medical or human use of RAM (including research use) must be physicians who meet specific training and experience requirements that are dependent on the category of medical use, as defined in 10 CFR 35 subparts D, E, F, G, H, and K. These training and validation requirements for physicians authorized to use RAMs were amended by the NRC in 2005. The following current categories of medical use are:

1. 35.100 Uptake, dilution, and excretion studies;
2. 35.200 Imaging and localization studies;
3. 35.300 Unsealed material for which a written directive is required;
4. 35.500 Sealed sources for diagnosis;
5. 35.400 Manual brachytherapy sources;
6. 35.600 Remote after loader units and gamma stereotactic radiosurgery units;
7. 35.1000 Other medical use.

There are two primary routes to demonstrate qualification as an AU. The first is by means of certification by a medical specialty board recognized by NRC and listed on the NRC website (http://www.nrc.gov/materials/miau/med-use-toolkit/spec-board-cert.html). The second route is by meeting the structured educational program, supervised work experience, and preceptor attestation requirements in the appropriate subpart that is documented on NRC form 313A. The required training and experience, including board certification, must have been obtained within the 7 years preceding the date of the application, or the individual must document having had related continuing education, retraining, and experience since obtaining the required training and experience.

Once an individual is approved and named as an AU on an NRC or agreement state RAMs license, that individual will satisfy the requirements to be named and practice under any other RAMs license for the same uses as already approved.

The training and experience requirements for a physician to be considered an AU for use of a linear accelerator for external beam therapy are set by the state and vary across the United States.

Any medical or human use of RAM or ionizing radiation-producing equipment, either clinical or research, must have associated with its use an AU (that meets the applicable

TABLE 1   Maximum Permissible Radiation Dose Limits (US)

|  | Limit per year |
| --- | --- |
| Occupational worker | |
| Whole body | 5 rem (50 mSv) |
| Lens eye | 15 rem (150 mSv) |
| Skin/extremities | 50 rem (500 mSv) |
| Embryo/fetus | 0.5 rem (5 mSv) |
| General public | 0.1 rem (1 mSv) |

training and experience requirements) that is responsible for the radiation safety and regulatory compliance aspects of the use.

## 4.6  Radiation Dose Limits

As described earlier, there are potential adverse health effects that can occur from exposure to ionizing radiation, whether it is in the form of external irradiation from diagnostic X-rays or internal irradiation from introduction of radioactive substances into the body. These range from deterministic effects such as erythema and cataracts, which occur from very high doses of radiation above a certain threshold, to stochastic effects such as cancer and hereditary disorders, which are thought to occur in the absence of a dose threshold. Irradiation of the embryo/fetus also carries risks of malformation, mental impairment, and childhood cancer. Therefore, the intentional exposure of humans to ionizing radiation at any dose for research purposes carries some risk of detriment or harm. While there are current federal radiation dose limits (10 CFR 20) set by the NRC for occupational exposure to adults, minors, embryo/fetus of pregnant worker and exposure to members of the general public as shown in Table 1, there are no regulatory radiation dose limits for individuals undergoing medical procedures (diagnostic or therapeutic) or for human research subjects. This applies to both exposures from ionizing radiation-producing equipment and RAM. One exception to this is for research conducted under a radioactive drug research committee (RDRC) involving radioactive drugs that are not approved by the FDA. Detailed information about the operation of RDRCs is provided below and in Chapter 2, "Investigational New Drug and Device Exemption Process."

The federal dose limits, along with the average exposure to background radiation in the United States, are often used as a comparison when evaluating a research protocol to assess the radiation dose to research subjects and the corresponding risk. Another source of guidance on this topic is ICRP publication 62 "Radiological Protection in Biomedical Research" [30]. In addition to discussing the design, assessment, justification, and oversight of biomedical research involving subject exposure to ionizing radiation, it provided a categorization of radiation dose to research subjects and a corresponding quantification of risk of harm and the level of societal benefit necessary to justify the research, as shown in Table 2. It should be noted that in this table, the risk is the total detriment from the exposure: namely, the sum of the probability of fatal cancers, nonfatal cancers, and serious hereditary disease resulting from the radiation dose. For research involving children, the detriment is assumed to be 2 to 3 times greater than for adults; and for people over age 50 years, the detriment is only about one-fifth

TABLE 2   Categories of Levels of Benefit and Corresponding Levels of Risk

| Level of societal benefit | Risk level corresponding to the benefit | Risk category (total risk—see text) | | Corresponding effective dose range for adults (mSv)[b] |
|---|---|---|---|---|
| Minor | Trivial | Category I | ~$10^{-6}$ or less | <0.1 |
| Intermediate to moderate | Minor to intermediate | Category II | | |
| | | Category II[a] | ~$10^{-5}$ | 0.1–1 |
| | | Category II[b] | ~$10^{-4}$ | 1–10 |
| Substantial | Moderate | Category III | ~$10^{-3}$ or more | >10[a] |

In the case of children, they should be reduced by a factor of 2 or 3.
[a]*To be kept below deterministic thresholds except for therapeutic experiments.*
[b]*These figures can be increased by a factor of 5–10 for those older than 50 years.*
*Based on ICRP 62.*

to one-tenth of that for younger adults. The lowest risk category is on the order of one in a million and is in the region in which most people are content to dismiss the risk as trivial. This dose level of less than 0.1 mSv (10 mrem) corresponds to the amount of dose delivered by natural background radiation in a few weeks. In the middle category, the risk is on the order of one in 10,000 to one in a 100,000 and is at the level at which people start to express some concern, although this level of risk is readily accepted in a wide range of circumstances. In dose terms, this corresponds to the level of dose received by most radiation workers and average annual doses received by all members of the public from natural, manmade, and medical sources. In the highest category, the risk is on the order of one in a 1000 or greater and is in the region in which people tend to regard as verging on the unacceptable for continued or repeated exposures. This dose level approaches the current annual dose limit for occupational exposure.

## 4.7 Radioactive Drug Research Committee

FDA regulations (21 CFR part 361.1) permit the research use, in human subjects, of radioactive drugs that are not currently the subject of an approved investigational new drug (IND) application, if reviewed and approved by an institutional RDRC, provided that certain specific requirements are met. The RDRC is established under the authority and in accordance with these regulations and serves to initially and continually review such research studies to ensure their compliance with the provisions of 21 CFR 361.1. Other conditions for the research to be approved by the RDRC include:

1. The research must be intended to obtain basic information regarding the metabolism (including kinetics, distribution, and localization) of a radioactively labeled drug or regarding human physiology, pathophysiology, or biochemistry, but not intended for immediate therapeutic, diagnostic, or similar purposes or to determine safety and effectiveness of the drug in humans for such purposes.
2. The research study is determined by the committee that scientific knowledge and benefit is likely to result, and the radiation exposure is justified by the importance of the information it seeks to gain.

3. Research subjects shall be at least 18 years of age and legally competent. Exceptions are permitted only in those special situations when it can be demonstrated that the use of subjects less than 18 years of age presents a unique opportunity to gain information not currently available, and the study is not of significant risk to the subject.
4. The number of subjects included in the study shall be sufficient, but no greater than necessary to gain the basic information. Inclusion of more than 30 subjects in the research study must be scientifically justified and requires advance notification of the FDA.
5. The dose to be administered must be known to not cause any clinically detectable pharmacological effect based on data available from published literature or other valid human studies.
6. Women of childbearing potential must state in writing that she is not pregnant, or, on the basis of a pregnancy test, be confirmed as not pregnant, before she may participate in the study.
7. The quality of the radioactive drug used in the research study shall meet appropriate chemical, pharmaceutical, radiochemical, and radionuclide standards of identity, strength, quality, and purity as needed for safety and be of such uniform and reproducible quality as to give significance to the research study conducted.
8. The package, label, and labeling of the radioactive drug must meet the requirements of federal, state, and local laws on RAMs.
9. The investigators listed on the research study are qualified by training and experience so as to provide reasonable insurance that scientific knowledge and benefit will result from the study.
10. The investigator is authorized to use the specific radionuclide for research under a RAMs license issued by the NRC or agreement state.
11. The amount of radioactive drug to be administered shall be such that the subject receives the smallest radiation dose with which it is practical to perform the study without jeopardizing the benefits to be obtained from the study. Under no circumstances may the radiation dose to an adult research subject from a single study or cumulatively from a number of studies conducted within 1 year exceed the limits in Table 3. The radiation dose to an individual subject consists of the sum total of all sources of radiation associated with the research protocol, including the following:
   a. The radiation absorbed dose from the radioactive drug, including any significant contaminant or impurity;

TABLE 3    RDRC Limits of Radiation Dose for Adults

| Organ or system | Single dose sieverts (rem) | Annual and total dose sieverts (rem) |
| --- | --- | --- |
| Whole body | 0.03 (3) | 0.05 (5) |
| Active blood-forming organs | 0.03 (3) | 0.05 (5) |
| Lens of the eye | 0.03 (3) | 0.05 (5) |
| Gonads | 0.03 (3) | 0.05 (5) |
| Other organs | 0.05 (5) | 0.15 (15) |

RDRC, radioactive drug research committee.

b. Radiation doses from any X-ray or other radioactive drug procedures that are part of the research study (i.e., would not have occurred but for participation in the study);

c. For research subjects under 18 years of age at their last birthday, the radiation doses shall not exceed 10 percent of the limits described above.

The RDRC must be approved by the FDA and have membership to include: (1) a physician recognized as a specialist in nuclear medicine; (2) a person qualified by training and experience to formulate radioactive drugs; and (3) a person with special competence in radiation safety and radiation dosimetry.

## 4.8 Increased Controls

In 2005, the NRC issued the increased controls (IC) order to licensees for certain sources of RAM to enhance their security so that the risk of theft, sabotage, or unauthorized use is minimized. In conjunction, the agreement states issued the same requirements to applicable materials licensees within their regulatory jurisdictions. One of the devices commonly used in research that was captured under this order was Cs-137 self-shielded irradiators. Among the requirements of that order were: (1) Limit access to only individuals who have been determined to be trustworthy and reliable (T&R)—the requirements for this determination involve a background investigation, including fingerprinting and Federal Bureau of Investigation (FBI) identification and criminal records check; (2) Control physical access to the device with security and alarm systems; and (3) Be able to monitor, detect, and assess theft of RAM, and coordinate response with local law enforcement. This order was codified by regulation in 2013 in 10 CFR 37 "Physical Protection of Category 1 and Category 2 Quantities of Radioactive Material." Each licensee of a Cs-137 self-shielded irradiator must establish, implement, and maintain a security program that is designed to monitor, detect, assess, and respond to an actual or attempted unauthorized access to the radioactive source.

## 5. KEY PERSONNEL AND UNIVERSITY COMMITTEES DESIGNATED TO IMPLEMENT REGULATORY MANDATES

The use of RAMs requires licensing by the NRC or an agreement state, and the use of ionizing radiation-producing devices requires that the devices be registered with the state. An institution possessing a license or registration is required by regulation to establish a formal RPP. The size and complexity of that program will be determined by the types of radiation sources and uses under the license or registration. Research activities using these sources may be conducted in a variety of departments, such as biological sciences, chemistry, geology, physics, engineering, health sciences, and affiliated medical facilities. The RPP must ensure that all sources of licensed RAM and radiation-producing equipment that fall under its responsibility are used optimally and safely. It must also ensure that these sources of radiation are used in compliance with the applicable federal and state regulations and institutional licenses. The main principle of the RPP is application of ALARA. Following the ALARA principle means making efforts to maintain exposures to radiation at a minimum (and resulting potential health risks) by taking into consideration the state of technology, economic factors, benefits to the public, and other societal considerations.

## 5.1 Radiation Safety Officer

Educational, medical, and research institutions typically assign the overall responsibility for regulatory compliance and radiation safety matters to an individual identified as the RSO. The RSO is required to be named on the RAMs license and radiation-producing device registration. To be effective, the RSO must have adequate training and experience to be qualified for the day-to-day administration and enforcement of the RPP. For medical (human) use licensees, there are specific regulatory requirements for the training and experience that an individual must satisfy to qualify to be named as an RSO (10 CFR 35.50), and the CRCPD SSRCR has suggested qualifications for an RSO overseeing the use of radiation-producing equipment (Part B—registration (licensure) of radiation machine facilities, (services) and associated healthcare professionals, appendix C).

The institution (management) must provide the RSO with the sufficient time and physical and financial resources to perform his/her duties and establish in writing the authority and responsibilities of the RSO (10 CFR 35.24(b)). The RSO must be delegated with the authority to immediately stop any operation involving the use of RAM or a radiation-producing machine in which health and safety may be compromised or may result in noncompliance with regulations.

The RSO is typically a full-time employee of the institution; however, for small programs, the RSO may be a consultant.

The RSO is responsible for managing the radiation safety program at all levels of the organization, identifying radiation safety problems, initiating, recommending, or providing corrective actions, verifying implementation of corrective actions, and ensuring compliance with regulations and license conditions.

## 5.2 Radiation Safety Committee

An RSC is usually established for large radiation safety programs and is required by regulation for certain types of RAMs licenses, especially for medical use licensees when two or more modalities are being performed (10 CFR 33.13, 10 CFR 35.24). The RSC is responsible for establishing the policies and procedures of the RPP and serves as the final authority in matters pertaining to decisions concerning approval or disapproval of uses and users and addressing any compliance issues. The committee should include a representative of management, the RSO, a nursing representative (if the license is for medical use), and other persons representing the major types of uses of RAM and ionizing radiation-producing devices. The chair of the committee is usually appointed by senior management. The RSC will usually meet quarterly and maintain written minutes of the meeting.

### 5.2.1 *Authority of the Radiation Safety Committee*

The RSC is usually delegated with the following authorities and responsibilities:

1. Establish policy and standards of practice for the RPP;
2. Review a summary of the occupational radiation dose records and provide recommendations on ways to maintain doses ALARA;.
3. Review the RPP to determine that all activities are being conducted in accordance with radiation safety policy, license conditions, and regulatory requirements;

4. Review and grant approval/disapproval, on the basis of safety and with regard to training and experience, individuals applying to become an AU;
5. Review and grant approval/disapproval, on the basis of safety, regulatory compliance, and the ALARA philosophy, for all new types or modalities of uses of RAMs and radiation-producing equipment;
6. Review radiation safety incidents, issues, and violations and recommend corrective actions;
7. Approve all RAMs licensing actions, as necessary.

## 5.3 Radiation Safety Office

Depending on the size and complexity of the RPP, additional radiation safety staff may be necessary to conduct the program. Each institution is somewhat unique in its structure and organization and requires an evaluation of the functions to be performed and the corresponding time requirements. Guidelines have been published on the recommended minimum radiation safety staffing levels for various categories of medical institutions [31].

The radiation safety office, under the direction of the RSO, is staffed with personnel (clerical, technologists, and health or medical physicists) who possess the necessary training and experience to perform the required radiation safety duties to implement the policies and procedures of the radiation safety program as approved by the RSC. The responsibilities of the radiation safety office include:

1. Maintain RAMs licenses and X-ray machine registrations and prepare and submit license renewals and amendments;
2. Provide radiation safety training to occupationally exposed workers and ancillary personnel;
3. Provide for personnel radiation monitoring of external exposures and conduct bioassay measurements to assess the uptake of RAM and determine the corresponding radiation dose;
4. Arrange for the receipt, survey, delivery, and transfer of shipments of RAM;
5. Maintain an inventory of all RAMs;
6. Perform routine radiation surveys and audits of laboratories using RAM;
7. Perform radiation safety review and design of experimental procedures;
8. Collect, process, and dispose of radioactive waste;
9. Calibrate portable radiation-detection instruments;
10. Perform routine leak tests on sealed sources and detector cells;
11. Perform radiation safety and regulatory compliance checks or surveys of ionizing radiation-producing equipment;
12. Perform audits of gamma irradiator safety and security systems;
13. Investigate incidents involving radiation or RAM;
14. Provide emergency response to radioactive spills and contamination incidents;
15. Maintain all radiation safety records as required by regulation.

## 5.4 Authorized Users

PIs and clinicians using or supervising the use of RAMs or radiation-producing machines for their work must be approved as an AU. Initial applications to become an AU are reviewed on the basis of the individual's training and experience and availability of adequate facilities and resources to use the requested sources of radiation safely. An AU will usually be required to have a college degree at the bachelor level or equivalent training and experience in the physical or biological sciences or engineering and at least 40 h of training and experience in the safe handling of RAMs, the characteristics of ionizing radiation, units of radiation dose and quantities, radiation-detection instrumentation, and biological hazards of exposure to radiation appropriate to the type and forms of byproduct material or radiation-producing equipment to be used. Requests for authorization are typically approved for a specific period, usually one to three years.

For continuing work, a renewal request must be submitted prior to expiration of an authorization. This is to ensure that each authorization is periodically reviewed and reflects current usage. In general, only faculty members are eligible to become an AU. An AU must comply with the conditions of their authorization for the use of radiation sources within a defined protocol or work activity. The responsibilities of the AU include:

1. Supervising all personnel using RAM and/or radiation-producing machines under the conditions of the authorization;
2. Maintaining compliance with the policies and procedures of the RPP;
3. Maintaining the security of all RAM;
4. Reporting promptly to the RSO any accident, incident, or emergency involving RAM or radiation-producing machines;
5. Maintaining a current inventory of all RAM;
6. Performing radiation and contamination monitoring as required by commitments to the RPP;
7. Providing adequate use-specific safety training for all radiation workers under the authorization;
8. Submitting amendment request to the RSC prior to any changes in the location(s) of RAM and radiation-producing machine use and experimental design;
9. Maintaining records of inventory, receipt and disposal, and laboratory surveys;
10. Arrange for disposal or transfer of all RAMs promptly on termination of the authorized use or application.

## 5.5 Radiation Workers

While the RAM license and RPP will hold the AU responsible for the use of RAM under their authorization, the actual hands-on work will usually be conducted by others working under the "supervision" of the AU. These individuals (research associates, technicians, co-investigators) must be adequately trained in the necessary protocol or experimental procedure and the associated radiation safety precautions and will also need to be identified on the AU application. While the RSO or radiation safety office staff will usually provide the necessary initial and refresher general radiation safety training, the AU will be responsible for providing the specific instruction for the required job duties. The AU may delegate essential duties to others, but not the overall responsibility for the use of radioactive material. The RSO will often have special training requirements for certain experimental procedures (I-125 iodinations, H-3 labeling with sodium borohydride) and using radiation-producing equipment (X-ray machines, gamma irradiators).

## 5.6 Use of Radiation Sources with Animals

Animal research involving the administration of RAM or irradiation from gamma or X-ray sources will need to be identified on a protocol-by-protocol basis for review by the RSC. This will be in addition to the protocol submission and review requirements by the Institutional Animal Care and Use Committee (IACUC), as outlined in Chapter 3 (Animal subjects). Radiation safety concerns for the use of RAM in animals include proper containment to avoid the spread of contamination, exposure to animal care technicians, proper labeling of cages and instruction on special radiation safety precautions to be followed, and procedures for disposal of the animal carcass, bedding, and other contaminated materials. Radiation safety concerns associated with the irradiation of animals, either from radiographic procedures or from gamma X-ray irradiators, are usually focused on delivering the appropriate radiation dose for the animal and on transportation of the animal to and from the location where the irradiation procedure occurred. For diagnostic X-ray procedures, the number, type, and exposure technique should be such that there is little likelihood of inducing any acute effect from the radiation dose. With gamma and X-ray irradiators for which the intention is to deliver a high radiation dose to the animal for the purpose of inducing changes in the cell and tissue survival, the prescribed dose and fractionation must be justified to produce the desired effects.

## 5.7 Security Requirements

Self-shielded gamma irradiators containing one or more sealed sources of Cs-137 are used for irradiating biological samples (subcellular components, cells, tissues, and live animals) to relatively high doses of radiation to study its effects in a variety of applications. Due to the high level of radioactivity contained in the sealed sources (above 27 Ci), the NRC instituted the requirements for IC in 2005 for all irradiator licensees. The IC requirements were imposed to enhance the security surrounding the use of gamma irradiators to prevent the theft and misuse of the source in a terroristic event, either as a radioactive dispersal device (dirty bomb) or as an improvised exposure source. One of the IC requirements is to restrict the access to the gamma irradiator to only those individuals who have been determined to be "trustworthy and reliable" (T&R). If an individual is not T&R approved, they may only use the gamma irradiator when they are "escorted" by someone who is T&R approved. The NRC defines an "escort" to mean the person is in visual contact with the escorted individual. For an individual to be determined to be T&R, the institution must perform a background check that includes employment verification, reference checks, and fingerprinting for FBI identification and criminal records checks. The T&R determination is usually performed by the institution's human resources department, radiation safety office, or combination of both. The check can take from several weeks to several months, especially for those foreign born or who are not US citizens, and cost upward of several hundred dollars, depending on what all is checked by the institution.

Several manufacturers now have X-ray irradiators that can be used in place of a Cs-137 gamma irradiator for irradiation of both cells and animals, thus eliminating the IC security requirements. Due to the lower photon energy of the X-ray irradiators, there may be some issues with comparison of results with experiments using Cs-137.

## 5.8 Human Subject Research

In most medical research institutions, all protocols involving the human use of RAMs and/or radiation-producing equipment are subject to RSC review, in addition to review by the IRB. The IRB review process is described in detail in Chapter 1, Human Subjects. This layer of review is usually focused at the appropriateness of the use of the radiation, the total radiation dose being delivered to the research subject, and the wording of statements of radiation risk from participation in the research protocol.

In smaller institutions this protocol review may be conducted by the RSO alone. In larger institutions, a human use subcommittee (HUSC) is usually established to expedite the review of human use protocols. This committee will be made up of members with expertise in radiology, nuclear medicine, radiation oncology, and radiation dosimetry/physics. The RSO will also usually be a member of the subcommittee. The HUSC will establish a formal application and protocol review process that the PI will need to follow, similar to that of the IRB. After completion of the protocol review by the HUSC, the response back to the PI will generally result in one of the following actions:

1. *Full approval:* Research study complies with the applicable regulations; no comments, concerns or suggested modifications.
2. *Approval pending investigator acceptance of directed changes:* Research study generally complies with applicable regulations; investigator must address minor modifications or items of clarification in the submitted protocol to effect full approval.
3. *Reconsideration:* Research study may be permitted under the applicable regulations; however, significant deficiencies in the research protocol must be addressed and/or the research protocol must be significantly modified to effect full approval.
4. *Disapproval:* Research study cannot be performed under the applicable regulations and/ or no scientific knowledge and benefit are likely to result from the study.

Review of the research by the HUSC may be in series or parallel to that of the IRB.

As discussed in the previous section, the FDA regulations (21 CFR 361.1) permit the research use, in human subjects, of radioactive drugs that are not currently approved by an investigational new drug (IND) or a new drug application (NDA), provided that certain specific conditions are met. An institutional RDRC is established under the authority and in accordance with these FDA regulations to allow local review and approval of such studies. Although it reviews and approves research studies involving the use of radioactive drugs, the activities of the RDRC are not regulated by any type of RAMs license granted by the NRC or agreement state. The RDRC is distinct from all other human research study review committees (e.g. IRB, HUSC); however, the FDA regulations do not prohibit the institution from involving the RDRC in other policy matters. Hence, to facilitate the review and approval of research studies involving the use of all radioactive drugs/devices and radiation-producing equipment, the members of the RDRC will also serve in the capacity of the HUSC.

### 5.8.1 Research Protocols Involving the Use of Standard Procedures That Emit Ionizing Radiation for Routine Medical Management

Biomedical research studies frequently involve the use of (1) a standard diagnostic procedure (e.g., nuclear medicine procedure, chest X-ray, CT, angiography) in a routine clinical manner and frequency for research subject screening and/or to evaluate a therapeutic response; or (2) a standard radiation therapy procedure indicated for medical management of the patient. Such uses of standard clinical care procedures will not require review and approval by the HUSC.

Standard clinical care is defined as the typical or routine management of the patient, that is, the number and type of radiological procedures that a patient would typically receive as part of the standard clinical care. This would not include individuals (e.g., healthy volunteers) who are not receiving the diagnostic procedure in association with the diagnosis or treatment of a disease or condition.

### 5.8.2 Research Protocols that Involve the Evaluation or Research Use of an Ionizing Radiation-Emitting Device or Drug

Biomedical research studies directed at the evaluation or research use (not related to the clinical management of the subject) of a drug or device that emits ionizing radiation must be reviewed by the HUSC. This would also include the modification of standard diagnostic or therapeutic clinical procedures such that the specific parameters (e.g., technique factors, total dose or dosage, fractionation scheme) of the radiation procedure(s) are defined by the research protocol. Examples of the different type of research use of radiation-producing equipment or RAM include:

1. Research evaluation or use of an FDA-approved device;
2. Research evaluation or use of a device that is the subject of an FDA-approved investigational device exemption (IDE);
3. Research evaluation or use of an unapproved device;
4. Research evaluation or use of an FDA-approved radiopharmaceutical prepared and administered in accordance with the approved product labeling;
5. Research evaluation or use of an FDA-approved radiopharmaceutical prepared using a nonapproved (i.e., not according to product labeling) method and/or administered by a nonapproved (i.e., not according to product labeling) route;
6. Research evaluation or use of a radioactive drug which is the subject of an FDA-approved IND exemption;
7. Research evaluation or use of a radioactive drug that is not FDA-approved.

Diagnostic or therapeutic procedures involving the internal or external administration of RAM or radiation from RAM must be performed by or under the supervision of a physician or AU who meets the required training and clinical experience required by the NRC or equivalent agreement state regulations.

The AU, who may be the PI, is also responsible for ensuring compliance with conditions of the protocol and other procedures related to the safe use of radiation sources. Commonly, however, the PI may not be authorized to use radionuclides in humans and, therefore, will enlist a physician who is an AU as a co-investigator to cover the human use procedures involving RAM. For diagnostic or research procedures involving the uptake dilution, excretion, imaging, or localization of RAM, the physician must be board certified in diagnostic radiology or nuclear medicine, or meet equivalent training and experience. For procedures involving the therapeutic administration of RAM or radiation there from, the physician must be board certified in nuclear medicine or radiation oncology, or meet equivalent training and experience. For protocols involving the diagnostic or interventional use of radiation-producing equipment, the physician must meet the applicable state medical licensing board requirements.

## 5.9 Organization Structure

The management and reporting for the RPP within an institution will vary in proportion to the size and complexity of activities being performed. The highest priority is for the RSO or RSC to have direct-line report to executive management. As with any compliance oversight function, the RPP must have the support and cognizance from a level of management that can reach all areas of the institution.

In most university medical research institutions, the RSC and RSO are part of the environmental health and safety department. In other institutions, it may be a division within the radiology department, or it may be part of a larger compliance office along with similar regulatory-mandated compliance committees such as the IRB, IACUC, and conflict of interest.

## 5.10 Lasers

Any institution using potentially hazardous laser systems is responsible for providing a safe work environment for personnel. A laser safety program will usually be developed, depending on the number and type of laser systems involved. The responsibility for the program is generally delegated to a safety department (environmental health, industrial hygiene, radiation) within the organization [31]. Individuals responsible for the laser safety program must be knowledgeable of the standards and regulations associated with laser use. There are few regulations for the use of lasers, and one must check with their state radiation protection agency for any registration or use requirements. Standards and recommendations for the safe use of lasers are provided by the American National Standards Institute standard Z136.8 [32].

Lasers are divided into a number of classes depending on the power or energy of the beam and the wavelength of the emitted radiation. Laser classification is based on the laser's potential for causing immediate injury to the eye or skin and/or potential for causing fires from direct exposure to the beam or from reflections from diffuse reflective surfaces [33].

Qualitative description of laser classes follows:

1. *Class 1 lasers*
   Class 1 lasers are considered to be incapable of producing damaging radiation levels and are therefore exempt from most control measures or other forms of surveillance. Example: laser printers.
2. *Class 2 lasers*
   Class 2 lasers emit radiation in the visible portion of the spectrum, and protection is normally afforded by the normal human aversion response (blink reflex) to bright radiant sources. They may be hazardous if viewed directly for extended periods. Example: laser pointers.
3. *Class 3 lasers*
   Class 3a lasers are those that normally would not produce injury if viewed only momentarily with the unaided eye. They may present a hazard if viewed using collecting

optics, for example, telescopes, microscopes, or binoculars. Example: HeNe lasers above 1 mW, but not exceeding 5 mW radiant power.

Class 3b lasers can cause severe eye injuries if beams are viewed directly or specular reflections are viewed. A class 3 laser is not normally a fire hazard. Example: visible HeNe lasers above 5 mW, but not exceeding 500 mW radiant power.

4. *Class 4 lasers*

Class 4 lasers are a hazard to the eye from the direct beam and specular reflections and sometimes even from diffuse reflections. Class 4 lasers can also start fires and can damage skin.

The laser safety program will generally include registration of lasers and laser workers, laser safety inspections, training, preparation of required laser warning signs, and investigation of any suspected injury involved with laser use. A "laser safety officer" is the individual responsible for monitoring laser use and safety. PIs will be responsible for wearing appropriate personal protective equipment, attending training, training their staff, and developing policies and procedures for their particular laser activities. The PI is also responsible for assuring all laser users under their supervision are properly trained and conduct laser activities in a safe manner. All laser users are expected to wear appropriate personal protective equipment.

## 6. COMMON COMPLIANCE CHALLENGES

### 6.1 Laboratory Use of Radioactive Materials

The use of RAM by an AU is limited to the specific isotopes, possession limits, locations, and experimental procedures, which have been approved by the RSC in response to the AU's application. No work may begin with radioactive materials until the listed requirements have been met. Similarly, ongoing use of radioactive material in the laboratory must continue to comply with all of the applicable radiation safety policies and procedures of the RPP. Much information supplied in the initial application changes over time; therefore, applications must be reviewed and updated periodically to ensure that the information on file is current. Authorization to use radionuclides will be granted for intervals not to exceed several years, at which time they must be renewed (or terminated); however, an amendment application must be submitted at any time the type of radionuclide, activity limits, or experimental protocol changes significantly.

Persons taking extended leave, such as sabbatical leave or for illness, who intend to have research or studies using RAM continue during their absence, must usually designate a qualified co-worker or preferably another AU to assume radiation safety responsibility during their absence. Persons terminating their use of RAMs must promptly notify the RSO prior to the termination so that the laboratories can be surveyed and down-posted prior to returning them to general use. If the AU intends to transfer RAMs to another institution, the RSO has the responsibility to oversee the packaging and transfer of the radionuclides. If laboratory equipment used in conjunction with RAMs is to be transferred to another institution, then the RSO must certify the equipment as free of RAMs prior to packing and shipping.

The RSO will typically perform periodic audits and surveys of all areas where sources of RAM are used to monitor and assure compliance with the applicable radiation safety policies and procedures. Documentation of the audit/survey results will be maintained by the RSO. The AU will be notified of any contamination or other program violations with a request for corrective action. The following is a list of the more common laboratory safety policies that are violated:

1. *Use of radioactive material in radiation laboratories*
   "Radiation laboratories" are considered to be restricted areas, where access is controlled to protect individuals from exposure to radiation and RAMs. The laboratory will have a "caution radioactive materials" label on the door or entrance area. Materials may only be used and stored in specifically designated and approved areas.
2. *Laboratory contamination surveys*
   Radiation workers are typically required to perform and document laboratory surveys to identify areas of radiation contamination and exposure. These surveys are usually required in addition to those performed by the RSO. The frequency with which the surveys must be performed is dependent on the amount of RAM and type of use and range from weekly to quarterly. The RSO will audit the laboratory survey records when performing their routine audit.
3. *Equipment repair and disposal*
   All laboratory equipment in which RAM is stored or processed (refrigerators, freezers, water baths, centrifuges, etc.) must be labeled with a "caution radioactive materials" label. Prior to repair, modification, placement into storage, or disposal, the equipment must be monitored for contamination by the RSO.
4. *Food and drink in radiation laboratories*
   Eating, drinking, smoking, storage/preparation of food, and application of cosmetics are not permitted in radiation laboratories to minimize the risks of ingesting potentially harmful agents into the body. The presence of coffee mugs, drink containers, food in refrigerators or cold rooms, coffeemakers, and microwave ovens provides evidence that eating and drinking may be occurring in the restricted area.
5. *Security of radioactive material*
   The use and storage of RAMs must either be under the constant surveillance and immediate control of a radiation worker or secured from unauthorized removal and access. Radioisotope laboratories are to be locked when unoccupied if there are unsecured sources of RAM. In unlocked and unoccupied laboratories, stock vials and nonexempt sealed sources must be secured in a locked container, such as a cabinet, refrigerator, shield, hood, or storage box. Any individual who is unknown to laboratory personnel or who is unfamiliar with the work practices in the laboratory should be "challenged" on entry into areas in which materials are unsecured.

## 6.2 Use of Radiation-Producing Machines

All machines that generate ionizing radiation are subject to regulation by the RSC.

This includes all clinical or research X-ray machines (radiographic, fluoroscopic, bone densitometers, etc.), analytical X-ray machines, electron microscopes, and particle accelerators.

Devices that produce significant external radiation fields may require specialized shielding to be installed. All shielding designs must usually be approved by the RSO prior to the start of construction. Whenever radiation-producing machines are purchased, transferred, or disposed, the RSO must be notified by the responsible individual prior to installation or disposal of the equipment. This individual will also be responsible for its safe operation and use. The RSO will survey each machine and the facility in which it is installed for compliance with applicable state regulations. Any items of noncompliance noted as a result of audits performed by the RSO must be corrected within a reasonable period following notification.

## 6.3 Human Use Research Involving Radioactive Material or Ionizing Radiation-Producing Equipment

In most medical research institutions, all protocols involving the human use of RAMs and/or radiation-producing equipment are subject to review and approval by the institutional RSC. It is well known that radiation exposure involves a risk of health impairment or injury, depending on the dose received. To protect patients or healthy volunteers who participate in research from excessive or unacceptable risk, the World Medical Assembly issued the Declaration of Helsinki—Ethical Principles for Medical Research Involving Human Subjects [34], which established the principles for design, justification, evaluation, and oversight of biomedical research involving humans. Radiation effects in humans fall into two general categories, deterministic effects and stochastic effects. A deterministic effect is a somatic effect resulting from cell killing and loss of tissue or organ function that increases in severity with increasing radiation dose above a certain threshold dose. Examples of this type of effect are skin erythema, cataract formation, and sterility. If the radiation exposure is kept below this threshold dose, the risk of injury in an individual is essentially zero. A stochastic effect results from damage to the DNA of a cell and is one in which the probability of the effect occurring continuously increases with increasing dose, while the severity of the effect remains independent of the magnitude of the radiation dose. A stochastic effect is assumed to occur in the absence of a dose threshold, so there is some risk of harm even at low doses. Examples of these effects are cancer and hereditary disorders. Therefore, the intentional irradiation of human subjects to ionizing radiation for the purpose of biomedical research carries a potential risk or detriment of harm. In planning a clinical research study, investigators should first consider whether it is necessary to use procedures that emit radiation to obtain the desired information. Any study requiring the use of procedures that emit ionizing radiation must produce the needed information at minimum radiation doses to human subjects, and the use of the radiation-emitting procedures in the research study must be defensible in terms of clinical and scientific relevance.

## 6.4 Ethical Aspects

Research involving the irradiation of human subjects must demonstrate a net benefit. In the case of biomedical research, the benefit to society from the increase in knowledge must outweigh the potential harm to the individual. When the research project is of direct diagnostic or therapeutic benefit to the individual patient volunteer, a specific potential benefit exists for this subject. However, when the research project exposes patients or healthy volunteers for which there is no direct benefit to the subject, there must be an expectation of increased scientific knowledge in general that will result in a societal benefit to future patients or others. In the research protocol design, it is important to consider the use of other methods not involving exposure to radiation if it is possible to obtain the same or equivalent information. In this consideration, the potential harm from the alternative method and any limitation in research results should not be overlooked. Statistical analysis should also be performed to ensure that the number of subjects participating in the research project is restricted to the minimum number necessary to obtain the necessary information with sufficient accuracy.

## 6.5 Radiation Dose Limits

While there are federal and state radiation dose limits for occupational exposures and for exposures to the general public, there are no regulatory dose limits for radiation exposures to patients for medical procedures or to volunteers participating in biomedical research. In all research protocols, the radiation dose (or administered activity) to a subject must be kept as low as possible, while still obtaining the required information or desired effect. This is application of the optimization or ALARA principle. Lowering the dose to a point at which the necessary information is lost or insufficient can cause the risk to not be accompanied by the desired benefit, which is contrary to the optimization principle. Radiation dose limits for human subjects are subject to approval by the RSC, which must balance the benefit with the risk. Most institutions will adopt the occupational dose limits that are shown in Table 1 as the dose constraint for research subjects. Others may apply the FDA dose limits for RDRC approval, as shown in Table 3. These radiation dose limits will apply to the total dose from all radionuclide procedures and all diagnostic radiology (X-ray) procedures related to the research study. It may also apply together with doses from other research studies in which the subject may be participating or has participated in during the current year. Some institutions will not permit radiation workers from participating as research subjects because of their occupational exposures, although there are no regulatory requirements to exclude such individuals. Larger radiation doses may be considered by the RSC when research subjects have limited life expectancy and the applicant adequately justifies the procedure and the importance of the anticipated scientific contribution.

The ICRP recommends setting the dose limit or level of risk to the corresponding level of societal benefit from the research study as shown in Table 2. Along with these dose constraints, the ICRP also recommends the research proposal be evaluated by an independent "ethics committee" made up of individuals with expertise in diagnostic radiology, radiotherapy, nuclear medicine, experimental use of radioactive compounds, and radiation protection. The committee's decision on requiring changes in the research design and methods or negative opinion for the research to proceed should be binding.

In research involving radiotherapy, all of the dose limits described above are readily exceeded. In these cases, an evaluation needs to be made on how much the therapeutic regimen differs in total dose or dosage and fractionation scheme from what is considered to be standard of care. It is important to have an individual with expertise in radiation oncology on the RSC reviewing these types of protocols.

The RDRC provides a convenient avenue for approval of research using radioactive drugs not approved by the FDA if used under certain conditions. The FDA dose limits for approval by the RDRC are similar to the federal and state occupational dose limits and generally allow for the conduction of PET studies involving novel radiotracers using C-11, N-13, O-15, and F-18. However, with the advent of PET/CT scanners and the requirement to include any X-ray procedure doses that are part of the research, the FDA dose limits can be quickly exceeded if the protocol involves multiple scans. Similarly, with the pediatric dose limits set at 10 percent of those for adults, it is very difficult to perform PET/CT studies on children under the RDRC.

## 6.6 Determination of Radiation Dose

The radiation dose to the research subject from all radiological procedures incurred from participation in the research protocol will need to be calculated or determined. In radiation protection, the ED concept has been developed to specify the amount of radiation dose which is quantitatively related to the probability of stochastic effects in the body for all types of radiation exposures, regardless of whether the radiation is incident on the body or emitted by radionuclides within the body. The unit for measuring ED is the Sv or rem. For consideration of deterministic effects to specific organs or tissues in the body, the absorbed dose (AD) is a unit of measure describing the average amount of radiation energy absorbed over the mass of the organ or tissue. The unit of AD is the Gy or rad. In most research studies, the ED will be the most appropriate measure of the subject radiation risk; however, if the research involves interventional radiology procedures or radiotherapy, the possibility of deterministic effects may exist and the AD will be an important quantity to measure for the likelihood of these effects. The ED and mean AD quantities should be based on the method of calculation as set forth by the Medical Internal Radiation Dose Committee (MIRDC) or the ICRP. Individual organ ADs and total body EDs for certain radiographic and nuclear medicine procedures are available in the published literature. The Radiation Dose Assessment Resource (http://www.doseinfo-radar.com/RADARDoseRiskCalc.html) and the Duke Radiation Safety Committee (http://www.safety.duke.edu/radsafety/consents/irbcf_asp/default.asp) websites offer online medical procedure radiation dose calculators and consent language generators.

## 6.7 Radiation Risk Statement

The radiation risks from participation in the research study must be addressed in the consent form with the other risks associated with the study. The risks must be clearly identified and explained so that they are understood by the individual enabling them to make an informed decision regarding whether or not to participate in the research. People typically misperceive radiation risks due to the fact that the topic of radiation risk is rather technical in nature and requires a specialized language (with specific units, terms, etc.) and a knowledge base requiring some specific education [35]. Many members of the general public have perspectives that are largely subjective rather than technical or scientific because of the media, which tend to sensationalize issues and present fictional portrayals of radiation exposure such as the "Hulk" and "Spiderman," in which radiation exposure caused supernatural powers. These misperceptions will often create an inherent fear of radiation and the assumption that all radiation is equally harmful.

Most institutions will compare the total ED from participation in the study to annual natural background radiation or occupational radiation dose limits [36]. The controversy lies in how to state or quantify the actual risk, especially for exposures less than the occupational limits for which there is great uncertainty in the level of harm, and estimates are based on a linear extrapolation from the high dose risk data. Examples of statements that are typically used include:

1. *For whole-body radiation exposures with an ED <10 mSv (1000 mrem):*
"Participation in this research study involves exposure to radiation from (*specify respective procedure(s) to be performed*). The amount of radiation exposure that you will receive from this (*these*) procedure(s) is equivalent to a uniform whole body dose of _____ mSv (a "mSv" is a unit of radiation dose), which is approximately (*indicate multiplication factor, fraction, or percentage of*) of the average radiation dose (3 mSv) that each member of the general public receives per year from naturally occurring radiation sources. There is no known minimum level of radiation exposure that is recognized as being totally free of the risk of causing genetic defects (abnormal cells) or cancer. However, the risk associated with the amount of radiation exposure that you will receive from participation in this study is considered to be negligible."

2. *For a whole-body radiation exposures with an ED of 10–50 mSv (1000–5000 mrem):*
"Participation in this research study involves exposure to radiation from (*specify respective procedure(s) to be performed*). The amount of radiation exposure that you will receive from this (*these*) procedure(s) is equivalent to a uniform whole-body dose of _____ mSv (a "mSv" is a unit of radiation dose), which is approximately (*indicate fraction or percentage of*) the annual radiation dose (50 mSv) permitted to radiation workers by federal regulations. There is no known minimum level of radiation exposure that is recognized as being totally free of the risk of causing genetic defects (abnormal cells) or cancer. However, the risk associated with the amount of radiation exposure that you will receive from this study is considered to be low and comparable to everyday risks."

3. *For a whole-body radiation exposures with an ED >50 mSv:*
"Participation in this research study involves exposure to radiation from (*specify respective procedure(s) to be performed*). The amount of radiation exposure that you will receive from this (*these*) procedure(s) is equivalent to a uniform whole-body dose of _____ mSv (a "mSv" is a unit of radiation dose), which is approximately (*indicate multiplication factor*) the annual radiation dose (50 mSv) permitted to radiation workers by federal regulations. Excess cancer and hereditary risk associated with this level of radiation exposure is estimated to be (*specify BEIR VII estimate*)."

For statement "3", a numerical estimate is calculated for the increased risk for incidence or mortality of cancer and/or hereditary detriment based on the appropriate radiation risk coefficients from the BIER VII "Health Risks from Exposure to Low Levels of Ionizing Radiation" [2].

Comparison of the ED to other diagnostic X-ray or nuclear medicine procedures, such as a chest X-ray, may be appealing with respect to comparison to something with which the subject may be familiar; however, this really does not portray the magnitude of risk, and it can heighten concern if the ED is orders of magnitude greater than a chest X-ray (ED of a chest X-ray is approximately 0.05 mSv). In situations in which the radiation dose received is higher than routine diagnostic studies, such as with interventional X-ray procedures or radiotherapy, the risk statement must be crafted for the individual situation. This is especially important if there is the likelihood of radiation-induced deterministic effects.

## 6.8 Pregnancy

In the United States, radiation exposure of a pregnant female in biomedical research is not specifically prohibited. However, because of the potential embryo/fetal risks from radiation exposure, their involvement in research should only be conducted if pregnancy is an integral part of the research and there is no other means to gain the desired scientific information. For protection of the embryo/fetus, strict controls should be placed on the use of radiation in these cases, and the potential benefit must far outweigh the potential harm. In general, pregnant subjects may not participate in research, and so the pregnancy status of a female subject in their childbearing years must be determined, either by clinical history or highly sensitive tests performed within a short timeframe prior to the exposure. Women who are breastfeeding should not be involved in research involving the administration of a radioactive drug.

## 6.9 Research in Children

Research studies involving children will require special consideration and review to assure that the proposed benefit substantially exceeds the risk. The review process should be supported by an independent qualified pediatric consultant to the RSC, HUSC, or RDRC. Consideration must be given to the increased radiation risk, which may be a factor of 2 to 3 times higher than in adults. Also, the appropriate dose constraint level will need to be determined (natural background radiation, minor occupational limits, adult occupational dose limits) unless the research is being conducted under the RDRC, in which the dose limits will be 10 percent of the adult levels.

# 7. ADDRESSING NONCOMPLIANCE

## 7.1 Institutional Inspections

Both the NRC and agreement states will oversee compliance of RAMs licensees through its inspection, investigation, and enforcement programs. Inspections involve unannounced visits by the NRC or agreement states personnel to each licensed facility on a periodic basis, ranging from once a year to once every four years, depending on the hazard level of RAMs and scope of the license. Special reactionary inspections are also performed to follow up on, and in response to, notification of a particular incident or event. Inspections are intended to ensure that licensed programs are conducted in accordance with regulatory requirements, with specific conditions of the license and with the health and safety requirements of workers, patients, and the general public. Inspectors will use direct observations of work activities, interviews with workers, and reviews of licensee records to determine compliance with the regulatory requirements. Enforcement actions may be taken against licensees when violations of regulations or license conditions are identified. Such violations range from severity level IV for those of minor concern, such as incomplete documentation of records, to severity level I for the most significant, with potential for personnel health and safety impact [37]. Sanctions can include more frequent inspections, release of negative publicity to the media, civil fines and penalties, and license revocation. More significant violations are candidates for escalated enforcement. A predecisional enforcement conference may be conducted with a licensee and regulatory agency officials before making an enforcement decision if escalated enforcement action appears to be warranted. Civil penalties are normally assessed for severity level I and II violations; however, the press release provided to the media on the enforcement action by the regulatory agency can be damaging to the institution. The NRC or agreement states may also issue orders to modify, suspend, or revoke a license or to cease and desist from a given practice or activity. While enforcement actions are typically accessed against the institution (licensee), deliberate acts of negligence or attempts to conceal a violation by an individual can result in personal fines or, in very serious cases, criminal prosecution. While the regulations governing the use of sources of ionizing radiation are fairly consistent across the country, the degree to which they are interpreted and enforced by the inspection process varies greatly from state to state, and even within different regions of a state.

## 7.2 Radiation Safety Audits and Surveys

All AU will be subjected to periodic audits and radiological surveys by the RSO or radiation safety office. The RSO will inspect each radioisotope laboratory by performing radiation exposure rate and surface contamination surveys, along with evaluating general radiation safety conditions and reviewing logbooks of RAMs use and required user surveys. AUs are expected to be in compliance at all times with the institutional RPP requirements. Violations of good laboratory practice leading to unnecessary exposure or violations of applicable safety policy will be brought to the attention of the AU. Violations of the RPP requirements may result in disciplinary action by the RSC. The level of response by the RSC depends on the severity of the violation, which may range from a simple warning to immediate termination of all licensed activities and revocation of approval to order and use radioisotopes or radiation-producing equipment. Minor violations, which merit only a warning, may escalate to a more serious level if subsequent inspections reveal no corrective action and repeated violations of the same item are observed. In emergent situations, the RSO has the authority from executive management to terminate all licensed activities of an AU if it is determined that serious threat to public health and safety and/or regulatory noncompliance is involved. In situations of continued operation of radiation-producing machines that fail to meet applicable regulations regarding their safe use, the RSO is also authorized to require immediate cessation of use of the machine and to take any other actions as necessary to ensure safe conditions. Such a move by the RSO would also be presented to and reviewed by the RSC.

## 7.3 Inspections of Human Subject Research Involving Radioactive Material or Ionizing Radiation Producing Machines

Medical programs authorized to conduct research involving the use of radioactive drugs or radiation-emitting devices in humans may require FDA approval. In addition, approval to conduct research studies also requires input from an IRB, an RDRC, or other appropriate committee(s), including the RSC. The NRC or agreement states will review the interaction between the RSC and the IRB and/or RDRC to assure compliance with the requirements in 10 CFR 35.6 that all research is conducted, supported, or regulated by another federal agency that has implemented "federal policy for protection of human subjects." The FDA will also conduct inspections of an institution's RDRC to assure that it is in compliance with the requirements governing RDRC approval in 21 CFR 361.1. Human subject research involving RAM or ionizing radiation-producing machines must still comply with all other applicable medical use regulations for that modality of RAMs or X-ray equipment, unless specifically exempted by the appropriate regulatory agency.

## 7.4 Medical Event and Notification Reporting Requirements

The NRC and AS regulations have reporting requirements for situations in which there is a deviation or error in the dose or dosage of radiation administered to a patient or research subject. This is called a "medical event," which was termed a "misadministration" prior to 2002. The criteria of a medical event include:

1. Administration of a dosage of RAM to a patient that differs from the prescribed dosage by 20 percent or more, or falls outside of the prescribed dosage range; and the radiation dose to the patient differs from that which would have resulted from the prescribed dosage by more than 5 rem EDE, 50 rem to an organ or tissue, or 50 rem shallow dose equivalent to the skin.
2. A dose that exceeds 5 rem EDE, 50 rem to an organ or tissue, or 50 rem shallow dose equivalent to the skin from any of the following:
   a. Administration of the wrong radioactive drug
   b. Administration of a radioactive drug by the wrong route
   c. Administration of a radioactive drug to the wrong patient.

There are also reporting and notification requirements for an unintended dose to an embryo/fetus or a nursing child. These criteria include:

1. A dose to an embryo/fetus that exceeds 5 rem that is the result of an administration of a radioactive drug to a pregnant patient, unless the dose to the embryo/fetus was specifically approved.
2. A dose to a nursing child that is a result of an administration of a radioactive drug to a breastfeeding patient that:
   a. Exceeds 5 rem EDE; or
   b. Has resulted in unintended permanent functional damage to an organ or physiological system of the child, as determined by a physician.

The licensee must notify by telephone the NRC or agreement states no later than the next calendar day after discovery of the medical event or dose to an embryo/fetus or nursing child. The licensee must also submit a written report to the appropriate NRC regional office within 15 days after discovery of the medical event or dose to an embryo/fetus or nursing child that describes the event and corrective action taken to prevent a recurrence.

## 8. CONCLUSION

Radiation protection regulations are developed and implemented for a number of appropriate reasons, including furthering protection and safety of humans, attempts to improve safety for individuals engaged in radiation-related activities, national security issues, and in response to the infrequent, but often high-profile, failures to adequately monitor or implement certain radiation protection functions. However, each of these new regulations brings with it additional oversight and auditing activities that add to the faculty and institutional compliance burden, with a resultant decrease in faculty productivity and consumption of institutional resources. Often, the demands of the new regulations are not in concert with the radiation exposure or risk that it attempts to prevent. Research institutions face certain struggles as they attempt to balance their vital compliance and stewardship obligations and responsibilities while trying to enhance the research productivity of an already overburdened faculty and staff. Institutions should review their existing policies, procedures, and practices and look for opportunities to integrate any new compliance requirements into existing systems, tools, and processes; avoiding duplicate, redundant, or unnecessary work is critical [38].

# References

[1] National Council on Radiation Protection and Measurements. Ionizing radiation exposure of the population of the United States. 2009. NRCP Report No. 160.

[2] National Academy of Sciences/National Research Council. Health risks from exposure to low levels of ionizing radiation BEIR VII phase. Washington (DC): National Academy Press; 2006. 2.

[3] International Commission on Radiological Protection. The 2007 recommendation of the international commission on radiological protection. Ann ICRP 2007;103(37):2–4.

[4] International Commission on Radiological Protection. Biological effects after prenatal irradiation (embryo and fetus). Publication 90, Ann. ICRP 2003;33(1–2).

[5] National Council on Radiation Protection and Measurements. Limitation of exposure to ionizing radiation. Bethesda (MD): National Council on Radiation Protection and Measurements; 1993. NRCP Report No. 116.

[6] International Commission on Non-Ionizing Radiation Protection. Guidelines for limiting exposure to time-varying electric, magnetic, and electromagnetic fields (up to 300 GHz). Health Phys 1998;74(4):494–522.

[7] Jones Cynthia Gillian. A review of the history of U.S. radiation protection regulations. Health Phys 2008;88(2):105–24.

[8] Clark C. Radium girls: women and industrial health reform, 1910–1935. Chapel Hill: University of North Carolina Press; 1997.

[9] Walker JS. Permissible dose: a history of protection in the twentieth century. Berkeley: University of California Press; 2000.

[10] Taylor LS. X-ray measurements and protection. Washington (DC): U.S. Department of Commerce; 1913–1964. NBS Special Publication 625; U.S. National Bureau of Standards; 1981.

[11] Kocher DC. Perspective on the historical development of radiation standards. Health Phys 1991;61(4):519–27.

[12] Meinhold C, Lauriston S. Taylor lecture: the evolution of radiation protection—from erythema to genetic risks of cancer to. Health Phys 2004;87(3):240–80.

[13] U.S. Nuclear Regulatory Commission. Protecting people and the environment. A short history of nuclear regulation;. 1946–2009 (NUREG/BR-0175, Revision 2); 2010.

[14] National Committee on Radiation Protection and Measurement. Permissible dose from external sources of ionizing radiation including maximum permissible exposure to man. National bureau of handbooks, vol. 59. 1954. NRCP Report No. 17.

[15] National Academy of Sciences/National Research Council. Committee on the biological effects of radiation: a report to the public. Washington (DC): National Academy of Sciences/National Research Council; 1956.

[16] National Committee on Radiation Protection and Measurement. Maximum permissible exposure to man. National bureau of standards handbook, vol. 59. Washington (DC): U.S. Department of Commerce; Addendum U.S; 1958.

[17] International Commission on Radiological Protection. Report on amendments during 1956 to recommendations of the International Commission on Radiological Protection. Radiology 1958;70:261–2.

[18] Conference of Radiation Control Program Directors, Inc. The first twenty-five years. CRCPD 1993;93(4).

[19] Health Physics Society. Occupational radiation safety standards and regulations are sound. Position Statement of the Health Physics Society. Bio 13–0. 2010.

[20] http://www.nrc.gov/materials.html [accessed 27.02.14].

[21] http://www.nrc.gov/about-nrc/state-tribal/agreement-states.html [accessed 27.02.14].

[22] http://www.crcpd.org/about/about.aspx [accessed 27.02.14].

[23] http://www.fda.gov/Radiation-EmittingProducts/default.htm [accessed 27.02.14].

[24] https://www.osha.gov/index.html [accessed 27.02.14].

[25] U.S. Nuclear Regulatory Commission. Consolidated guidance about material license. Program-specific guidance about academic, research and development, and other licenses of limited scope. Including gas chromatographs and X-ray fluorescence analyzers. NUREG-1556, vol. 7. 1999.

[26] U.S. Nuclear Regulatory Commission. Consolidated guidance about material licenses. Program-specific guidance about licenses of broad scope. NUREG-1556, vol. 11. 1999.

[27] U.S. Nuclear Regulatory Commission. Consolidated guidance about material licenses. Program-specific guidance about 10 CFR part 36 irradiator licenses. NUREG-1556, vol. 6. 1999.

[28] U.S. Nuclear Regulatory Commission. Consolidated guidance about material licenses. Program-specific guidance about medical use licenses. NUREG-1556, vol. 9. 2008. Rev.2.

[29] http://www.crcpd.org/SSRCRs/default.aspx [accessed 27.02.14].

[30] International Commission on Radiological Protection. Radiological protection in biomedical research. Ann ICRP 1992;22(3). ICRP Publication 62.

[31] Miller KL. CRC handbook of management of radiation protection programs. 2nd ed. CRC Press LLC; 1992.

[32] American national standard for safe use of lasers in research, development, or testing. Laser Institute of America. ANSI; 2012. Z136.8.

[33] http://www.stanford.edu/dept/EHS/prod/researchlab/radlaser/laser/procedures/classes.html [accessed 28.02.14].

[34] http://www.wma.net/en/30publications/10policies/b3/ [accessed 27.02.14].

[35] Health Physics Society. Specialist in radiation safety. Risk/benefit of medical radiation exposure. Classic, K. HPS; 2011.

[36] Frank Jr PC. An attempt to standardize the radiological risk in an institutional review board consent form. Investig Radiol 1993;28(6):533–8.

[37] http://www.nrc.gov/about-nrc/regulatory/enforcement/program-overview.html [accessed 28.02.14].

[38] National Council of University Research Administrators (NCURA). NCURA senior research summit: aligning services, resources and institutional mission to enhance faculty research productivity and competitiveness. Research management review. J Natl Counc Univ Res Adm 2009;16(2). [Special issue].

# Controlled Substances: Maintaining Institutional Compliance

*Patrick A. Lester[1], Katherine A. Shuster[2], Portia S. Allen[1], Gerald A. Hish Jr.[3], Daniel D. Myers Jr.[1,4]*

[1]Unit for Laboratory Animal Medicine, University of Michigan, Ann Arbor, MI, USA; [2]Safety Assessment and Laboratory Animal Resources, Merck, Kenilworth, NJ, USA; [3]Department of Comparative Medicine, University of Washington, Seattle, WA, USA; [4]Conrad Jobst Vascular Research Laboratories, University of Michigan, Ann Arbor, MI, USA

## 1. INTRODUCTION

Controlled substances are used in a variety of research settings, from discovery and bench top research, to basic and applied research using animal models. Research conducted within academia, contract research organizations, pharmaceutical companies, compounding pharmacies, analytical laboratories, and others relies on the use of controlled substances. Their application in research may be federally mandated or necessary based on scientific objectives and goals. Complete understanding of the laws and regulations requiring and regulating the application of controlled substances in research is critical for all users to ensure regulatory compliance. Federal laws and regulations governing animal research mandate the use of appropriate sedatives, anesthetics, and analgesics if animals will experience more than slight or momentary pain or distress, unless scientific justification for withholding these pharmaceuticals is provided and approved by the institutional animal care and use committee (IACUC). This requirement is outlined in the Animal Welfare Act [1], Animal Welfare Regulations [2], specifically Title 9 Code of Federal Regulations (CFR) §2.31, and the Animal and Plant Health Inspection Service, Animal Care Policy #3, which addresses proper veterinary care of research animals [3]. Although the Animal Welfare Regulations do not apply to mice of the genus *Mus* and rats of the genus *Rattus* bred for the purposes of research, any institution conducting Public Health Service (PHS)-sponsored activities must comply with the *US Government Principles for the Utilization and Care of Vertebrate Animals Used in Testing, Research, and Training,* [4] the *PHS Policy on Humane Care and Use of Laboratory Animals* [5], and the *Guide for the Care and Use of Laboratory Animals* (NRC 2011) [6]. These three documents outline the need for proper use of sedatives, anesthetics, and analgesics in all animals used in

PHS-supported research that undergo more than momentary or slight pain or distress. Additionally, nearly 900 international institutions are accredited by the Association for Assessment and Accreditation of Laboratory Animal Care (AAALAC) International [7]. AAALAC accreditation necessitates implementation of the *Guide for the Care and Use of Laboratory Animals* (NRC 2011) [6]. All of the aforementioned regulating documents also require animal euthanasia to be humane and painless, following the recommendations of the American Veterinary Medical Association *Guidelines for the Euthanasia of Animals* [8]. These guidelines consider the intravenous or intraperitoneal overdose administration of barbiturates and barbituric acid derivatives, or other nonbarbiturate anesthetic compounds under certain conditions, to be acceptable and humane methods of animal euthanasia. Because many controlled substances function as sedative, anesthetic, analgesic, and euthanasia agents, their essential utility in animal research is apparent.

Controlled substances have application in research beyond sedation, anesthesia, analgesia, and euthanasia in research animals. These substances, many of which are commonly abused by humans, may be administered to animals to model human addiction and abuse behavior, allowing for behavioral and physiological evaluation of the addiction and identification of potential therapeutic modalities [9–11]. Complementary in vitro research may also use these compounds [12]. Amphetamines, phencyclidine, and others have been used to model various psychiatric disorders, such as schizophrenia and obsessive-compulsive disorder [13,14]. These models have led to the identification of interventional psychopharmacologic agents, many of which are controlled substances. For example, methylphenidate is used for the treatment of attention-deficit hyperactivity disorder [15]. Testosterone and testosterone-related compounds, or androgens, are schedule III controlled substances; thus, bench top, in vitro, and animal research using these compounds require knowledge of controlled substance regulations. Bench top research in pharmaceutical design, synthesis, and development may result in the clandestine production of analogs of currently controlled substances or novel bioactive molecules with variable potentials for abuse [16]. Additionally, analytical laboratories commonly use controlled substances as reference standards.

Whether controlled substances are used in animal, in vitro, or bench top research, a clear understanding of the laws and regulations surrounding their use is required, because the paradigm by which research institutions manage controlled substance use is highly variable. Particularly in academia, controlled substance licensing and legal obligation may be placed at the level of the principal investigator, the laboratory animal resources unit, the institution as a whole, or a combination of those models. Laws and regulations will also vary based on the category of the business and how it is licensed by the corresponding state and registered with the Drug Enforcement Administration (DEA). This chapter will review the various oversight agencies, regulations, and guidance documents available for the use of controlled substances in research, and discuss methods to maintain institutional regulatory compliance, prevent diversion, and protect public health.

## 2. HISTORICAL PERSPECTIVES

### 2.1 1906 Food and Drug Act

Prior to the passage of this act, the states controlled the regulation of food and drugs produced domestically, and there was no federal oversight. The US Pharmacopoeia (USP) was first published in 1820 by a group of physicians and pharmacists to create a formulary of current drugs along with information on purity, strength, and quality [17]. Pharmacists then created the National Formulary in 1888 to cover standards for drugs not listed in the USP. The Division of Chemistry was created in 1862 by the appointment of Charles M. Wetherill to the Department of Agriculture [17]. This organization was the predecessor to the current US Food and Drug Administration (FDA).

In 1883, the new chief of the Division of Chemistry, Harvey Washington Wiley, was a strong proponent of federal legislation to regulate drugs. In a dramatic demonstration, he recruited young men to form a "poison squad" [18]. They ingested substances that were currently being used as food coloring agents and preservatives (e.g., formaldehyde, boric acid), and over time, the young men displayed gastrointestinal side effects [17]. Around the same time, Upton Sinclair published his landmark book, "The Jungle," which exposed the appalling and unsanitary conditions of the meat packing industry [17]. These two events lead to public outcry and passage of the 1906 Food and Drug Act (also called Wiley's Law) [19]. This law prohibited the manufacture and interstate commerce of adulterated or misbranded food and drugs. The USP and the National Formulary were used as the official standards for drugs, and a drug or food was considered adulterated or misbranded if it contained harmful or addictive substances (e.g., morphine, opium, cocaine) and these ingredients were not listed on the label [19,20].

This law was a huge step forward, but there were also problems. During this time, there were a lot of "cure-all" drugs on the market for various conditions (e.g., baldness, cancer) [17]. Most of these drugs were worthless, but prosecuting the individuals selling them was difficult and usually only resulted in small fines. In the United States vs. Johnson, the Supreme Court ruled in favor of a manufacturer and stated the therapeutic claims were a matter of opinion [17,21]. This series of events lead to the passage of the Sherley Amendment in 1912. This amendment banned false therapeutic claims, but placed the burden of proof on the government rather than the manufacturer [17,19]. This made it difficult to prosecute manufacturers because the government had to prove in court that the manufacturer knowingly attempted to defraud the consumer.

## 2.2 Harrison Tax Act of 1914

This piece of legislation was to "provide for the registration of, with collectors of internal revenue, and to impose a special tax on all persons who produce, import, manufacture, compound, deal in, dispense, sell, distribute, or give away opium or coca leaves, their salts, derivatives, or preparations, and for other purposes" [22].

This act also required a prescription from a physician, dentist, or veterinary surgeon if the amount of narcotics in a product exceeded the allowable limit [22]. Pharmacists, physicians, or veterinary surgeons whom dispensed narcotics were required to keep detailed records for a period of two years [22].

## 2.3 1938 Food, Drug, and Cosmetic Act

The FDA assembled a collection of products that showed the limitations of the 1906 Food and Drug Act. These included products such as Lash-Lure, an eyelash dye that caused injuries to women's eyes, including one case of permanent blindness; Radithor, a radium-containing tonic that caused a protracted and painful death for consumers of it; and Banbar, an ineffective cure for diabetes [23]. A reporter touring the exhibit called it "The American Chamber of Horrors" [23]. This led to the creation of a new bill, but it stalled in Congress until a serious incident occurred in 1937. A drug company marketed a sulfa drug for pediatric patients called Elixir Sulfanilamide [23]. The product was untested, and the solvent used was an extremely toxic chemical analog of antifreeze [23]. More than 100 people died, including many children. The public outcry that arose helped push the bill through Congress, which became the 1938 Food, Drug, and Cosmetic Act. This law brought cosmetics and medical devices under federal control and required that drugs be labeled with directions for safe use. It required premarket approval for new drugs and mandated that the manufacturer prove to the FDA that a drug was safe [21]. This set the burden of proof on the manufacturer rather than the government and therefore eliminated the Sherley Amendment. It also set food standards and authorized factory inspections [21]. The FDA was also able to use injunctions as a tool to enforce the law [23]. In 1951, the Durham–Humphrey Amendment was passed. This set requirements that specific drugs be labeled as for sale by prescription, only used under medical supervision [17].

## 2.4 Kefauver–Harris Amendments of 1962

In the late 1950s, Senator Estes Kefauver held hearings to gather more information on drug costs and the science backing effectiveness and label claims [24]. After 17 months, he presented his bill, which called for FDA review of efficacy claims, monitoring of pharmaceutical advertising, and ensuring that all medications had generic names [24]. He also wanted pharmaceutical companies to show the comparative effectiveness of similar drugs and to change some of the patenting laws to ensure competitive markets [24].

In 1960, a FDA medical officer named Frances Kelsey was assigned to review an application for a drug called thalidomide. It was marketed as a sleeping pill by a German company, but had also been shown to be effective as a treatment for morning sickness in pregnant woman [25]. Dr. Kelsey did not believe that the safety data the company presented was complete and refused to approve the drug for sale in the United States until they provided additional safety data. Despite pressure from the company, Dr. Kelsey continued to refuse to approve the drug application, although the drug was approved in other countries [25]. In 1961, reports emerged from Europe linking thalidomide ingestion during pregnancy with severe birth defects (e.g., phocomelia) in infants [25]. When this story was published, the public interest in drug regulation increased substantially, and the Kefauver–Harris Drug Amendments were passed in 1962.

Under this law, the manufacturer had to prove the drug was safe and effective for its intended use, and it required that the FDA approves the marketing application (it had 180 days to do so) before the drug could be marketed to the public [26]. Previously, the drug application would be automatically approved if the FDA did not act within 60 days of the application's submission. There was a requirement for informed consent of any humans participating in drug studies [26]. Finally, the amendments formalized good manufacturing practices, required that adverse events be reported to the FDA, and made the FDA responsible for prescription drug advertising (which previously had been the responsibility of the

Federal Trade Commission) [26]. These amendments were the first step in creating the current system of pharmaceutical research (preclinical, phase 1, phase 2, and phase 3 clinical trials) [27].

## 2.5 Drug Abuse Control Amendments of 1965

This law covered depressant and stimulant drugs that had the potential to cause a threat to public health and safety. It included barbiturates and any derivatives, amphetamines and any derivatives, and any other type of drug that has the potential for abuse due to its depressant or stimulant effect on the central nervous system or its hallucinogenic effect [27]. This was an amendment to the 1938 Federal Food, Drug, and Cosmetic Act and therefore gave the FDA control over these types of drugs [27]. This was the first federal law to directly prohibit a drug.

## 2.6 Controlled Substances Act of 1970

This law requires that every person who manufactures, distributes, dispenses, imports, or exports any controlled substances must register with the DEA, which was also created under this law and resides in the Department of Justice [28]. It also establishes drug schedules (I–V) with different ordering and storage requirements in place for drugs in schedules I and II (DEA Form 222 to order these drugs) compared with drugs in schedules III–V [28]. The schedule classifications are listed below, with examples of drugs in each schedule:

Schedule I
1. The drug or other substance has a high potential for abuse, the drug or other substance has no currently accepted medical use in treatment in the United States, and there is a lack of accepted safety for use of the drug or other substance under medical supervision.
2. Examples: lysergic acid diethylamide (LSD), heroin, peyote
Schedule II
1. The drug or other substance has a high potential for abuse, the drug or other substance has a currently accepted medical use in treatment in the United States or a currently accepted medical use with severe restrictions, and abuse of the drug or other substances may lead to severe psychological or physical dependence.
2. Examples: Cocaine, morphine, fentanyl
Schedule III
1. The drug or other substance has a potential for abuse less than the drugs or other substances in schedules I and II, the drug or other substance has a currently accepted medical use in treatment in the United States, and abuse of the drug or other substance may lead to moderate or low physical dependence or high psychological dependence.
2. Examples: Ketamine, buprenorphine, pentobarbital euthanasia solutions that are combined with other substances not in schedule II
Schedule IV
1. The drug or other substance has a low potential for abuse relative to the drugs or other substances in schedule III, the drug or other substance has a currently accepted

medical use in treatment in the United States, and abuse of the drug or other substance may lead to limited physical dependence or psychological dependence relative to the drugs or other substances in schedule III.

2. Examples: Diazepam, chloral hydrate, phenobarbital

Schedule V

1. The drug or other substance has a low potential for abuse relative to the drugs or other substances in schedule IV, the drug or other substance has a currently accepted medical use in treatment in the United States, and abuse of the drug or other substance may lead to limited physical dependence or psychological dependence relative to the drugs or other substances in schedule IV.

2. Examples: Medications with small amounts of codeine

## 2.7 International Treaties

### 2.7.1 Single Convention on Narcotic Drugs of 1961 [29]

This United Nations (UN) convention helps provide organized international control to help reduce the illegal trafficking of narcotics as well as to encourage member nations to provide medical assistance to those suffering from narcotic addiction. This document does recognize that there are important medical and research uses for these substances, so there is no attempt to ban them from appropriate use. Narcotics covered by this convention are listed in schedules (I–IV), and they are updated as needed. It also provides for the creation of an International Narcotics Control Board. The board implements and enforces the convention as well as provides annual reports of its work to the UN parties and secretary-general.

### 2.7.2 Convention on Psychotropic Substances of 1971 [30]

This UN convention helps provide organized international control to help reduce the illegal trafficking of psychotropic substances. It also has provisions to encourage member nations to develop programs to prevent addiction and provide medical assistance to those suffering from addiction. Psychotropic substances in the convention are listed in schedules (I–IV) and are updated as needed. A substance may be added to the list if it has the ability to produce a state of dependence and central nervous system stimulation or depression, resulting in hallucinations or disturbances in motor function or thinking or behavior or perception or mood. The International Control Board has the same responsibilities as in the Single Convention on Narcotic Drugs of 1961.

### 2.7.3 United Nations Convention Against Illicit Traffic in Narcotic Drugs and Psychotropic Substances of 1988 [31]

This UN convention was developed to promote cooperation among member nations to address the issues involved in illicit trafficking of narcotics and psychotropic substances more effectively. It also provides additional funding for the International Narcotics Board to effectively carry out its mandated responsibilities from the Single Convention on Narcotic Drugs of 1961 and Convention on Psychotropic Substances of 1971.

## 2.8  1988 Omnibus Drug Act

This law created the Office of National Drug Control Policy and established the following provisions [32]:

1. New and increased penalties related to drug trafficking, the creation of new federal offenses and regulatory requirements, changes in criminal procedures, and increases in funding for drug law enforcement;
2. Organized and coordinated federal antidrug efforts;
3. Reduction of drug demand by increased prevention efforts and treatment for drug addiction;
4. Reduction of drug production overseas and of international trafficking in illicit drugs;
5. Penalties intended to put added pressure on drug users (user accountability).

## 2.9  1996 Comprehensive Methamphetamine Control Act [33]

The federal government recognized that methamphetamine use in the 1990s had increased dramatically and that it was associated with permanent brain damage with long-term use. Its use had also been associated with an increase in violent crimes, deaths, and criminal activity associated with illegal importation. This law placed restrictions on the sale of list 1 chemicals (see Section 2.11 below) or equipment that can be used in the manufacture of methamphetamine. It increased the penalties for the trafficking of methamphetamine and any precursor chemicals. It also placed restrictions on the over-the-counter sales of medications that contained ephedrine, pseudoephedrine, or phenylpropanolamine because these substances can be used in the production of methamphetamine. Finally, it established provisions to provide education and training for law enforcement officials and wholesale and retail distributors or precursor chemicals and supplies.

## 2.10  Combat Methamphetamine Act of 2005 [34]

This law further restricted sales of over-the-counter medications that contained ephedrine, pseudoephedrine, or phenylpropanolamine. It required retailers to place them behind the counter, restrict the amount sold per customer, and keep a logbook of the sales with information on the amount sold, the purchaser's name and address, and the date of the sale. Restrictions were also placed on mail orders of these medications. This act also increased the penalties for smuggling methamphetamine or precursor chemicals, established programs for addicts, increased the penalties for individuals exposing minors to methamphetamine production, and further regulated the importation and distribution of precursor chemicals.

## 2.11  List Chemicals [35]

In 1988, the Chemical Diversion and Trafficking Act was passed, which placed 41 chemicals under DEA regulation. These laws provide a system of regulatory controls and criminal penalties to prevent diversion of chemicals which are precursors to illegal drugs, without preventing access to them for legitimate purposes. The chemicals are separately classified (list I and list II) based on their use and significance in the manufacture of illegal drugs. Examples of list I chemicals include ephedrine, iodine, red phosphorus, white phosphorus, and pseudoephedrine. Examples of list II chemicals include toluene, potassium permanganate, acetone, and ethyl ether.

## 3. RELEVANT REGULATORY/OVERSIGHT AGENCIES, REGULATIONS, AND GUIDANCE DOCUMENTS

Regulations regarding controlled substances are mandated both at the state and federal level. For example, most states require special licensing for researchers, research institutions, or laboratories using controlled substances, while registration is mandatory by the United States Department of Justice, DEA.

### 3.1 State Controlled Substance Regulations

State laws regarding controlled substances are enforced by each individual state board of pharmacy. Contact information for state boards of pharmacy can be found on the National Association Boards of Pharmacy (NABP®) Website (http://www.nabp.net). Each state board of pharmacy issues a set of controlled substance administrative rules or regulations based on the laws of the state, which outline controlled substances, drug schedules, requirements for licensing, security, inventory, prescriptions, dispensing, reporting, and other special circumstances. State boards of pharmacy may enforce stricter regulations compared to federal controlled substance regulations, but cannot override existing federal regulations. Controlled substance administrative rules and regulations may vary between states. For example, some states may not require additional licensure in addition to federal registration with the DEA. In addition, some states may regulate certain legend drugs such as ephedrine as controlled substances, although they are not controlled at the federal level. Furthermore, most states have mandatory prescription and dispensing drug monitoring programs (e.g., Michigan Automated Prescription System) or may require additional controlled substance inventory reporting compared to the DEA. Many states use the following types of licenses to regulate controlled substances: medical practitioner, pharmacy, research, analytical laboratory, manufacturer, wholesaler, or distributor. Discussion of different state laws and regulations regarding controlled substances is beyond the scope of this chapter. As a result, readers are strongly encouraged to contact their specific state board of pharmacy and review all mandatory laws and regulations pertinent to their profession and location of business or laboratory.

### 3.2 Federal Controlled Substance Regulations

The federal regulatory agency for oversight of controlled substances is the US Department of Justice, DEA. Federal controlled substance regulations are enforced by the DEA and apply to practitioners, medical facilities, manufacturers, importers, exporters, dispensers, and distributors of controlled substances, including regulated chemical precursors to controlled substances. The DEA registration is predicated on first satisfying all state licensing requirements for controlled substances. President Richard Nixon formed the DEA in 1973 to centralize the enforcement and regulation of controlled substances as outlined in the Controlled Substance

Act of 1970. The DEA's main priorities include disrupting illegal growing, manufacturing, or trafficking of illicit controlled substances and preventing diversion of legitimate pharmaceutical controlled substances from lawful medicinal or research usage to illicit drug markets.

### 3.2.1 DEA Organization

According to the March 2013 DEA Factsheet, the DEA has more than 200 domestic offices that work in conjunction with federal, state, and local law enforcement and more than 80 international offices. The DEA employs more than 5000 special agents to investigate and mitigate illegal domestic and international controlled substance trafficking and distribution. More than 600 diversion investigators, within the DEA Office of Diversion Control (http://www.deadiversion.usdoj.gov), provide compliance oversight and enforce federal regulations regarding the legitimate use of controlled substances for medicinal and scientific research purposes, with the goal to prevent diversion into illicit markets. Diversion investigators are primarily responsible for ensuring medical facilities, pharmacies, manufactures, distributors, importers, exporters, practitioners, researchers, and analytical laboratories comply with the Controlled Substance Act of 1970 and Title 21 CFR §§1300–1321. Failure to comply with state and federal controlled substance regulations can lead to administrative civil or criminal prosecution. In addition, the DEA employs chemists and research specialists to assist special agents and diversion investigators.

### 3.2.2 Food and Drug Administration

The DEA works in conjunction with the FDA, Department of Health and Human Services (DHHS) when determining the abuse potential of drugs and which drugs have valid medicinal use. The Controlled Substance Act, 21 USC §811 or Title II of the Comprehensive Drug Abuse Prevention and Control Act of 1970 Pub. L. 91-512 created five classifications or schedules in which drugs with potential for abuse, such as narcotics, stimulants, depressants, hallucinogens, anabolic steroids, and chemicals used in their production, would be classified. Drug schedules outlined in 21 USC §811 were described earlier in this chapter.

According to 21 USC §811, either the DEA or the FDA may initiate a petition (e.g., new drug application) to modify, add, or delete the schedule of a drug. In addition, special interest groups, individuals, medical boards, or local government agencies may petition the DEA to change the abuse schedule of a drug. Once a petition is obtained, the DEA contacts the DHHS to review the abuse potential of the drug in question. The FDA's mission is to protect public health, and thus it performs a medical and scientific review of the drug in question with regard to its abuse and dependence potential vs. any medical benefits. In addition, the National Institute of Drug Abuse (NIDA) may perform a concurrent review and assist the FDA with the evaluation and review process. The FDA's final evaluation is sent to the secretary of the DHHS, who reviews the data and makes a recommendation as to whether a drug should be classified as a controlled substance and the schedule of abuse to which it will be assigned based on its ability to produce physical and psychological dependence. Alternatively, a drug may be recommended for exclusion or removal from controlled substance status. According to 21 USC §811(c), the following factors should be reviewed to determine a drug's abuse potential and whether it should be classified as a controlled substance: "(1) Its actual or relative potential for abuse. (2) Scientific evidence of its pharmacological effect, if known. (3) The state of current scientific knowledge regarding the drug or other substance. (4) Its history or current pattern of abuse. (5) The scope, duration, and significance of abuse. (6) What, if any, risk there is to the public health. (7) Its psychic or physiological dependence liability. (8) Whether the substance is an immediate precursor of a substance already controlled under this title." The final recommendation is sent to the attorney general and by delegation to the DEA for a final decision regarding controlled substance scheduling. If the DHHS determines a drug should not be scheduled, the attorney general and DEA cannot grant a scheduled classification. In addition to the formal FDA review process, some drugs may be scheduled to conform to international treaty obligations. Furthermore, the DEA has the ability to schedule immediate precursors to a controlled substance with the same or higher schedule as the controlled substance drug.

### 3.2.3 Schedule I Controlled Substances

Schedule I drugs or chemicals may be used in research, especially in the area of addiction and drug abuse research. According to 21 USC §823 (f), practitioners or researchers that need to use schedule I controlled substances for clinical research, preclinical research, or analytical research must registered with the DEA to engage in such research. Registration to perform research with schedule I drugs is separate and in addition to registration to perform research with schedule II–V drugs. In such instances, the DEA refers to the secretary of DHHS to determine the qualifications and competency of the researcher and the scientific merit of the proposed research. Both the FDA and the DEA, working in conjunction, will determine the best safety mechanisms to prevent diversion and protect public health while permitting research activities to promote medical science. The attorney general and DEA may deny registration for research with schedule I controlled substances if the applicants meet criteria as outlined in 21 USC § 824. Most states require licensure for performing research with schedule I drugs, which is separate and in addition to licensing for performing research with schedule II–V drugs.

## 4. KEY REGULATORY MANDATES

### 4.1 Title 21 CFR, Chapter II—DEA, Department of Justice, (Parts 1300–1321)

The primary regulatory controlled substance mandates that research institutions and researchers must follow are outlined in 21 USC §§801–971 and Title 21 CFR, Chapter II—DEA, Department of Justice, (Parts 1300–1321). Readers are strongly advised to review all regulations and consult with their local DEA office regarding registration or compliance questions. Title 21 CFR Parts 1300–1321 are divided into the following: Part 1300 Definitions; Part 1301 Registration of Manufacturers, Distributors, and Dispensers of Controlled Substances; Part 1302 Labeling and Packaging Requirements for Controlled Substances; Part 1303 Quotas; Part 1304 Records and Reports of Registrants; Part 1305 Order Forms; Part 1306 Prescriptions; Part 1307 Miscellaneous; Part 1308 Schedules of Controlled Substances; Part 1309 Registration of Manufacturers, Distributors, Importers and Exporters of List 1 Chemicals; Part 1310 Records and Reports of Listed Chemicals and Certain Machines; Part 1311 Digital Certificates; Part 1312 Importation and Exportation of Controlled Substances; Part 1313 Importation and Exportation of Precursors and Essential Chemicals; Part 1314 Retail Sale of Scheduled Listed Chemical Products; Part 1315 Importation and Production Quotas for Ephedrine, Pseudoephedrine, and Phenylpropanolamine; Part 1316 Administrative Functions, Practices, and Procedures; Part 1321 DEA Mailing Addresses. Researchers or laboratories planning to store, administer, or import schedule II–V controlled substances should especially review and familiarize themselves with Title 21 CFR Parts 1300 (Definitions), 1301 (Registration), 1304 (Records), 1305 (Order Forms), 1307 (Miscellaneous-Disposal), 1308 (Schedules of Controlled Substances), 1312 (Importing or exporting), and 1316 (Administrative Functions, Practices, and Procedures) because these pertain to the most common and necessary compliance information for academic and industry research practices. In addition, Title 21 CFR § 1300.01 describes important definitions as they relate to controlled substances, while Title 21 CFR §1300.02 describes common definitions regarding list chemicals.

### 4.1.1 *Drug Enforcement Administration Registration for Research Laboratories and Researchers*

Title 21 CFR §1301.11(a) outlines key information regarding registration requirements and states, "Every person who manufactures, distributes, dispenses, imports, or exports any controlled substance or who proposes to engage in the manufacture, distribution, dispensing, importation or exportation of any controlled substance shall obtain a registration unless exempted by law or pursuant to §§1301.22 through 1301.26." As a result, federal controlled substance registration is mandatory for all research activities involving controlled substances. Per Title 21 CFR §1301.13(a), "No person required to be registered shall engage in any activity for which registration is required until the application for registration is granted and a Certificate of Registration is issued by the Administrator to such person."

### 4.1.2 *Separate Registrations for Separate Locations*

According to Title 21 CFR §1301.12(a), "A separate registration is required for each principal place of business or professional practice at one general physical location where controlled substances are manufactured, distributed, imported, exported, or dispensed by a person." This is a key regulation that mandates that each laboratory location where controlled substances are stored must be registered with the DEA. Most states have similar regulations requiring licensing for each principal place of business. It is highly recommended that a research institution or researcher contact their state board of pharmacy and local DEA office to determine where and how best to register their laboratory research location(s). In some cases, this may require registering the entire institution, a department, research building, room, or individual researcher. The registration location(s) may also depend on the physical street addresses in a decentralized institution. Depending on the size and scope of an academic research institution, individual researcher or individual laboratory registrations are usually recommended to maximize inventory and record-keeping compliance while ensuring security practices and personnel screening to prevent diversion. Industry-based research organizations generally will register their entire location or company. Title 21 CFR §1301.12 (b) outlines locations that do not require additional registration: "The following locations shall be deemed not to be places where controlled substances are manufactured, distributed, or dispensed." Title 21 CFR §1301.12 (b) (3) states, "An office used by a practitioner (who is registered at another location in the same State or jurisdiction of the United States) where controlled substances are prescribed but neither administered nor otherwise dispensed as a regular part of the professional practice of the practitioner at such office, and where no supplies of controlled substances are maintained." In select cases, if a practitioner-researcher uses their practitioner DEA registration for nonclinical research, the address of the laboratory where the controlled substances are stored must be registered. A practitioner-researcher cannot have a single DEA registration if they store controlled substances (acquired with their registration) at two locations, such as the laboratory and a private clinic. In this instance, both addresses must be registered with the DEA. Prescriptions for controlled substances may be written at any location within the state they are registered. A full discussion of registration requirements for bulk manufacturing and importation–exportation of controlled substances is beyond the scope of this chapter and are outlined in Title 21 CFR §§1309 and 1312.

### 4.1.3 Registration for Independent and Coincident Activities

Title 21 CFR §1301.13(e) outlines the specific categories of registration, which are deemed independent of each other, the required registration fees, and any coincident activities associated with the registration categories. A separate registration is required if one engages in more than one group of independent activities, unless outlined in coincident activities [36]. Title 21 CFR §1301.13(e)(ii) provides important information regarding practitioner coincidental activities for schedule II–V controlled substances and states, "May conduct research and instructional activities with those substances for which registration was granted, except that a mid-level practitioner may conduct such research only to the extent expressly authorized under state statute." In select cases, and if approved by the state board of pharmacy where the practitioner resides, a practitioner may use her practitioner DEA 224 registration to administer and store controlled substances at the laboratory location. This is generally limited to academic institutions with multiple practitioner-researchers. However, it is generally agreed that a separate researcher registration for the laboratory address should be obtained in addition to the practitioner registration. Some institutions may have internal policies that mandate both registrations, regardless if controlled substances are only stored at the laboratory location. Coincidental activities also apply to research using schedule II–V controlled substances as outlined in Title 21 CFR §1301.13(e)(v), which states, "May conduct chemical analysis with controlled substances in those schedules for which registration was issued; manufacture such substances if and to the extent that such manufacture is set forth in a statement filed with the application for registration or reregistration and provided that the manufacture is not for the purposes of dosage form development; import such substances for research purposes; distribute such substances to persons registered or authorized to conduct chemical analysis, instructional activities or research with such substances, and to persons exempted from registration pursuant Title 21 CFR §1301.24; and conduct instructional activities with controlled substances."

### 4.1.4 Schedule I Controlled Substance Registration

Researchers or laboratories requiring the use of schedule I controlled substances must apply for a specific schedule I researcher registration. This registration is separate and in addition to registration for schedule II–V controlled substances.

In addition, applicants must submit a protocol per Title 21 CFR §1301.18 to the DEA to receive approval. Clinical investigations involving schedule I controlled substances require additional approval from the DHHS or FDA, as described in Title 21 CFR §§1301.18(b) and 1301.32.

Title 21 CFR §1301.18 outlines the specific protocol form requirements and types of information (e.g., purpose, names of schedule I controlled substances, location of proposed research, security provisions, manufacturing or importing, and institutional approvals). Moreover, the following coincident activities are allowed with a schedule I research registration provided the activities are outlined in the approved protocol per Title 21 CFR §1301.13(e)(1)(v): "A researcher may manufacture or import the basic class of substance or substances for which registration was issued, provided that such manufacture or import is set forth in the protocol required in Title 21 CFR §1301.18 and to distribute such class to persons registered or authorized to conduct research with such class of substance or registered or authorized to conduct chemical analysis with controlled substances."

### 4.1.5 Drug Enforcement Administration Registration Exemptions—Laboratory Personnel

Agents or employees of a DEA registered practitioner are not required to obtain separate registration when acting in the usual course of his/her business or employment [37].

## 4.2 State Controlled Substance Licensing

In general, state boards of pharmacy have licensing regulations that mimic the federal regulations. Readers are encouraged to contact their local state regulatory boards and the DEA for additional guidance. State board of pharmacy contact information is located on the National Association Boards of Pharmacy (NABP®) Website at http://www.nabp.net.

## 4.3 DEA—Records and Reports

Title 21 CFR §1304.03(a) mandates that all registrants including researchers and research laboratories maintain appropriate records to remain in full compliance with federal regulations. A single record-keeping system for all activities at each registered location is preferred. It is extremely essential that accurate and readily retrievable records of controlled substances be maintained at all times. Federal regulations do not stipulate that practitioners must maintain prescription records. However, dispensing records must be maintained. The vast majority of veterinary practitioners and researchers do not directly dispense controlled substances in a research or laboratory setting. In select cases, a state board of pharmacy may allow a practitioner (e.g., veterinarian) of a research institution to directly dispense controlled substances to individual research laboratories for medicinal animal usage (similar to a veterinary clinic dispensing controlled substances to a client or owner). In these cases, federal regulations as outlined in Title 21 CFR §1304.03(b) mandate that an individual practitioner must keep all records of controlled substances in schedules II, III, IV, and V that are dispensed and not prescribed in the lawful course of professional practice. Additional state laws and regulations regarding labeling and reporting of dispensing logs may apply. Such practices in a research setting generally require approval from the corresponding state board of pharmacy and local DEA office. Records can be subdivided into inventory, continuing (purchase and administration), and disposal categories.

### 4.3.1 Inventory Records

According to Title 21 CFR §1304.04(a), inventory and other records as required per Title 21 CFR §1304.04 must be maintained and remain available for inspection and copying by DEA diversion investigators for at least two years from the date of such inventory or records.

Laboratories and researchers must keep all records at the registered location unless they have received special permission from the DEA for an alternative storage location. In addition, all records of controlled substances in schedule I or II must be maintained separately from schedules III, IV, and V records and in such a manner that they are readily retrievable from ordinary business records of the registrant [38]. For individual research laboratories, this is most easily accomplished by keeping schedule I and II records in a separate binder or using a divider to separate schedules I and II records from schedules III–V records if retained in a single binder. All controlled substance records should be securely stored at all times.

Separate inventories are required for each registered location and each registered independent activity [39]. General inventory requirements are outlined in Title 21 CFR §1304.11(a): "Each inventory shall contain a complete and accurate record of all controlled substances on hand on the date the inventory is taken, and shall be maintained in written, typewritten, or printed form at the registered location. An inventory taken by use of an oral recording device must be promptly transcribed." "The inventory may be taken either as of opening of business or as of the close of business on the inventory date and it shall be indicated on the inventory." [39].

There are three types of inventory records required per Title 21 CFR §1304.11, initial inventory, biennial inventory, and inventory for newly scheduled substances.

#### 4.3.1.1 INITIAL INVENTORY

The initial inventory must be performed on the date the registrant first commences business (manufacture, distribution, dispensing, or research activities) with controlled substances. Furthermore, absence of controlled substances does not eliminate the need to perform an initial inventory per Title 21 CFR §1304.11(b): "In the event a person commences business with no controlled substances on hand, he/she shall record this fact as the initial inventory." Each researcher registrant or registered institution must perform an initial inventory as soon as they receive their DEA registration, even if a "zero inventory" is reported.

#### 4.3.1.2 BIENNIAL INVENTORY

A biennial (every two years) inventory is required after the initial inventory, and the registrant must take a new inventory of all stocks of controlled substances on hand at least every two years. According to the Title 21 CFR §1304.11(c), "The biennial inventory may be taken on any date which is within two years of the previous biennial inventory date."

#### 4.3.1.3 NEW CLASSIFICATION INVENTORY

Noncontrolled substances that are reclassified by the DEA as new controlled substances must be included in a registrants inventory (if on hand) on the effective date of their scheduling [40]. Afterward, any newly classified controlled substances will be reported in the biennial inventory. Additional inventory regulations for manufacturers and distributors are outlined in Title 21 CFR §§1304.11(e)(1–2).

### 4.3.2 *Inventory Criteria*

Researchers and research laboratories must familiarize themselves with specific inventory reporting criteria as outlined in Title 21 CFR §1304.11 (e)(3), which states, "Each person registered or authorized to dispense, conduct research, or act as a reverse distributor with controlled substances shall include in the inventory the same information required of manufacturers pursuant to paragraphs (e)(1)(iii) and (iv) of this section. In determining the number of units of each finished form of a controlled substance in a commercial container which has been opened, the dispenser, researcher, or reverse distributor shall do as follows: (i) If the substance is listed in Schedule I or II, make an exact count or measure of the contents, or (ii) If the substance is listed in Schedule III, IV or V, make an estimated count or measure of the contents, unless the container holds more than 1000 tablets or capsules in which case he/she must make an exact count of the contents."

Inventory requirements outlined in Title 21 CFR §1304.11(e)(1)(iii) are described as, "For each controlled substance in finished form the inventory shall include: (A) The name of the substance; (B) Each finished form of the substance (e.g., 10-milligram tablet or 10-milligram concentration per fluid ounce or milliliter); (C) The number of units or volume of each finished form in each commercial container (e.g., 100-tablet bottle or 3-milliliter vial); and (D) The number of commercial containers of each such finished form (e.g. four 100-tablet bottles or six 3-milliliter vials)," and described in Title 21 CFR §1304.11(e)(1)(iv): "For each controlled substance not included in paragraphs (e)(1)(i), (ii) or (iii) of this section (e.g., damaged, defective or impure substances awaiting disposal, substances held for quality control purposes, or substances maintained for extemporaneous compoundings) the inventories shall include: (A) The name of the substance; (B) The total quantity of the substance to the nearest metric unit weight or the total number of units of finished form; and (C) The reason for the substance being maintained by the registrant and whether such substance is capable of use in the manufacture of any controlled substance in finished form."

### 4.3.3 Continuing Records

In addition to inventory reports, every registrant required to maintain records per Title 21 CFR §1304.03 must maintain current, complete, and accurate records of each controlled substance manufactured, imported, received, sold, delivered, exported, or disposed [41].

It states, "In recording dates of receipt, importation, distribution, exportation, or other transfers, the date on which the controlled substances are actually received, imported, distributed, exported, or otherwise transferred shall be used as the date of receipt or distribution of any documents of transfer (e.g., invoices or packing slips)" [42]. Furthermore, per Title 21 CFR §1304.22(c) Records for dispensers and researchers, "Each person registered or authorized to dispense or conduct research with controlled substances shall maintain records with the same information required of manufacturers pursuant to paragraph (a)(2)(i), (ii), (iv), (vii), (ix) of this section" including "(i) The name of the substance"; "(ii) Each finished form (e.g., 10-milligram tablet or 10-milligram concentration per fluid ounce or milliliter) and the number of units or volume of finished form in each commercial container (e.g., 100-tablet bottle or 3-milliliter vial)"; "(iv) The number of units of finished forms and/or commercial containers acquired from other persons, including the date of and number of units and/or commercial containers in each acquisition to inventory and the name, address, and registration number of the person from whom the units were acquired"; "(vii) The number of commercial containers distributed to other persons, including the date of and number of containers in each reduction from inventory, and the name, address, and registration number of the person to whom the containers were distributed" and "(ix) The number of units of finished forms and/or commercial containers distributed or disposed of in any other manner by the registrant (e.g., by distribution of complimentary samples or by destruction), including the date and manner of distribution or disposal, the name, address, and registration number of the person to whom distributed, and the quantity in finished form distributed or disposed."

### 4.3.3.1 ORDERING AND PURCHASING—DEA FORM 222

Schedule I and II controlled substances must be ordered using DEA Form 222 order forms [43]. In addition, orders for schedule I or II controlled substances may be submitted electronically via the Controlled Substances Ordering System (CSOS) if all requirement are met (CFR §1305.21). Most individual researchers will use DEA Form 222 due to smaller order volumes compared to pharmacies, wholesalers, and distributors that primarily use electronic CSOS ordering.

DEA Form 222 is a triplicate form with three attached copies (copy 1, copy 2, and copy 3). DEA Form 222 is issued by the DEA to registered individuals in mailing envelopes containing either seven or 14 forms [44]. DEA Form 222 is serially numbered and issued with the name, address, and registration number of the registrant [45]. Each DEA Form 222 must remain intact until submitted. Furthermore, additional DEA Forms 222 must be requested online from the DEA Diversion Control Website and must be kept in a secure and locked location to prevent diversion. Missing forms must be reported to the DEA [46].

### 4.3.3.2 POWER OF ATTORNEY

"A registrant may authorize one or more individuals, whether or not located at his or her registered location, to issue orders for Schedule I and II controlled substances on the registrant's behalf by executing a power of attorney for each such individual, if the power of attorney is retained in the files, with executed Forms 222 where applicable, for the same period as any order bearing the signature of the attorney. The power of attorney must be available for inspection together with other order records." [47] The registrant may revoke any power of attorney at any time by executing a notice of revocation [48]. A sample power of attorney and notice of revocation are listed in Title 21 CFR §1305.05 (c). A power of attorney must be kept on file and readily retrievable during a DEA inspection. Although federal law allows for power of attorney to be granted, not all state controlled substance laws and regulations allow a power of attorney to be used for a DEA Form 222. In some instances, the power of attorney must possess a state controlled substance license and also be registered with the DEA to qualify. As a result, readers are encouraged to contact their state regulatory agency or board of pharmacy to verify power of attorney requirements.

The registrant or power of attorney completes the top brown (copy 1) or "Purchaser" section of the triplicate form, with only one item entered for each line [49]. After signing and dating copy 1 of the triplicate form, the registrant or power of attorney removes and retains the blue (copy 3) portion of the form while keeping copy 1 and copy 2 with carbon paper attached. The purchaser mails or submits the attached copy 1 and 2 to the supplier. "A supplier may fill the order, if possible and if the supplier desires to do so, and must record on Copies 1 and 2 the number of commercial or bulk containers furnished on each item and the date on which the containers are shipped to the purchaser. If an order cannot be filled in its entirety, it may be filled in part and the balance supplied by additional shipments within 60 days following the date of the DEA Form 222. No DEA Form 222 is valid more than 60 days after its execution by the purchaser." [50] The supplier forwards the DEA Form 222 copy 2 (green) at the close of the month during which the order was filed to the DEA, while retaining copy 1 for their records [51]. On receipt of controlled substances, the purchaser must complete the "Packages Received" and "Date Received" sections on copy 3. Copy 3 is retained with the registrant's records for two years. All DEA Forms 222 must remain accounted for, including nonexecuted, executed, and voided forms. If the registration of any purchaser terminates (because the purchaser dies, ceases legal existence, discontinues business or professional practice, or changes the name or address as shown on the purchaser's registration) or is suspended or revoked, all unused DEA Form 222 order forms must be sent back to the nearest DEA office for destruction [52].

## 4.4 Security

"All applicants and registrants shall provide effective controls and procedures to guard against theft and diversion of controlled substances." [53] Practitioners and nonpractitioners authorized to conduct research or chemical analysis must store controlled substances in a securely locked, substantially constructed cabinet [54]. In addition, "Carfentanil, etorphine hydrochloride and diprenorphine shall be stored in a safe or steel cabinet equivalent to a U.S. Government Class V security container" [55].

### 4.4.1 Security Controls

"The registrant shall not employ, as an agent or employee who has access to controlled substances, any person who has been convicted of a felony offense relating to controlled substances or who, at any time, had an application for registration with the DEA denied, had a DEA registration revoked or has surrendered a DEA registration for cause." [56] To avoid hiring an employee likely to commit a drug security breach, the following questions should be asked during an employer's screening program: "Question (1) Within the past five years, have you been convicted of a felony, or within the past two years, of any misdemeanor or are you presently formally charged with committing a criminal offense? (Do not include any traffic violations, juvenile offenses or military convictions, except by general court-martial.) If the answer is yes, furnish details of conviction, offense, location, date and sentence. Question (2) In the past three years, have you ever knowingly used any narcotics, amphetamines or barbiturates, other than those prescribed to you by a physician? If the answer is yes, furnish details." [57] Furthermore, it is highly recommended that employers or registrants perform employee candidate background checks (by local courts, law enforcement agencies, or background screening companies) to screen for previous controlled substance-related offenses or convictions. Additional security precautions include maintaining an up-to-date authorized personnel (direct access to controlled substances) log, restricting access to the controlled substance storage cabinet to only authorized personnel, minimizing laboratory traffic flow near the storage area, and ability to reset locks, keys, or combinations if authorized personnel are terminated or if a loss/theft is suspected or reported. It is imperative that controlled substances never be left unattended. In addition, controlled substances requiring refrigeration should be stored in a locked container securely fastened within a refrigeration unit unless the refrigeration unit can be locked from the outside.

## 4.5 Theft and Loss

"The registrant shall notify the Field Division Office of the Administration in his/her area, in writing, of the theft or significant loss of any controlled substances within one business day of discovery of such loss or theft. The registrant shall also complete, and submit to the Field Division Office in his area, DEA Form 106 regarding the loss or theft" [58].

### 4.5.1 Significant Loss

"When determining whether a loss is significant, a registrant should consider, among others, the following factors: (1) the actual quantity of controlled substances lost in relation to the type of business; (2) the specific controlled substances lost; (3) whether the loss of the controlled substances can be associated with access to those controlled substances by specific individuals, or whether the loss can be attributed to unique activities that may take place involving the controlled substances; (4) a pattern of losses over a specific period, whether the losses appear to be random, and the results of efforts taken to resolve the losses; and, if known, (5) whether the specific controlled substances are likely candidates for diversion; and (6) local trends and other indicators of the diversion potential of the missing controlled substance" [59]. Routine record reconciliation to verify up-to-date accuracy of current inventories and administration records should be performed to minimize record-keeping discrepancies. This also allows the registrant to determine standards for significant loss or to prevent potential diversion from personnel. The frequency of record reconciliation will depend on size of inventory and frequency of administration. Weekly to monthly record reconciliation is a good starting point for most individual researchers.

## 4.6 Disposal of Controlled Substances

A researcher or practitioner may dispose of out-of-date, damaged, or otherwise unusable or unwanted controlled substances by transferring them to a reverse distributor who is registered with the DEA and authorized to receive such materials [60]. In select cases, a researcher may transfer or distribute (without being registered to distribute) a small amount of controlled substances to another DEA registrant authorized to receive such controlled substances [61]. In these cases, the total number of dosage units to be transferred or distributed cannot exceed 5% of the total number of dosage units of all controlled substances distributed and dispensed by the researcher-practitioner during the same calendar year [62]. As a result, most academic laboratories with small controlled substance inventories will only be allowed to transfer or distribute a small quantity each year to another registered individual. As a result, distributions or transfers between registered researchers are discouraged. Distributions or transfers to reverse distributors are not bound by the 5% rule. Distributions or transfers of schedule II controlled substances require the use of DEA Form 222, whereas distributions or transfers of schedule III–V controlled substances can be documented by use of an invoice. All disposal records and distribution transfer records must be maintained for a minimum of two years from the date of transaction.

## 4.7 DEA Inspections

DEA diversion investigators may make random, unannounced inspections to registered research facilities. It is strongly recommended that the principal investigator or researcher licensed and registered to store and administer controlled substances at the laboratory familiarize themselves with DEA inspection entry procedures as outlined in Title 21 CFR 1316.05. In addition, all laboratory personnel should be prepared in case the registrant researcher is not in the vicinity when DEA diversion investigators arrive for inspection. All laboratory personnel should know who to contact and what to expect during a DEA inspection.

On their arrival, DEA diversion investigators will present a Notice of Inspection (DEA Form-82) to the registrant or authorized personnel in charge of the laboratory. In addition, DEA diversion investigators will present a written informed consent for inspection to be signed by the registrant or agent in charge [63]. The registrant or agent in charge of the laboratory may refuse to sign the written notice of consent, but the DEA will then seek an administrative or search warrant signed by a judge prior to their return. Consent for inspection is voluntary and can be withdrawn at any time during the inspection [63]. The DEA diversion inspectors may request to see registrations, inventory (initial and/or biennial) records, DEA Forms 222, administration records, disposal records, authorized personnel logs, storage areas, and security systems. During the inspection, an accountability audit may be performed to review record accuracy. Invoices for schedule III–V drugs must include the date the controlled substances were received, quantity received, and initials or signature of person receiving controlled substances. Houck provides an excellent and detailed review of the DEA inspection process [64].

Once the DEA diversion inspectors have arrived, the institution's office of general counsel, office of research compliance, and corresponding department chair should be notified in case additional assistance is needed during the inspection. Noncompliance with controlled substance regulations discovered during an inspection may result in a letter of admonition, referral to a state regulatory agency, registration revocation, civil fines, and criminal prosecution. Civil fines relating to record keeping can reach $10,000 per violation [65].

## 5. KEY PERSONNEL AND UNIVERSITY COMMITTEES DESIGNATED TO IMPLEMENT REGULATORY MANDATES

### 5.1 Office of Research Compliance

In an academic setting, the office of research compliance or corresponding office responsible for coordinating research policies, conduct, and compliance should be integrally involved with establishing institutional nonclinical research controlled substance policies. It is essential that the office of research compliance or equivalent office coordinate controlled substance compliance with institutional stakeholders such as department chairs, research cores or institutes, animal care program, IACUC, occupational health and environmental safety, medical school, affiliated healthcare clinical regulatory office, local law enforcement, state regulatory boards, and the DEA. As one can surmise, there are many parties and agencies that must effectively collaborate to develop a quality controlled substance compliance program tailored to the institution's research and clinical programs. If resources allow, a research controlled substance compliance coordinator or office should manage the program for the institution. This individual or team would assist researchers and principal investigators with proper licensing, registration, security details, record-keeping guidance, disposal, and license or registration modifications. In addition, the controlled substance compliance coordinator can serve as a liaison with other institutional stakeholders, state regulatory boards, and the DEA regarding regulatory questions or compliance concerns.

## 5.2 Institutional Animal Care and Use Committee

In the United States, an IACUC must routinely review and assess institutional compliance with the Animal Welfare Act, PHS Policy, and the Guide for the Care and Use of Laboratory Animals. In these efforts, the IACUC must ensure researchers follow all local laws and federal regulations including controlled substances regulations. The IACUC should assist the Office of Research Compliance or equivalent in setting institutional policies and guidelines regarding controlled substance compliance. These policies may involve implementing controlled substance compliance training programs, laboratory and drug storage site inspections, internal record-keeping audits, maintaining a database of researchers with state controlled substance licenses and DEA registrations, and tracking controlled substance orders and storage areas. Because the IACUC must approve all animal-related research protocols, the IACUC office should have the capability to evaluate which researchers require controlled substances and the types and dosages of controlled substances as outlined in animal use protocols. Furthermore, the IACUC in conjunction with the institutional official and office of research compliance or equivalent may suspend or halt animal research activities if controlled substance noncompliance is suspected or determined.

## 5.3 Occupational Safety and Environmental Health

The occupational safety and environmental health (OSEH) or equivalent institutional department responsible for ensuring and promoting occupational safety and environmental compliance should play an active role in maintaining institutional controlled substance compliance. Depending on the organization of the institution, OSEH may be involved with all aspects of the controlled substance compliance program, including maintaining or assisting with licensing and registration, procurement or ordering of controlled substances, security plans, training, and disposal, or just a subset of the program such as managing controlled substance training, disposal, and reverse distribution practices. If OSEH manages the entire controlled substance program, a controlled substance coordinator or director should be employed to serve as the liaison for the institution and coordinated activities between other institutional departments, state regulatory boards, and federal agencies. Many institutions prefer to have controlled substance activities for nonclinical research managed by their OSEH department because the OSEH or equivalent office generally has safety, regulatory, and waste disposal processes already in place. In addition, most researchers associate OSEH with regulatory compliance and waste management of hazardous materials.

## 5.4 Laboratory Animal Care Veterinarians

Laboratory animal veterinarians and animal care program directors historically have supplied and managed controlled substance activities for nonclinical research due to their inherent responsibilities for managing animal care and health and regulatory compliance.

Most controlled substances used in laboratory animals are for anesthesia, analgesia, and euthanasia purposes. Additional uses of controlled substances include analytical laboratory or chemical analysis and direct research of the controlled substances themselves either in vitro or in vivo. In addition, many laboratory animal veterinarians maintain active practitioner licenses and possess active DEA registrations. For facilities at a single location, a laboratory animal veterinarian may use their practitioner controlled substance license and DEA registration to order, store, and administer controlled substances to animals under their direct care either for surgical purposes or acute medical treatment. This may involve the direct administration of controlled substances by veterinarians or veterinary technicians employed by the animal care unit or department. In this scenario, the laboratory animal veterinarian would maintain all controlled substance inventory, administration, and disposal records related to laboratory animal medical care, while individual researchers or departments would maintain their own state controlled substance licenses and DEA registrations for approved research.

Laboratory animal veterinarians must not distribute or transfer controlled substances ordered with their DEA registration to other researchers for research use, especially if the controlled substances will be stored at multiple separate locations within the institution. In select cases, a veterinarian may dispense small amounts of controlled substances for anesthesia, analgesia, or euthanasia to individual researchers, but these processes must mimic state regulations for dispensing (e.g., veterinary practitioner clinic dispensing to clients), including prescription directions and maintaining dispensing records. In addition, some states require that all dispensed controlled substances be reported to a central state managed database for diversion prevention and control. As a result, laboratory animal veterinarians should avoid dispensing or distribution of controlled substances unless their state regulatory boards and the DEA approve such practices.

## 5.5 Office of Clinical Regulatory Affairs and General Counsel

Many academic research institutions have associated medical schools, health centers, or hospitals. Academic health centers generally have an office of clinical affairs or comparable health center regulatory compliance office to monitor medical activities and assist physicians with training and regulatory administrative processes. Medical practitioners (e.g., physicians, dentists, and veterinarians) generally maintain an active state license and are registered with the DEA to prescribe or administer controlled substances as part of their clinical responsibilities. Furthermore, multiple states have controlled substance regulations that allow for coincidental research activities similar to federal regulations. As a result, in select cases, a practitioner may choose to use his or her practitioner controlled substance license and DEA registration for nonclinical research purposes, especially if they only prescribe controlled substances as part of their clinical duties and do not order controlled substances using their DEA registration for a secondary location (e.g., private clinic or office). The coincidental use of their practitioner state controlled substance license and DEA registration must be coordinated with the academic health center's office of clinical affairs or equivalent office, which generally provides administrative oversight for professional licensing and registration. This is essential because the hospital or associated health center may have clinical controlled substance policies that are separate and in addition to nonclinical research controlled substance policies set by the institution's research compliance department. Researcher-practitioners must be made aware of all institutional controlled substance policies and how these policies apply in different areas of the academic institution (e.g., hospital vs. nonclinical research laboratories). As a result, the office of clinical affairs or equivalent should be included in a comprehensive controlled substance program in addition to nonclinical research regulatory compliance offices.

Because controlled substance compliance involves multiple state and federal regulations, legal counsel should always be sought, especially when developing institutional compliance policies. Because controlled substance noncompliance may be associated with civil, administrative, or criminal penalties, the office of general counsel or legal affairs should provide guidance during implementation of institutional policies and during federal or state inspections.

## 5.6 Institutional Health Care Center or Hospital Pharmacy

Researchers registered with the DEA may obtain controlled substances from multiple distributors, wholesalers, their institutional health care pharmacy, or the NIDA (depending on specific research aims). In such instances, controlled substance orders must be documented on an invoice or DEA Form 222 (schedule I or II controlled substances). In select cases, an institutional health care or hospital pharmacy may distribute controlled substances to individual researchers with an active DEA registration. Because these orders are considered a distribution, they must remain in compliance with the 5% statute [62]. As a result, the institutional hospital or academic health center pharmacy must have a sufficient annual controlled substance volume to distribute or supply controlled substances to registered researchers. To prevent medication dispensing errors, human hospital pharmacies should only supply human FDA-approved controlled substances (e.g., ketamine, pentobarbital, or buprenorphine) to nonclinical research laboratories. As a result, drugs approved by the FDA for veterinary use (e.g., anesthetics and euthanasia solutions) must be acquired from a veterinary distributor or wholesaler. All transfers or distributions from the institutional hospital or health center pharmacy to individual researcher laboratories must be documented using an invoice or DEA Form 222. Both the hospital or health center pharmacy and registered researcher must keep records of all distributions.

## 5.7 Department Chairs and Unit Directors

Department chairs and unit directors are key stakeholders when implementing institutional controlled substance regulatory mandates since they provide leadership and share a responsibility for ensuring research under their direction is in full compliance. The institutional Office of Research Compliance and/or the research controlled substance compliance coordinator (if applicable) should meet regularly with department chairs and unit directors to discuss institutional and departmental goals regarding controlled substance policies and methods for implementation. In addition, department chairs and unit directors should be included in controlled substance compliance training and in any discussions regarding DEA inspections, internal audits, theft or loss, or any reports of noncompliance by their research investigators.

## 5.8 Department of Public Safety or Local Law Enforcement

Institutions should partner with local law enforcement agencies when developing an institutional controlled substance compliance program. Involvement of local law enforcement augments security practices and provides a rapid method of communication when reporting or suspecting diversion, theft, or loss. In some instances, institutions or health centers may have their own internal security practices or personnel. However, policies should be drafted to outline whom to contact in case of suspected diversion, loss, or theft of controlled substances in both the clinical and nonclinical research settings. Local law enforcement may also assist with personnel background checks to verify if any current or previous controlled substances convictions may exclude laboratory personnel from working with controlled substances.

## 5.9 State and Federal Regulating Agencies

Each institution or individual researcher should contact or review their corresponding state regulatory board or board of pharmacy and DEA field office for general information regarding controlled substance regulations, licensing, registration, modifications, record-keeping, security, and disposal. In large academic research institutions, it is not uncommon to have unique questions on how to apply or interpret controlled substance regulations in the nonclinical research setting. In these cases, it is best to consult with the appropriate regulatory agencies for additional guidance to ensure conformance and compliance with all state and federal controlled substance regulations. Common questions relate to modifications to existing state controlled substance licenses and DEA registrations and the logistics related to moving a laboratory to a new address either within the same institution or to a new institution. Other questions may relate to determining significant loss, reporting theft, documentation requirements for continual records, or discovery of orphaned controlled substances during a laboratory renovation.

# 6. COMMON COMPLIANCE CHALLENGES

## 6.1 Development of Controlled Substance Compliance Program

There must be commitment on multiple institutional levels to establish a quality controlled substance compliance program. Although the principal investigator or researcher registrant is ultimately responsible for ensuring controlled substance security and compliance in the laboratory, institutions should provide ample oversight and training regarding registration, security, ordering, record-keeping, and disposal to ensure full compliance with all controlled substance laws and regulations. From an institutional standpoint, the following are concepts and practices that can have a positive impact for solving compliance challenges: developing an institutional controlled substance policy, providing guidance with registration and licensing; collaborating and aligning controlled substance compliance policies with associated institutional health centers (if applicable); establishing universal security practices; developing a controlled substance training program; collaborating with an OSEH department to ensure proper disposal; and implementing institutional inspection and mock audit programs.

### 6.1.1 Developing an Institutional Controlled Substance Policy

For most academic institutions, the offices of research compliance and occupational safety or equivalent should provide leadership to develop institution-wide controlled substance policies for nonclinical research. These efforts should be coordinated with other institutional stakeholders with the goal to incorporate controlled substance policies in the human or veterinary clinical setting. The final policy should outline expectations for the use of controlled substances in nonclinical research, clinical research, and clinical medicine. Policy collaboration with institutional health centers is important because some practitioners performing nonclinical research may have the option to use their practitioner DEA registration for clinical prescribing and for obtaining controlled substances for their nonclinical research laboratories (e.g., controlled substances used for analgesia and anesthesia of laboratory animals or in vitro research). Furthermore, the institutional controlled substance compliance policy may require that all practitioners or researchers using controlled substances in nonclinical research obtain separate controlled substance research licenses and corresponding DEA researcher registrations for their laboratories. Institutional training requirements and expectations regarding controlled substance compliance should be documented in the institutional controlled substance compliance policy.

### 6.1.2 Licensing and Registration Compliance

Controlled substance state licensing and federal registration requirements can be complicated, especially when medical practitioner faculty provide clinical services and perform nonclinical research or maintain laboratories at the same institution. As a result, an institution should dedicate personnel or resources to assist and coordinate licensing and registration for both the clinical and research settings. Such personnel can serve as a liaison or link to state regulatory boards and DEA field offices when additional licensing or registration guidance is required. Assistance with licensing and registration can be accomplished in multiple ways and may involve direct communication with a controlled substance compliance coordinator or development of a website with application information and links to state regulatory offices and the DEA Office of Diversion Control (http://www.deadiversion.usdoj.gov/). Additional information, regarding supplemental application materials, fees, and state fingerprinting requests, can greatly assist with streamlining the licensing and registration process while preventing errors and delays associated with application processing.

#### 6.1.2.1 MODIFICATIONS TO LICENSING AND DEA REGISTRATION

At some point, researchers may retire, cancel their controlled substance license or DEA registration, update schedule codes, or relocate their research laboratory (within the same institution or to another institution). All of these modifications require specific steps to be followed, which may include several weeks to months for processing and approval. According to federal regulations, "Any registrant may apply to modify his/her registration to authorize the handling of additional controlled substances or to change his/her name or address, by submitting a letter of request to the Registration Unit, Drug Enforcement Administration" [66]. As a result, researchers must schedule time in advance for approval prior to relocating their laboratory. This can be a major compliance challenge if the laboratory has initiated their moving plans prior to coordinating and approval with the corresponding state regulatory board and the DEA. If the new location has not been approved, the current controlled substance inventory may have to remain at the old location until disposal can be arranged with a reverse distributor. State regulatory boards usually have similar regulations regarding controlled substance research license modifications.

### 6.1.3 *Aligning Institutional Compliance Policies*

In large decentralized academic institutions, the basic science departments, medical school, and institutional health centers may have separate physical addresses and separate compliance or regulatory policies. For example, controlled substance licensing and registration policies for medical practitioners may be coordinated by the institution's health center office of regulatory compliance while controlled substance policies for nonclinical research laboratories may be coordinated by individual research departments, the research compliance office, or the occupational safety and environmental health department. In addition, the institutional pharmacy department may coordinate disposal of controlled substance waste in the hospital or health center, while the department of OSEH may coordinate disposal of controlled substances for nonclinical research laboratories. As a result, institutions must make an active effort to align their internal controlled substance policies and determine which departments or offices will be responsible for implementation and maintaining compliance oversight.

### 6.1.4 *Establishing Security Practices—Preventing Diversion, Loss, or Theft*

Institutions must have multiple level security practices in place to prevent controlled substance diversion, theft, or loss. Although the final security controls are the primary responsibility of the licensed and registered researcher, the institution should provide access to local law enforcement, real-time surveillance, secure entry or badge access mechanisms, and personnel background check support. Furthermore, researchers must be trained or provided guidance on the importance of maintaining up to date and accurate records including inventory, purchasing (invoices and DEA Form 222), administration, and disposal records. The DEA expects accurate and readily retrievable records during a DEA inspection: "*Readily retrievable* means that certain records are kept by automatic data processing systems or other electronic or mechanized recordkeeping systems in such a manner that they can be separated out from all other records in a reasonable time and/or records are kept on which certain items are asterisked, redlined, or in some other manner visually identifiable apart from other items appearing on the records." [67] Failure to supply all mandatory records or discrepancies in controlled substance records found during an inspection may lead to civil, administrative, or criminal penalties. Record-keeping discrepancies can be avoided or caught early with frequent reviews of all records. In addition, licensed and registered researchers should maintain current personnel logs for those individuals with access to controlled substances storage cabinets. Personnel logs must be continually updated with corresponding changes to combinations or key access to controlled substance storage locations. Compliance challenges generally occur when researchers do not employ or designate a laboratory manager to maintain or review controlled substance policies, security, or records for the laboratory on a frequent and continual basis. Large laboratories with multiple personnel are at increased risk for diversion or record-keeping discrepancies if practices are not uniform and consistent. Institutions should monitor and review shipping practices from outside vendors to laboratories. There is a potential for loss or diversion if the registered laboratory location (documented on the DEA registration) is different than the actual delivery site (e.g., packages are dropped off at a central location for tertiary delivery within the institution). Using shipping companies who provide online tracking services and require recipients to sign on delivery can prevent transit or delivery losses. The DEA expects that all packages will be delivered to the registered location.

Special arrangements including reviews of security and chain of custody policies may be required by the DEA if direct delivery to laboratories is not available. In such instances, it is best to consult with a DEA Field Office.

## 7. ADDRESSING NONCOMPLIANCE

Controlled substance noncompliance should be addressed at multiple levels within an institution. Individual registrants should be made aware that state and federal regulations supersede institutional policies and that civil and criminal prosecution is a possibility for controlled substance noncompliance, diversion, theft, and loss. As a result, controlled substance compliance must be taken seriously, and institutions should invest in resources to assist researchers with promoting and maintaining compliance with all controlled substance regulations. The best method to address noncompliance is through planning, prevention, and awareness. Having an institutional policy outlining controlled substance compliance expectations is a key first step. Having an institutional controlled substance compliance coordinator will greatly assist researchers with general licensing and registration, training, security requirements, and record-keeping questions, and can serve as a liaison with regulating agencies regarding compliance questions, inspections, or concerns. Noncompliance concerns must be immediately addressed and should include institutional stakeholder discussions with the compliance coordinator, the institutional office coordinating research regulatory affairs, department chairs, local law enforcement and security, IACUC, and office of general counsel. In the event of actual theft or significant loss, local law enforcement must be notified immediately along with any state regulating agency and the DEA. In some instances, post-approval monitoring or institutional audits can be performed, especially for laboratories with multiple personnel or those using large quantities of controlled substances especially with higher abuse schedules. Institutions must be prepared to suspend or terminate a researcher's research controlled substance privileges when controlled substance diversion or negligent noncompliance is suspected or documented or places risk on the public, researcher, laboratory personnel, or institution.

## References

[1] Title 7 USC §§ 2131-2159.
[2] Title 9 CFR §§ 1.1 – 4.1. http://www.gpo.gov/fdsys/browse/collectionCfr.action?collectionCode=CFR&search Path=Title+9&oldPath=&isCollapsed=true&selectedYearFrom=2013&ycord=0.
[3] Policy#3: Veterinary care. http://www.aphis.usda.gov/animal_welfare/policy.php?policy=3 [accessed 18.02.14].
[4] US government principles for the utilization and care of vertebrate animals used in testing, research, and training. http://grants.nih.gov/grants/olaw/references/phspol.htm#USGovPrinciples [accessed 18.02.14].
[5] Health Research Extension Act of 1985, Public Law 99–158. Animals in research [accessed 18.02.14]
[6] National Research Council. Guide for the care and use of laboratory animals. 8th ed. Washington, DC: The National Academies Press; 2011.
[7] Association for Assessment and Accreditation of Laboratory Animal Care International. http://www.aaal ac.org/; 2014 [accessed 09.02.14].
[8] American Veterinary Medical Association Panel on Euthanasia. AVMA guidelines for the euthanasia of animals: 2013 Edition. 2013. https://www.avma.org/KB/Policies/Documents/euthanasia.pdf [accessed 09.01.14].

[9] Heard K, Cleveland NR, Krier S. Benzodiazepines and antipsychotic medications for treatment of acute cocaine toxicity in animal models—a systematic review and meta-analysis. Human Exp Toxicol 2011;30:1849–54.

[10] Advances in the neuroscience of addiction. In: Kuhn C, Koob G, editors. Frontiers in Neuroscience. 2nd ed. Boca Raton, FL: CRC Press; 2010. http://www.ncbi.nlm.nih.gov/books/NBK53356/.

[11] Lynch WJ, Nicholson KL, Dance ME, Morgan RW, Foley PL. Animal models of substance abuse and addiction: implications for science, animal welfare, and society. Comp Med 2010;60:177–88.

[12] Waterhouse BD. Methods in drug abuse research: cellular and circuit level analyses. Boca Raton, FL: CRC Press; 2010.

[13] Levin ED, Buccafusco JJ. Animal models of cognitive impairment. Boca Raton, FL: CRC Press; 2010.

[14] Nestler EJ, Hyman SE. Animal models of neuropsychiatric disorders. Nature Neurosci 2010;13:1161–9.

[15] Dela Peña I, Kim B-N, Han DH, Kim Y, Cheong JH. Abuse and dependence liability analysis of methylphenidate in the spontaneously hypertensive rat model of attention-deficit/hyperactivity disorder (ADHD): what have we learned? Arch Pharm Res 2013;36:400–10.

[16] Lemke TL, Williams DA. Foye's principles of medicinal chemistry. Baltimore, MD: Lippincott Williams & Wilkins; 2012.

[17] FDA Review.org, a project of The Independent Institute. http://www.fdareview.org/history.shtml - fifth [accessed 03.02.14].

[18] FDA's Origin & Functions—FDA's Origin. http://www.fda.gov/AboutFDA/WhatWeDo/History/Origin/ucm124403.htm [accessed 03.02.14].

[19] FDA's origin & functions—FDA history—part I. http://www.fda.gov/AboutFDA/WhatWeDo/History/Origin/ucm054819.htm [accessed 03.02.14].

[20] Legislation—Federal Food and Drugs Act of 1906. http://www.fda.gov/regulatoryinformation/legislation/ucm148690.htm [accessed 03.02.14].

[21] Promoting safe and effective drugs for 100 years. http://www.fda.gov/aboutfda/whatwedo/history/productregulation/promotingsafeandeffectivedrugsfor100years/default.htm [accessed 03.02.14].

[22] Harrison Narcotics Tax Act, 1914—full text. http://www.erowid.org/psychoactives/law/law_fed_harrison_narcotics_act.shtml [accessed 03.02.14].

[23] FDA's origin & functions—FDA history—part II. http://www.fda.gov/aboutfda/whatwedo/history/origin/ucm054826.htm [accessed 03.02.14].

[24] Greene JA, Podolsky SH. Reform, regulation, and pharmaceuticals—the Kefauver–Harris amendments at 50. New Engl J Med 2012;367:1481–3.

[25] News & events—50th anniversary of the Kefauver-Harris drug amendments of 1962—interview with FDA historian John Swann. http://www.fda.gov/drugs/newsevents/ucm320927.htm [accessed 03.02.14].

[26] Consumer updates—Kefauver–Harris amendments revolutionized drug development. http://www.fda.gov/ForConsumers/ConsumerUpdates/ucm322856.htm [accessed 03.02.14].

[27] Drug Abuse Control Amendments of 1965, Public Law 89-74, 79 STAT 226. Enrolled acts and resolutions of Congress, compiled 1789–2011. Department of State; 1965.

[28] Legislation—Controlled Substances Act. http://www.fda.gov/regulatoryinformation/legislation/ucm148726.htm [accessed 03.02.14].

[29] Single convention on narcotic drugs. http://www.unodc.org/unodc/en/treaties/single-convention.html [accessed 03.02.14].

[30] Convention on psychotropic substances. http://www.unodc.org/unodc/en/treaties/psychotropics.html [accessed 03.02.14].

[31] Convention against the illicit traffic in narcotic drugs and psychotropic substances. http://www.unodc.org/unodc/en/treaties/illicit-trafficking.html [accessed 03.02.14].

[32] Text of H.R. 5210 (100th): Anti-Drug Abuse Act of 1988 (passed Congress/enrolled bill version). http://www.govtrack.us/congress/bills/100/hr5210/text [accessed 03.02.14].

[33] Public Law 104-237—Comprehensive Methamphetamine Control Act of 1996. http://www.gpo.gov/fdsys/pkg/PLAW-104publ237/content-detail.html [accessed 03.02.14].

[34] CMEA (The Combat Methamphetamine Epidemic Act of 2005)—general information. http://www.deadiversion.usdoj.gov/meth/cma2005.htm [accessed 03.02.14].

[35] Title 21 CFR—PART 1310-Section 1310.02 Substances covered. http://www.deadiversion.usdoj.gov/21cfr/cfr/1310/1310_02.htm - a [accessed 03.02.14].

[36] Title 21 CFR §1301.13(e). http://www.deadiversion.usdoj.gov/21cfr/cfr/1301/1301_13.htm [accessed 10.02.14].
[37] Title 21 CFR § 1301.22(a). http://www.deadiversion.usdoj.gov/21cfr/cfr/1301/1301_22.htm [accessed 10.02.14].
[38] Title 21 CFR §§1304.04(e-f). http://www.deadiversion.usdoj.gov/21cfr/cfr/1304/1304_04.htm [accessed 10.02.14].
[39] Title 21 CFR §1304.11(a). http://www.deadiversion.usdoj.gov/21cfr/cfr/1304/1304_11.htm [accessed 10.02.14].
[40] Title 21 CFR §1304.11 (d). http://www.deadiversion.usdoj.gov/21cfr/cfr/1304/1304_11.htm [accessed 10.02.14].
[41] Title 21 CFR §1304.21(a). http://www.deadiversion.usdoj.gov/21cfr/cfr/1304/1304_22.htm [accessed 10.02.14].
[42] Title 21 CFR §1304.21(d). http://www.deadiversion.usdoj.gov/21cfr/cfr/1304/1304_22.htm [accessed 10.02.14].
[43] Title 21 CFR §1305.04. http://www.deadiversion.usdoj.gov/21cfr/cfr/1305/1305_04.htm [accessed 10.02.14].
[44] Title 21 CFR §1305.11 (a). http://www.deadiversion.usdoj.gov/21cfr/cfr/1305/1305_11.htm [accessed 10.02.14].
[45] 21 CFR § 1305.11(d). http://www.deadiversion.usdoj.gov/21cfr/cfr/1305/1305_11.htm [accessed 10.02.14].
[46] Title 21 CFR §1305.16. http://www.deadiversion.usdoj.gov/21cfr/cfr/1305/1305_16.htm [accessed 10.02.14].
[47] Title 21 CFR §1305.05(a). http://www.deadiversion.usdoj.gov/21cfr/cfr/1305/1305_05.htm [accessed 10.02.14].
[48] Title 21 CFR §1305.05(b). http://www.deadiversion.usdoj.gov/21cfr/cfr/1305/1305_05.htm [accessed 10.02.14].
[49] Title CFR §1305.12(b). http://www.deadiversion.usdoj.gov/21cfr/cfr/1305/1305_12.htm [accessed 10.02.14].
[50] Title CFR §1305.13(b). http://www.deadiversion.usdoj.gov/21cfr/cfr/1305/1305_13.htm [accessed 10.02.14].
[51] Title 21 CFR §1305.13(c). http://www.deadiversion.usdoj.gov/21cfr/cfr/1305/1305_13.htm [accessed 10.02.14].
[52] Title 21 CFR §1305.18. http://www.deadiversion.usdoj.gov/21cfr/cfr/1305/1305_18.htm [accessed 10.02.14].
[53] Title 21 CFR §1301.71. http://www.deadiversion.usdoj.gov/21cfr/cfr/1301/1301_71.htm [accessed 10.02.14].
[54] Title 21 CFR §§1301.75(a-b). http://www.deadiversion.usdoj.gov/21cfr/cfr/1301/1301_75.htm [accessed 10.02.14].
[55] Title 21 CFR §1301.75(d). http://www.deadiversion.usdoj.gov/21cfr/cfr/1301/1301_75.htm [accessed 10.02.14].
[56] Title 21 CFR §1301.76(a). http://www.deadiversion.usdoj.gov/21cfr/cfr/1301/1301_76.htm [accessed 10.02.14].
[57] Title 21 CFR §1301.90. http://www.deadiversion.usdoj.gov/21cfr/cfr/1301/1301_90.htm [accessed 10.02.14].
[58] Title 21 CFR §1301.76(b). http://www.deadiversion.usdoj.gov/21cfr/cfr/1301/1301_76.htm [accessed 10.02.14].
[59] Title 21 CFR §§1301.76 (b)(1-6). http://www.deadiversion.usdoj.gov/21cfr/cfr/1301/1301_76.htm [accessed 10.02.14].
[60] Title 21 CFR §1307.11(2). http://www.deadiversion.usdoj.gov/21cfr/cfr/1307/1307_11.htm [accessed 10.02.14].
[61] Title 21 CFR §1307.11(a). http://www.deadiversion.usdoj.gov/21cfr/cfr/1307/1307_11.htm [accessed 10.02.14].
[62] Title 21 CFR §1307.11(a)(1)(IV). http://www.deadiversion.usdoj.gov/21cfr/cfr/1307/1307_11.htm [accessed 10.02.14].
[63] Title 21 CFR 1316.08. http://www.deadiversion.usdoj.gov/21cfr/cfr/1316/1316_08.htm [accessed 10.02.14].
[64] Houck LK. Death, taxes, and DEA inspections: dealing with the inevitable. Food and Drug Law Institute – Update. November–December 2011 27–35. http://www.fdli.org [accessed 10.02.14].
[65] Title 21 USC 13 §842 (c)(B). http://www.deadiversion.usdoj.gov/21cfr/21usc/842.htm [accessed 10.02.14].
[66] Title 21 CFR 1301.51. http://www.deadiversion.usdoj.gov/21cfr/cfr/1301/1301_51.htm [accessed 10.02.14].
[67] Title 21 CFR 1300.01. http://www.deadiversion.usdoj.gov/21cfr/cfr/1300/1300_01.htm [accessed 10.02.14].

# Export Controls and US Research Universities

*Gretta Rowold[1], Jennifer A. Ponting[2]*

[1]Office of Legal Counsel, University of Oklahoma, Norman, OK, USA; [2]Office for Sponsored
Programs, Harvard University, Cambridge, MA, USA

## 1. SUMMARY

United States export controls have historically focused on physical exports leaving the United States for other destinations. However, these regulations have been increasingly used to govern the exportation of controlled technical data since the 1990s, including the creation of the "deemed export rule," which regulates the transfer of export-controlled technical data to foreign nationals in the United States.

Attempts to broaden regulatory jurisdiction to include traditionally academic activities such as publication of scholarly works, scientific communication among peers, and instruction of foreign students were met with legal challenges in the 1980s, ultimately resulting in the creation of a national policy on the transfer of scientific, technical, and engineering information. This chapter will explore the legal underpinnings of export controls, the deemed export rule, and key terms like fundamental research. The relevant regulations and federal agencies will be identified, and common export control challenges encountered in the academic environment will be discussed.

## 2. KEY DEFINITIONS

1. **Export controls**: Federal regulations that govern the exportation of items, technology, and, in some instances, services. The term "export controls" is typically used to denote the Export Administration Regulations (EAR), the International Traffic in Arms Regulations (ITAR), and the Foreign Assets Control Regulations (FACR). Related but distinct regulations govern importation of export-controlled items and technologies.
2. **Sanctions**: In international law, "sanctions" are a set of legal requirements imposed on a particular country (or groups or individuals within a country) with the intent to

procure improved behavior. Within the topic of export controls, the term "sanctions" is used somewhat ubiquitously. However, it is most often used to denote regulations administered by the Office of Foreign Assets Control (OFAC) within the US Department of Treasury.

3. **Deemed export**: The concept that release of export-controlled technical data to a foreign national can constitute an "export" under the EAR or ITAR.

4. **Foreign national**: Anyone who is not a US citizen by birth or naturalization, a lawful permanent resident (established by issuance of a permanent resident visa or "green card"), or a "protected person" under 8 USC 1324b (a) (3) (political refugees and asylum holders).

5. **Defense service**: The concept that the provision of certain services relating to defense articles on the US munitions list (USML) can be a regulated activity. This definition is currently being rewritten under the export control reform effort and, as of the date of this publication, has not been finalized.

6. **Fundamental research**: Basic and applied research in science and engineering, the results of which ordinarily are published and shared broadly within the scientific community, as distinguished from proprietary research and from industrial development, design, production, and product utilization, the results of which ordinarily are restricted for proprietary or national security reasons. Some universities' academic freedom policies require that they only perform fundamental research.

7. **Exemption**: A regulatory provision that excludes activity or transactions from regulation.

8. **License exception**: A regulatory provision that eliminates the need to obtain a license if certain predetermined conditions are met.

9. **Technology control plan**: An internal document that is used to control access to export-controlled technical data.

## 3. INTRODUCTION

Export control regulations can impact a broad variety of university activity and transactions. While export controls typically exclude or exempt most university research, certain types of activity can still expose a university to liability. Universities with robust sponsored research portfolios, particularly those with expertise in a field articulated on the Commerce Control List (CCL) or USML, should be mindful of export control obligations. Similarly, universities with a significant international presence may encounter regulated transactions or activity.

## 4. HISTORICAL PERSPECTIVES

The Arms Export Control Act (AECA) [1] and EAA [2] both contain provisions for the exportation of controlled technical data. The AECA regulates the exportation of technical data listed on the USML. Similarly, the EAA regulates the exportation of technical data found on the CCL. Both statutes appear to have originally been drafted to address the actual exportation of technical data to another country. However, implementing regulations began to reflect the application of these provisions to the release of controlled technical data in the United States (also known as a deemed export).

In the 1970s, export control policy received increased attention in response to concerns that Soviet attempts to acquire US hardware and technologies could erode the lead in weaponry and other key military systems that the United States enjoyed. Notable advances in Soviet weapons design seemed to demonstrate that the technological gap between the United States and Soviet Union was closing. Critics of high technology exports warned that the current US policy was subsidizing the Soviet advances in sophisticated weapons systems. At the same time, the intelligence community expressed concern that the Soviets were not only successfully acquiring US technology through conventional means, such as espionage, but also increasingly through acquisition of open-source information.

Two particularly vocal government officials, Admiral Bobby Inman (then deputy director of the Central Intelligence Agency (CIA)) and Frank Carlucci (then deputy secretary of defense and former deputy director of the CIA), focused their attention on the release of sophisticated technology and know-how from American universities, particularly through open scientific conferences and meetings and academic publications. Both asserted that security concerns should override any academic interest in dissemination of unclassified technical information. In 1976, the AECA was passed [1], and shortly thereafter, the first version of the ITAR was promulgated. Almost immediately, the scientific community was confronted with its provisions, causing many scientists and even the National Academies to express their concerns about government overreach [3].

## 4.1 Constitutional Challenges and Escalating Government Action

By 1978, the Office of Legal Counsel within the US Department of Justice (DOJ) had become embroiled in the controversy surrounding overly broad interpretations of export controls. In a series of memoranda and testimony, DOJ attorneys advised that export control regulations in their current form were an unconstitutional prior restraint on protected speech and needed to be revised [4]. Shortly after this advice was provided, the Ninth Circuit Court of Appeals held in *US v. Edler* that the ITAR definition of technical data, if read literally, was unconstitutional and overly broad [5]. Stating that "an expansive interpretation of technical data relating to items on the Munitions List could seriously impede scientific research and publishing and the international scientific exchange," the *Edler* court narrowed the scope of "technical data," holding that the regulations could only cover information "significantly and directly related to specific articles" on the USML. The court stated, "These limitations are necessary both to adhere to the purpose of the Act and to avoid serious interference with the interchange of scientific and technological information."

Citing the *Edler* holding and amid apparent assertions that the current regulations could be applied within the bounds articulated by the *Edler* court, DOJ continued to provide guidance advising that export control regulations themselves needed to be revised. Perhaps most telling were DOJ's intimations that the EAR and ITAR were both so fraught with constitutional issues that they were vulnerable to being overturned in their entirety [6].

In the aftermath of *Edler* and in response to the DOJ advice, the State Department issued its own interpretation of the surviving provisions of regulatory authority [7]. While acknowledging frustrations with attempts to regulate scientific communication, the State Department asserted that the ITAR do not cover "general mathematical engineering or statistical information, not purporting to have or reasonably expected to be given direct application to equipment in such categories" [8]. For information that could still be captured by the ITAR, the State Department assured exporters that an expedited licensing review process would be used to avoid any "burdensome delays" [7].

After interagency wrangling, the State Department ultimately requested the DOJ's review of proposed revisions to the ITAR. The DOJ responded that while the revised version of the ITAR was a significant improvement, "[E]ven as revised, it can have a number of unconstitutional applications" [9]. Notably, the DOJ felt that the proposed revisions did not sufficiently remedy the unconstitutionality of the ITAR when applied to "communications of unclassified information by a technical lecturer at a university or to the conversation of a United States engineer who meets with foreign friends at home to discuss matters of theoretical interest" [9]. Stating, "For obvious reasons, the best legal solution for the overbreadth problem is for the Department of State, not the courts, to narrow the regulations," the DOJ recommended that the State Department return to the drawing board and revise the ITAR further such that it could not apply to the protected types of speech identified [9]. At the same time, as these discussions with the State Department, the DOJ sent a memorandum to the Commerce Department conveying that like the ITAR, the EAR appeared to be an unconstitutional prior restraint as currently written [10].

Throughout this period, the Department of Defense (DoD) and the State Department began attempting to limit foreign national access to equipment at universities, including supercomputers in the United States funded by the National Science Foundation [11]. Citing national security concerns [12], university recipients were asked to limit access to the supercomputers by Soviet or Chinese users. When the NSF requested that the four university recipients sign agreements barring Soviet and Chinese users, the universities did not uniformly agree to comply.

DoD officials within the Reagan administration also escalated their attempts to curtail or censor scientific conferences, asking organizers to withdraw unclassified papers on topics they deemed sensitive or to limit attendees to US citizens only [13]. The perceived interference with scientific exchanges was disturbing enough that in 1981, the presidents of Stanford, California Institute of Technology, Massachusetts Institute of Technology, Cornell, and the University of California wrote to the secretaries of commerce, state, and defense, voicing their concern about attempts to apply export control regulations to teaching and research activity at universities. The presidents were "deeply concerned" about recent attempts to apply the ITAR and EAR to university activity. The letter urged the secretaries to refrain from extending the regulations in any manner that would make them applicable to university activity unless and until the ramifications, including the legal and constitutional issues of such an extension, could be thoroughly assessed [14].

Following up on its prior attempts to prompt the Departments of State and Commerce to amend their regulations to remedy the constitutional issues, the DOJ sent a memorandum reiterating its prior recommendations to the State Department. The memo clearly reflects that the State Department had attempted to exclude from the definition of technical data a broader array of public domain data, including scientific data. However, the DOJ felt, "[A]lthough the definitions of technical data in the prior and current drafts differ because of the exclusion in the current draft of information in the public domain and general mathematical or engineering information, we do not believe that this difference amounts to a substantive change in the coverage of the regulations" [15]. Also problematic was the State Department's reliance on exemptions from licensing requirements. As the DOJ explained, the State Department's approach to subjecting the flow of information to regulation and then exempting it from licensing requirements did nothing to remedy the ITAR's unconstitutional prior restraint on speech [15].

## 4.2 Development of a National Policy and Regulatory Changes

In March 1982, the Committee on Science, Engineering, and Public Policy (COSEPUP) of the National Academy of Sciences convened a Panel on Scientific Communication and National Security chaired by Dale R. Corson, physicist and president emeritus of Cornell University, partially to address the concerns of the academic community. The panel produced what is referred to as The Corson Report, which countered the idea that government funded research needed to be restricted or classified [16]. The report stated, "The long-term security of the United States depends in large part…on the vigorous research and development effort that openness helps to nurture" [16].

More specifically, the Corson Panel examined the EAR and ITAR and concluded that neither could be used to restrict scientific communication, with two narrow exceptions. First, when export-controlled technical data regulated under the ITAR were "significantly and directly related to" specific articles enumerated on the USML, the ITAR could be used to regulate transfers of the unclassified information. However, in instances in which the information could have both peaceful and military applications (which is generally the case in university settings), only situations in which the party involved had knowledge that the information would be used for a prohibited use could serve as grounds for prosecution. Second, commercial transactions involving unclassified technical data would not receive the same constitutional protections as scientific communication [16].

Outside of these two areas, the Corson Report concluded that constitutional protections were large for scientific communication (a term that encompasses scholarly exchanges, educational instruction, publication, and research). As evidence of the constitutional protections involved, the Corson Report stated that neither the ITAR nor EAR was suitable for restricting domestic publications [16].

## 4.3 National Security Decision Directive 189

In September 1985, years of debate and discussion culminated in the creation of a national policy on the government's ability to regulate and classify the products of federally-funded research. National Security Decision Directive 189 (NSDD-189) was hailed by both sides as significant progress in the debate on scientific communication and national security. NSDD-189 marked a shift away from the government's previous approach that more regulation of unclassified technology was needed (or that increased classification was necessary to protect national security) [17,18]. After the issuance of NSDD-189, researchers receiving federal funds would be put on notice of the likelihood of their research results being classified during the negotiation of the research contract.

Importantly, the policy states, "No restrictions may be placed upon the *conduct* or *reporting* of federally-funded fundamental research that has not received national security classification *except as provided in applicable U.S. statutes*" [19]. The reference to conduct appears to harken back to earlier attempts to control access to scientific equipment or facilities. The reference to reporting appears to remedy the interrupted meetings, conferences, symposia, and publications of the late 1970s and early 1980s.

The concluding sentence has also lead to considerable debate and confusion. Some parties contend that the EAR and the ITAR themselves provide authority for imposing export control regulation. However, this belies the history of the policy. The impetus for creation of NSDD-189 was whether or not the EAR or ITAR could be used to regulate scientific communication and research, particularly within the university setting. Interpreting the concluding sentence as holding that both the EAR and ITAR can override the protections afforded to fundamental research would in effect make the policy meaningless to all involved. Further, the policy specifies that statutory (not regulatory) authority is needed to override the protections afforded by the policy.

During the timeframe that the policy was being crafted, several statutes did, in fact, provide for the regulation and classification of research and technical know-how, even in a wholly private, industrial, or academic setting. In 1985, when NSDD-189 was published, the Defense Authorization Act allowed for DoD regulation of the exportation of controlled technical data in some circumstances [20]. Previously, in 1980, Congress used the Defense Authorization Act to subject DoD-funded research on very high-speed integrated circuits (VHSICs) to ITAR regulation, specifically limiting foreign national access to the research program and curtailing dissemination of program information at open meetings [21]. Prior to this congressional designation of ITAR restrictions, VHSIC research had been unclassified, and universities could publish their findings [22].

Furthermore, two other non-DoD statutes permit the classification and regulation of private know-how, and both pre-date the issuance of NSDD-189 and remain in full effect, notwithstanding the policy's provisions. The Atomic Energy Act allows for the classification of "Restricted Data," a category of information that is "born classified" regardless of whether it was generated by the government or private researchers [23]. Strict dissemination controls apply to "Restricted Data" until it is declassified pursuant to the act [23]. Similarly, the Invention Secrecy Act provides statutory authority for the government to classify or restrict the public release of technology owned by private inventors if such a release would cause damage to national security [24]. Neither of these statutory provisions is overridden or superseded by NSDD-189.

The proposition that the concluding sentence of NSDD-189 allows for the applicability of the EAR and ITAR to university activity is also undercut by the findings of the Corson Report. After researching both sets of regulations, the Corson Panel found that neither the EAR nor the ITAR could be used to regulate university research and scientific communication [16]. This language, when taken into consideration with the legal and political history of the policy, is a clear recognition of the policy's limitations to those areas of already mandated by statute.

While NSDD-189 has been hailed as a success by all parties involved in its creation, the last sentence creates some notable limitations on its applicability. First, the policy applies only to federally funded research. Non-federally funded research is not bound by its provisions. It also does not clearly account for export-controlled technical data that are required for the conduct of fundamental research, leading many to conclude that this category of information could remain regulated.

### 4.3.1 *The Creation of the Deemed Export Rule (1994)*

In 1996, the Bureau of Export Administration (BXA, the predecessor to the Bureau of Industry and Security) proposed the creation of a deemed export rule. Interestingly, the 1979 Export Administration Act (EAA) does not expressly recognize the deemed export concept [25]. In contrast, recognition that export control regulation should not be applied to scientific endeavors such as research, education, and publication is clearly expressed [26]. As efforts to reauthorize the EAA occurred over the years, attempts to create statutory authority for deemed exports were unsuccessful [25].

Even in the absence of statutory authority, the BXA was successful in promulgating a regulatory deemed export rule. In an interim final rule published in 1996, BXA stated that the EAR provided coverage of more than exports and that actions not typically understood to constitute an "export," such as the release of technology to a foreign national in the United States would be included in that term [27]. Section 734 went on to set forth the extent to which legal authority to regulate exports is implemented via the EAR [27]. Section 734 then codified an expanded interpretation of "export" as:

> "Export" means an actual shipment or transmission of items subject to the EAR out of the United States; or release of technology or software subject to the EAR to a foreign national in the United States [27].

This provision remains intact as of the date of this publication.

### 4.3.2 *US v. Roth [28]*

A historical summary of export controls and university research would not be complete without a discussion of the first prosecution of a university professor for violations of export control regulations. This case is an illustration of the limitations of NSDD-189 to protect all university activity from regulation. The case is often cited as a cautionary tale by regulatory agencies, enforcement agencies, and academia alike.

In May 2006, the US Federal Bureau of Investigation (FBI) executed search warrants on the offices and research laboratories of Dr John Reece Roth, a professor emeritus at the University of Tennessee Knoxville. Dr Roth had received research funding from the Air Force Research Laboratory. The research award contained a publication restriction, as well as the following language:

5352.227-9000 Export-Controlled Data Restrictions.

> (a) For the purpose of this clause, (1) Foreign person is any person who is not a citizen or national of the U.S. or lawfully admitted to the U.S. for permanent residence under the Immigration and Nationality Act, and includes foreign corporations, international organizations, and foreign governments; (2) Foreign representative is anyone, regardless of nationality or citizenship, acting as an agent, representative, official, or employee of a foreign government, a foreign-owned or influenced firm, corporation or person; (3) Foreign sources are those sources (vendors, subcontractors, and suppliers) owned and controlled by a foreign person; and (b) The Contractor shall place a clause in subcontracts containing appropriate export control restrictions, set forth in this clause. (c) Nothing in this clause waives any requirement imposed by any other U.S. Government agency with respect to employment of foreign nationals or export controlled data and information. (d) Equipment and technical data generated or delivered under this contract are controlled by the International Traffic in Arms Regulation (ITAR), 22 CFR Sections 121 through 128. An export license is required before assigning any foreign source to perform work under this contract or before granting access to foreign persons to any equipment and technical data generated or delivered during performance

(see 22 CFR Section 125). The Contractor shall notify the Contracting Officer and obtain written approval of the Contracting Officer prior to assigning or granting access to any work, equipment, or technical data generated or delivered under this contract to foreign persons or their representatives. The notification shall include the name and country of origin of the foreign person or representative, the specific work, equipment, or data to which the person will have access, and whether the foreign person is cleared to have access to technical data (DoD 5220.22-M, National Industrial Security Program Operating Manual (NISPOM)). (End of clause)

At the time this award was accepted, the university's administration lacked an individual or office specifically tasked with export controls compliance. No one specifically alerted Dr Roth to his obligations to comply with these provisions. After using two foreign graduate students on the research project, Dr Roth sought assistance from a newly appointed export compliance officer. On review of the research contract, the university realized that export control violations could be occurring. They advised Dr Roth to remove all foreign nationals from the research and not to take any project-related data to China while on an upcoming trip. Ultimately, the university self-disclosed what it believed were violation of export controls to the Directorate of Defense Trade Controls (DDTC).

Dr Roth was charged with 17 criminal counts, including 15 counts of violating the Arms Export Control Act. At jury trial, Dr Roth was convicted on all counts, including one count of conspiracy, 15 counts of exporting defense articles and services without a license, and one count of wire fraud. Dr Roth appealed, focusing on whether the district court correctly instructed the jury on the meaning of the term "willfully" in the Arms Export Control Act, 22 U.S.C. 2778(c), in which the court required the jury to find that petitioner voluntarily and intentionally violated a known legal duty, but did not require the jury to find that petitioner knew that the exported items were on the USML, 22 C.F.R. 121.1. The Sixth Circuit Court of Appeals affirmed the district court ruling, and the US Supreme Court declined to hear the case [28].

Notably, the government stipulated at trial that national security had not been damaged. There was no evidence presented that Dr Roth (or anyone else) actually accessed the technical data he took out of the United States on his laptop. A DoD witness testifying at trial admitted that the research results likely would have been approved for public release. The original Broad Agency Announcement published by DoD specified that portions of the research were for dual-use applications, something that Dr Roth unsuccessfully asserted in his trial. After the conviction, Will Mackey, the assistant US attorney who had successfully prosecuted Dr Roth, sought to allay fears that aggressive investigations of universities were becoming an enforcement priority. Instead, Mackey asserted, "This is the first case in which there was something that was brought to our attention that seemed to rise to a level that we thought could be proved that amounted to an intentional violation."

Perhaps most importantly, the research was federally funded, and the award contained specific access and dissemination controls, as well as a conclusive statement that the research was subject to the ITAR and foreign nationals required approval. Thus, the research appears to have fallen squarely outside the protections of NSDD-189. The case demonstrates that in those instances in which a university or its researchers accept federal research funding that contains specific access and dissemination controls, the applicability of export controls is possible, if not probable.

# 5. RELEVANT REGULATORY/OVERSIGHT AGENCIES, REGULATIONS, AND GUIDANCE DOCUMENTS

The Bureau of Industry and Security (BIS) within the Department of Commerce is tasked with administering the provisions of the EAR, which is codified in 15 C.F.R. 730–774. Statutory authority for the EAR is found in the EAA, which has been expired since 2001. Issuance of executive orders has allowed the provisions of the EAA to be carried out under the authority of the International Emergency Economic Powers Act (IEEPA). The BIS Website has an online training room that provides a free Webinar on the topic of deemed exports [29]. Additionally, supplement one to part 734 of the EAR contains frequently asked questions on a number of topics important to universities, including publication, fundamental research, deemed exports, and federal contract controls [30].

The directorate of defense trade controls within the State Department is responsible for administering the provisions of the ITAR. The ITAR is codified in 22 C.F.R. 120–130 and is implemented under the statutory authority of the Arms Export Control Act.

The OFAC within the Treasury Department is responsible for administering the provisions of the Foreign Assets Control Regulations (FACR), which are economic and trade sanctions imposed by a variety of executive orders and statutes. The FACR is codified in 31 C.F.R. 500–599.

Investigations of export control violations can be conducted by a number of federal agencies, sometimes with overlapping jurisdiction. The Office of Export Enforcement (OEE) is somewhat unique in that it is a federal law enforcement agency tasked solely with enforcing the EAR. For example, OEE agents are authorized to pursue criminal and administrative penalties and have the authority to issue subpoenas, execute search warrants, and seize goods [31].

In contrast, other federal agencies have broader investigatory authority that includes specific provisions of export controls. Customs and Border Protection (CBP) agents can investigate and seize illegal shipments, Immigration and Customs Enforcement can investigate visa violations, and the FBI has the authority to investigate counterintelligence matters, including economic espionage, theft of trade secrets (either of which may involve export controlled technologies), and violations of export control and intellectual property statutes [32].

## 5.1 Export Enforcement Coordination Fusion Center

Executive Order 13,558 created the Export Enforcement Coordination Center (E2C2), a multiagency center tasked with coordinating export control investigations [33]. Representatives from the enforcement agencies identified above, as well as from OFAC, DDTC, the National Nuclear Security Administration (NNSA), DoD, and others, coordinate their efforts in export control investigations, licensing, and outreach.

# 6. REGULATORY MANDATES

University export control programs maintain comprehensive policies that serve to both affirm the institution's commitment to fully complying with US Export Controls and Regulations and address those specific regulatory mandates that are identified as posing a high risk of requiring a license from the appropriate federal agency. In particular, universities must be cognizant of export regulations governing not only physical exports, but also the transfer of controlled technical information to foreign persons either in the United States or abroad. Additionally, universities must take care that activities, including travel, do not violate current OFAC sanctions, which prohibit certain transactions based on national policy concerns.

## 6.1 Physical Exports

It is well established that physical exportation of items identified on the CCL or USML is a regulated activity. OFAC sanctions may further regulate the physical export of items not found on either control list. Prior to physically exporting items or equipment, universities must determine whether or not a license is required for exportation. This includes classifying the item and determining where the item is being sent, to whom, and for what purpose [34].

If an item is determined to be subject to the ITAR, the university, as the shipper of record, must apply for a license from the Department of State. The license application requires that the university be registered with the DDTC and provide detailed information about the item, who will be using the item, and how it will be shipped to its destination. Similarly, if an item is controlled by the EAR (even those designated to be EAR99), a license may be required depending on the end-user or end-use. Shipping an item to an embargoed or sanctioned country may also necessitate a license under the applicable OFAC regulations.

It is important to note that physical exports do not have to be shipped; they can also be hand-carried out of the country or, in the case of controlled information, transmitted electronically to another country. Temporary exports of items subject to the EAR, either via shipment or hand-carry, may qualify for an exception from the licensing requirements, depending on the type of item, destination, duration of time and primary use while abroad, and whether the item will remain in the control of the US person taking or shipping such item.

## 6.2 Deemed Exports

In addition to restricting physical exports and transmissions, both the EAR and the ITAR include restrictions on deemed exports of controlled technology and related information. Under the EAR, any release of technology or source code subject to the EAR to a foreign national in the United States is deemed to be an "export" to the home country of the foreign national. "Technology" is defined as specific information necessary for the development, production, or use of a product controlled by the Commerce Department for export. Under the ITAR, the concept of deemed exports is described as disclosing technical data, which include any information required for the design, development, production, manufacture, assembly, operation, repair, testing, maintenance, or modification of defense articles, to a foreign person either in the United States or abroad [35]. "Technical data," as defined under the ITAR, expressly include classified information and information covered by a secrecy order, as well as software directly related to a defense article.

In a university setting, a deemed export may occur when a foreign national participates in a research project or program that involves export-controlled technology or technical data.

As set forth in NSDD-189, not all federally funded research qualifies as fundamental research and for exclusion from the applicable export regulations [36]. Universities should carefully review federally funded research awards for any attempt to place proprietary or national security restrictions on research results, because such restrictions will preclude application of the fundamental research exemption. If the funding instrument contains such restrictions and their removal cannot be successfully negotiated, the university is responsible for reviewing the award and determining the export control implications or more specifically, if an export control license will be required. While, by definition, restricted research is subject to regulation, depending on the activity and subject matter involved, the project may not involve export-controlled technical data or technology and therefore may not trigger any license requirements. If the project does involve controlled information and the university desires to involve any foreign nationals in the research, a license from the Department of Commerce or State may be required.

## 6.3 Defense Services

The ITAR defines a "defense service" as the provision of assistance (including training) or technical data to a foreign national anywhere in the United States or abroad in the connection with the design, development, engineering, manufacture, production, assembly, testing, repair, maintenance, modification, operation, demilitarization, destruction, processing, or use of a defense article [37]. Technical data as defined by the ITAR do not include information concerning general scientific or engineering principles commonly taught in schools, colleges, and other universities [38] or data that are in the public domain [39]. Defense services also include informal collaborations, conversations, or interchanges concerning technical data. It is worth noting that technical assistance using only public-domain information could still be considered a defense service, if it involves the integration of an ITAR-controlled component.

As of the date of this publication, proposed revisions to the definition of defense services would significantly limit the possibility of providing defense services with public-domain information. The proposed changes, which were published in April 2011, would redefine defense services in relevant part as follows:

1. The furnishing of assistance (including training) using other than public-domain data to foreign persons (see §120.16 of this subchapter), whether in the United States or abroad, in the design, development, engineering, manufacture, production, assembly, testing, intermediate or depot-level repair or maintenance (see §120.38 of this subchapter), modification, demilitarization, destruction or processing of defense articles (see §120.6 of this subchapter); or
2. The furnishing of assistance to foreign persons, whether in the United States or abroad, for the integration of any item controlled on the U.S. Munitions List (USML) (see §121.1 of this subchapter) or the Commerce Control List (see 15 CFR part 774) into an end item (see §121.8(a) of this subchapter) or component (see §121.8(b) of this subchapter) that is controlled as a defense article on the USML, regardless of the origin [40].

Notably, it appears that defense services could still be provided with public-domain information if integration activities are involved, because the phrase "using other than public domain data" was omitted from the second paragraph.

## 6.4 Office of Foreign Assets Control Sanctions

Determined based on foreign policy concerns, OFAC sanctions vary significantly from country to country and may include partial or total embargoes against certain countries, groups, or individuals [41]. These economic and trade sanctions generally apply to the activities of "U.S. persons" wherever located and broadly restrict financial transactions, travel, and general services involving the sanctioned country. As previously noted, OFAC sanctions may control the exportation of physical items, regardless of whether or not an item is on the USML or CCL.

One of the most difficult challenges for universities is the dissimilar application of sanctions across countries and the speed at which such sanctions can change or be updated. It is therefore crucial that universities remain cognizant of those countries currently under sanction, in addition to being aware of any export controls imposed under the EAR of the ITAR.

In addition to the country-specific sanctions programs, OFAC also maintains and publishes a list of individuals and companies owned or controlled by, or acting for or on behalf of, sanctioned countries, as well as individuals, groups, and entities designated under sanctions programs that are not country-specific [42]. Collectively, these individuals, groups and companies are referred to as "Specially Designated Nationals" or "SDNs." Universities and all other US persons are prohibited from doing business with any SDN without a license or specific government approval [43].

## 6.5 Other Considerations

### 6.5.1 Restricted Parties

In addition to the SDN, universities must be aware of additional agency-driven restricted parties lists, including the Denied Persons List, the Entity List, and the Unverified List, each of which are maintained by BIS, as well as the Department of State's Debarred Parties lists and those related to nonproliferation sanctions [44].

#### 6.5.1.1 BIS LISTS

Individuals and entities on the Denied Persons List have had their export privileges revoked or suspended by BIS. No exports to listed persons are permitted for the period of the denial, including any dealings with denied persons that involve items subject to the EAR [44]. The Entity List, which is also maintained by BIS, comprises those individuals and entities, including a number of universities and research institutions, identified as being involved in proliferation of missile technology, weapons of mass destruction, and related technologies. Participation by a university in any transactions with such persons may trigger licensing requirements supplemental to those found elsewhere in the EAR [45]. While transactions with parties on BIS's Unverified List are not barred, listed persons are ineligible to receive items controlled under the EAR by means of a license exception. Special due diligence is required prior to engaging with such entities, even when no license is required.

#### 6.5.1.2 STATE DEPARTMENT LISTS

Entities on either the Statutorily Debarred Parties or Administratively Debarred Parties lists compiled by the State Department cannot participate directly or indirectly in the export of defense articles, including technical data, or in the furnishing of defense services, for which a license or approval is required by the ITAR [46]. Listed parties include those individuals and entities who have been convicted of violating or conspiring to violate the AECA, or who have been debarred on a case-by-case basis as the result of enforcement proceedings arising from a violation of the AECA or the ITAR. Additionally, the State Department may impose nonproliferation sanctions against foreign individuals, entities, and governments that engage in nuclear proliferation activities.

### 6.5.2 Antiboycott Regimes

The United States maintains two separate antiboycott regimes managed by the Department of Commerce, as set forth in the EAR [47] and the Department of Treasury, as codified in the Internal Revenue Code [48]. While these laws were originally drafted to discourage US entities from furthering or supporting the boycott of Israel sponsored by the Arab League, they broadly apply to all boycotts imposed by foreign countries that are unsanctioned by the United States. The antiboycott laws and regulations prohibit or penalize cooperation with international economic boycotts in which the United States does not participate and effectively prevent US entities from being used to implement foreign agendas that are in conflict with US policy [50].

The Treasury Department requires individuals and organizations to report services performed in, with, or related to a boycotting country on the Treasury Department list. Similarly, the Commerce Department requires a quarterly report disclosing any requests to advance an unsanctioned foreign boycott. University programs that conduct any activities or business transactions in one of these countries should coordinate with their appropriate institutional tax officials to complete the reporting requirements [50,51].

### 6.5.3 Prohibited End Use

Part 744 of the EAR contains a catchall category of activities and transactions that may require a license even if other provisions of the EAR are inapplicable, including a provision for regulated activities "unrelated to exports" [49]. Thus, while the types of issues described in part 744 would likely only be encountered on rare occasion, this part has the ability to encompass activities or transactions in an academic setting that would not otherwise be subject to the EAR. Additionally, under part 744, BIS may inform persons, personally through specific notice, through an amendment to the EAR, or through a notice published in the Federal Register, that a given activity or transaction at hand requires a license. For these reasons, any analysis of the applicability of export controls should include the restrictions and licensing requirements contained in this part.

## 7. KEY PERSONNEL AND UNIVERSITY COMMITTEES

In December 2006, the US Government Accountability Office (GAO) released a report titled "EXPORT CONTROLS: Agencies Should Assess Vulnerabilities and Improve Guidance for Protecting Export-Controlled Information at Universities" that focused primarily on research activity and the foreign national population within the university community [52]. Although the extensive investigation that served as the basis for the report did not uncover any export violations at the university level, the report resulted in specific instructions to the Departments of State and Commerce "to improve their oversight of export-controlled information at universities...and direct their export control entities to strategically assess potential vulnerabilities in the conduct and publication of academic research through analyzing available information on technology development and foreign student populations at universities" [52].

Given the fact that a notable amount of university activity subject to export control compliance is research related, oversight of export control compliance has typically resided in a university's academic research office or, even more locally, in the office of sponsored programs. Despite the specific instructions that came out of the GAO report, the report's narrow focus did little to encourage universities to broaden the scope of their compliance regimes. Today, many resources remain in the research arm of the institution, which then consults with procurement, legal, travel, and human resources personnel as necessary to address compliance issues. However, because many of the liabilities stemming from export controls are admittedly not tied to research funding (physical exportation, visa issues, visiting scholars, international travel (including travel to Cuba), etc.), universities may opt to address export controls through the provost, office of legal counsel, and/or office of the president. Regardless of the structure of the office or administrative unit ultimately responsible for export controls, universities will rely on a network of individuals and offices to address these issues.

## 7.1 Sponsored Programs

Historically, most university programs have been housed administratively within research and/or sponsored programs, due primarily to the 2006 GAO report. Another contributing factor to this trend was the criminal prosecution of a University of Tennessee Knoxville professor for violations of export controls, described earlier in this chapter [28].

After Dr Roth's conviction, and in light of the GAO report, many universities justifiably turned their attention and resources to screening research awards. Sponsored research continues to create significant export control liability. Having a qualified and experienced export control officer involved in sponsored research efforts continues to be a "must-have" for most universities with sponsored research.

## 7.2 University Export Control Officer

Key to a university's compliance program is the role of university export control officer (ECO). Such individual has the authority and the responsibility for the implementation of export control policies and procedures throughout the university, rendering training and advice to faculty and staff in all export-related matters. Working closely with academic units and researchers, the ECO is responsible for identifying areas impacted by export control regulations and developing both general control procedures and protocol for specific university activities. The ECO monitors legislation and regulatory changes to ensure trainings and procedures remain up to date. The ECO may also be involved in the legal review and drafting of license applications and in the preparation of other regulatory submissions as required.

## 7.3 Empowered Official

An empowered official (EO) is the person designated by a university to represent the institution before export control regulators in matters related to registration, licensing, and other requests, including commodity jurisdiction requests and voluntary disclosures. The individual must be a US person and must be directly employed by the university in a position having authority for policy or management. He or she must further understand the provisions and requirements of the various export control statutes and regulations and the criminal liability, civil liability, and administrative penalties for violating the AECA and the ITAR [53].

Importantly, the EO must have the "independent authority" to inquire into "any aspect" of proposed exports, verify the legality of the transaction and the accuracy of the information involved, and withhold signature on applications or other approvals "without prejudice or other adverse recourse." This degree of authority and autonomy can be challenging to find in a university setting. In particular, few positions within a university can require access to all documents, records, and personnel that may hold information relevant to the legality or accuracy of the export transaction(s) at hand. Additionally, the ITAR requires that a refusal to provide authorization must be made "without prejudice or adverse recourse." Because export controls can often be perceived as costly to universities (not just in terms of liability, but also in terms of lost opportunities when research funding is turned away due to export control considerations), it is critical to designate individuals who would not be in a conflicted position if a decision to turn down revenue or assets (external research funding, donations of property and equipment, etc.) needs to be made.

## 7.4 University Export Control Committee

Due to the decentralized nature of universities, some institutions have adopted a committee-based approach to export control compliance. A university's export control committee is generally staffed by key stakeholders from various academic units and research offices, including the office of sponsored programs and the office of general counsel, and reports into the ECO or the university compliance office. The goal of the committee is to facilitate communication throughout the university community on the importance of export control compliance and to disseminate up-to-date information in a consistent manner. Additionally, committee members serve as (or have direct access to) the front lines of export-related activity, including travel, billing, shipping, and hiring activity. The idea is that committee members are in the strongest position to assist in the identification of potentially controlled activity and ensure that researchers are able to leverage the correct university resources in dealing with any issues that may arise. Although there are benefits to the committee model, many institutions do not use such a model and choose a more streamlined approach to export compliance. The successes and challenges for this model depend on the specific institution and risk allocations related to compliance and should only be a consideration when creating an export compliance program.

## 7.5 International Travel Office

Export control regulations are not triggered by the shipping of items or the transfer of technical information alone. Travel by university actors can also trigger the application of export control regulations, particularly when personnel are traveling with equipment or technology.

Licensing requirements are based on the type of items, destination, and ultimate purpose for transporting such items. For example, electronic devices that contain encryption technology or certain other software are subject to export controls. US Customs officials have the authority to search and seize any devices from US individuals traveling internationally and assess the information contained on such devices for potential export control violations. Many universities encourage employees traveling on university business to coordinate such activity through a centralized office so that country-specific travel information and guidance, including with respect to export control issues, may be provided. Such information may include entry and visa requirements, security warnings and regulatory guidance, as well as more general health and safety facts, including a list of country-specific restricted parties.

## 7.6 Other Important Offices and Resources

Even the most robust export compliance program relies on the resources and expertise from other university offices for day-to-day export control functions.

Physical exports of equipment represent a large portion of university export licensing activity. Further, violations of applicable regulations may result in prosecution of the university as an actor and not an individual researcher. The University of Massachusetts Lowell was fined $100,000 for shipping an EAR99 atmospheric testing device to Pakistan without a license [54]. Although EAR99 technology is a permitted export to Pakistan, the receiver was identified on the Commerce Department's Entity List as ineligible to receive any items subject to the EAR.

A university's centralized shipping office and/or formalized shipping procedures can aid in ensuring compliance with Foreign Trade Regulation requirements for physical exports, as well in identifying license requirements under the EAR and the ITAR. In addition to aiding with import compliance, the centralized procurement office may also assist in providing up-to-date information regarding OFAC trade embargoes and restricted party lists. A university's office of environmental health and safety may further provide specific resources on the shipping and receiving of biological, hazardous, and/or radioactive materials.

Due to the addition of a question concerning export control licenses on the US Citizenship and Immigration Service (USCIS) Form I-129, a university's office of international students or the equivalent is also now involved in export compliance. All US employers must complete Form I-129 when petitioning for a foreign worker to come to the United States temporarily to perform services under an H1-B visa or another specialty occupation visa [55]. As a result of the added question, university employers must now certify whether or not the proposed employee will require a deemed export license during the course of his or her employment at the university. Universities should seek specific information about the scope of work to be performed and any laboratories that an employee may be entering to analyze the potential for deemed export licenses. This requirement has been heavily scrutinized by the academic community due to the fact that USCIS has no responsibility for export control enforcement [56], and it is unlikely that the scope of work at the time of the visa application remains inert throughout an employee's tenure. The USCIS has clarified that the certification is to be based on the scope of work and deemed export licensing requirements at the time of visa application. Thus, for an employee who did not require a deemed export license initially, but later encounters a deemed export licensing requirement (due, e.g., to regulatory changes or modifications to the employee's scope of work or job responsibilities), the initial certification that no deemed export license is required remains valid and appropriate. The employer would need to obtain a deemed export license for the employee's work going forward, but there is no need to modify the initial visa application.

## 8. COMMON COMPLIANCE CHALLENGES

Export control regulations present unique challenges for universities as they strive to balance concerns about national security and regulatory compliance with traditional concepts of academic freedom and the unrestricted dissemination of research findings and results through publication. Below are some common issues encountered when analyzing and implementing export control laws and regulations.

### 8.1 Misapplication of the Fundamental Research Exemption or Exclusion

One of the biggest challenges for university export control programs is the misconception that all research and other university activity conducted on a university campus is exempt from export control regulation. This misconception is fueled by the reliance by universities on the fundamental research exemption or exclusion ("FRE"), which is codified in both the EAR [57] and the ITAR [39]. Although the FRE covers a wide scope of university activity, the application of the FRE is limited in many instances. For example, the FRE would not be applicable when dealing with: physical exports; use of a research sponsor's controlled proprietary technical data that are restricted from publication; use of certain encrypted software; research or other activity conducted abroad; the receipt of classified information, or the classification of research results; research with no intention to be published or that contains restrictions on publication; or research that restricts the involvement of foreign persons. The FRE would also not be applicable to research that was funded under a US government agency contract containing specific access and dissemination controls. The most common clauses restrict participation by foreign nationals on the sponsored project or restrict the university from disclosing information or results about the project.

Accordingly, the results of restricted research may be subject to control under the ITAR or the EAR. It is important to note that in both examples listed below, either the university or the researcher could accept restrictions that would invalidate the FRE. Side deals or other agreements beyond the scope of the final contract can constitute a publication restriction or access controls.

### 8.2 Faculty Travel

Faculty at many universities are afforded significant autonomy and discretion when planning and participating in international travel. This degree of independence can pose unique challenges from an export control perspective, because universities may not have notice of travel to another country until after the travel has occurred. Consequently, the university's ability to address licensing requirements is understandably limited. Many university training programs have focused on this vulnerability, particularly with activity that poses a significant chance of requiring a license, for example, travel to Cuba, Iran, North Korea, Sudan, or Syria and/or travel with university-owned equipment or research samples.

## 8.3 Global Research

Universities are increasingly going global. While research has traditionally been conducted at campuses in the United States, multinational collaborative research efforts are becoming the norm. While export controls have been crafted to avoid regulation of fundamental research, the applicability of these provisions to fundamental research being performed abroad has been questioned. The EAR notes that it is the type of research, particularly the intent and freedom to publish, that is dispositive of the fundamental research characterization. Institutional locus is not controlling [58].

The ITAR does not contain similar provisions, and many feel that the institutional locus of the research is relevant when analyzing fundamental research under the ITAR. Additionally, sanctions regulate the exportation of services to certain countries [59], and it remains unsettled whether this might include fundamental research activities.

## 8.4 Decentralization

A key challenge for many universities is the decentralized nature of their operations and activities. Implementing export compliance functions can be a daunting responsibility when many university functions that lead to regulated exports are decentralized and spread across many academic units, administrative offices, and even campuses. For example, while some universities have a centralized shipping office, the reality is that there is unlikely to be an all-encompassing requirement that all university personnel use the shipping office for international shipments. Consequently, tracking international shipments (noted above as a significant potential source of licensing requirements) is inherently decentralized. Benchmarking with other universities that share similar operations and risk tolerance can be used to support the development of an export compliance program while engaging key offices and stakeholders throughout the university. Elements of the compliance program as described above combined with a robust training resources go a long way in reducing risk and creating best practices.

# 9. ADDRESSING NONCOMPLIANCE

Monitoring and conducting internal audits of existing compliance programs is key to maintaining a successful program. Since September 11, 2001, government agencies have dramatically increased the investigation and successful prosecution of export regulation violations and, as previously mentioned, have focused much of their effort on the academic community. The penalties for these violations can be severe, including personal liability, monetary fines, and imprisonment. Any university individual who suspects a violation has occurred should immediately notify the university's designated point of contact for export control issues. The university should conduct an internal review of the suspected violation by gathering information about the circumstances, personnel, items, and communications involved. Universities may choose to use in-house counsel or external counsel to direct this review and to determine whether a violation of university policy and/or federal regulation has occurred.

During the investigatory stage, the university may decide to provide an initial notification about the suspected violation to the appropriate government agency [60]. If a violation has in fact occurred, the activity must be stopped immediately, next steps must be outlined, and a communication strategy must be put in place to ensure that any affected employees understand what, if any, details regarding the suspected violation may be shared or discussed. If an initial notification has occurred, the university should follow up with a formal voluntary disclosure made in accordance with the statutory requirements related to the violation. Both the State and Commerce Departments consider such disclosures a mitigating factor in the event an export control violation is determined to have occurred.

ITAR violations should be initially disclosed to the Directorate of Defense Trade Controls [61] immediately after a violation is discovered and followed by a written statement confirming: (1) a precise description of the nature and extent of the violation (e.g., an unauthorized shipment, doing business with a party denied US export privileges, etc.); (2) the exact circumstances surrounding the violation (including a thorough explanation of why, when, where, and how the violation occurred); (3) the complete identities and addresses of all persons known or suspected to be involved in the activities giving rise to the violation (including mailing, shipping, and email addresses, telephone and fax/facsimile numbers, and any other known identifying information); (4) Department of State license numbers, exemption citation, or description of any other authorization, if applicable; (5) the USML category and subcategory, product description, quantity, and characteristics or technological capability of the hardware, technical data or defense service involved; (6) a description of corrective actions already undertaken that clearly identifies the new compliance initiatives implemented to address the causes of the violations set forth in the voluntary disclosure, as well as any internal disciplinary action taken, and how these corrective actions are designed to deter those particular violations from occurring again; and (7) the name and address of the person making the disclosure and a point of contact, if different, should further information be needed [61].

Voluntary disclosures under the EAR are narrative in nature and should include an explanation of the internal review conducted and the measures that are being taken to minimize the likelihood that violations will occur in the future. The narrative account should include: (1) the kind of violation involved (e.g., a shipment without the required license, or dealing with a party denied export privileges); (2) an explanation of when and how the violations occurred; (3) the complete identities and addresses of all individuals and organizations, whether foreign or domestic, involved in the activities giving rise to the violations; (4) license numbers, if applicable; (5) the description, quantity, value in US dollars, and the Export Control Classification Number from the CCL or other classification of the items involved; (6) a description of any mitigating circumstances; and (7) all supporting documentation, such as, but not limited to, licenses, license applications, import certificates, and end-user statements, shipper's export declarations, air waybills and bills of lading, and other backup documentation [60].

Although less prescriptive than the Commerce or State Department, the Treasury Department encourages self-disclosure and likewise considers such disclosure a mitigating factor in the event of a violation. A self-disclosure should be in the form of a detailed letter sent, along with any supporting documentation, to the current director, Office of Foreign Assets Control, US Department of the Treasury, 1500 Pennsylvania Ave., N.W., Washington, DC 20220 [62]. While no blanket amnesty is provided by OFAC in the case of violation, the violation is reviewed using a totality of the circumstances standard, with consideration given to the quality of the entity's OFAC compliance program.

After a formal disclosure has been submitted, the university should wait for instructions from the relevant agency. The agency will determine either that there was no violation or that a violation has occurred, at which time the agency and the university will either receive a cautionary statement regarding compliance or a request to enter into settlement agreement negotiations. While, as noted above, voluntary disclosures are considered a mitigating factor in determining appropriate penalties, such disclosures do affect a university's reputation and may result in increased regulatory scrutiny, even when a violation is not affirmed.

Universities should consider establishing clear disciplinary action for those employees who decide to work with export-controlled data to prepare for a possible violation. An escalating scale of action can be used internally whether or not a formal disclosure occurs and could include targeted training, removal from current and future restricted research activities, written improvement plans linked to performance review and/or tenure review, and/or termination. Of course, the goal of any export control compliance program should be to prepare (or prevent) a violation before it occurs. The policies and procedures described herein present a well-rounded approach to university export control compliance that balances the risks of noncompliance with the openness and free interchange of information that is paramount to the academic community.

## References

[1] Arms Export Control Act, 22 U.S.C. § 2778, implemented by the International Traffic in Arms Regulations, 22 C.F.R. §§; 120–130; 1976.

[2] Export Administration Act, 50 U.S.C. App § 2401, implemented by the Export Administration Regulations, 15 C.F.R. §§ 730–774; 1979. [Note: On August 20, 2001, the EAA expired, and since that time, the EAR has been administered under the statutory authority of the International Emergency Economic Powers Act, Pub. L. No. 95-223, Exec. Order No. 13222, 3 C.F.R. 13,222(2002).]

[3] In August of 1977, a group of cryptography researchers received a letter stating that publishing in their field of study and participating in an open conference would violate the AECA and ITAR. See Shapley, D. and Kolata, G. Cryptology: Scientists Puzzle Over Threat to Open Research, Publication. Science September 30, 1977:1345. The interpretation of the ITAR set forth in the letter at issue was later refuted by the deputy director of the Office of Munitions Control at the State Department, who stated, "Publications and material available to the public are exempt from export control rules." See also Brown, M. Scientists Accuse Security Agency of Harassment Over Code Studies. The New York Times. October 18, 1977.

[4] The DOJ advised the science advisor to the President, Dr. Frank Press, "It is our view that the existing provisions of the ITAR are unconstitutional insofar as they establish a prior restraint on disclosure of cryptographic ideas and information developed by scientists and mathematicians in the private sector." OLC Memorandum to Frank Press, May 11, 1978, reprinted in The Government's Classification of Private Ideas: Hearings Before A Subcomm. Of the House Comm. On Gov't Operations, 96th Cong., 2nd Sess. 268 (1980) [Hereinafter Hearing Transcript.]

[5] 579 F.2d 516 (9th Cir. 1978).

[6] "[I]t appears that the government would have difficulty prohibiting the export of cryptographic information for scientific purposes…Thus, while the Ninth Circuit's decision is helpful in resolving First Amendment issues [because it takes a narrow construction]…we do not believe that it either resolves the First Amendment issues presented by restrictions on the export of cryptographic ideas or eliminates the need to reexamine the ITAR." See August 29, 1978, letter to Colonel Wayne Kay, Office of Science and Technology Policy, available via Hearing Transcript.

[7] Cryptography/Technical Data. Munitions Control Newsletter, Number 80, February 1980 published by Office of Munitions Control, U.S. Department of State.

[8] Hearing Transcript, supra at 705, "Concern has been voiced that ITAR provisions relating to export of technical data as applied to cryptologic equipment can be so broadly interpreted as to restrict scientific exchanges of basic mathematical and engineering research data…[The ITAR controls do] not include general mathematical engineering or statistical information, not purporting to have or reasonably expected to be given direct application to equipment in such categories. It does not include basic theoretical research data. It does, however, include algorithms and other procedures purporting to have advanced cryptologic application. The public is reminded that professional and academic presentations and information discussions, as well as demonstrations of equipment, constituting disclosure of cryptologic technical data to foreign nationals are prohibited without the prior approval of this office. Approval is not required for publication of data within the U.S. as described in 125.11(a)(1). Footnote 3 does not establish a prepublication review requirement."

[9] 5 U.S. Op. Off Legal Counsel 202; 1981.

[10] 5 U.S. Op. Off Legal Counsel 230, "The requirement to obtain a license applies a prior restraint to protected speech and is thus impermissible except in the most compelling circumstances. For example, we do not believe that the courts would uphold a requirement that a professor obtain a license before 'releasing' information to foreign students simply because the information may be used in the overhaul of certain kinds of computer chips. The same considerations suggest that an American scientist could not be barred in advance from informing his colleagues, some of whom are foreign nationals, of the results of an experiment that could help produce some other high technology item. Other examples could readily be imagined. In more general terms, the regulations cover a wide variety of speech that is constitutionally protected. We believe that they should therefore be substantially narrowed." 1981.

[11] Norman C. Supercomputer restrictions pose problems for NSF, Universities. Science July 1985;229:148.

[12] Goodwin I. APS Opposes proposed restrictions on NSF supercomputers. Phys Today December 1985;38(12):53.

[13] Kolata G. Export Control Threat Disrupts Meeting. Science September 1982;217:1233. Norman, C. Security Problems Plague Scientific Meeting. Science April 1985; 228: 471. Burnham, D. Pentagon Acts to Curb Science Parley Papers. New York Times. April 8, 1985. Sect. A15.

[14] Gast AP. The impact of restricting information access on science and technology. AAU. Massachusetts Institute of Technology, Vice-President for Research; 2003.

[15] 8 U.S. Op. Off. Legal Counsel, 7, 8.

[16] Panel on Scientific Communication and National Security Committee on Science, Engineering, and Public Policy National Academy of Sciences National Academy of Engineering Institute of Medicine. Scientific Communication and National Security. Report; 1982.

[17] Defense Science Board Task Force on Export of U.S. Technology, an Analyis of Export Control of U.S. Technology—A DOD Perspective (1976) (hereinafter the "Bucy Report"). The Bucy Report noted that while export controls had traditionally not been applied to university activity, the report recommended that scientific exchanges and training of citizens from communist countries should be controlled. pp. 38–39.

[18] Draft Executive Order 12,356 which attempted to relax the criteria for national security classification by omitting an exclusion for basic research. See Executive Order on Security Classification: Hearings Before a Subcomm. of the House Comm. on Government Operations, 97th Cong. 2d Sess. 241 (1982). The final version of the EO had the exclusion for basic research reinserted.

[19] [Online]. Available from: http://fas.org/irp/offdocs/nsdd/nsdd-189.htm.

[20] The 1984 DAA allowed the DoD to exempt from public disclosure via the Freedom of Information Act (FOIA) any unclassified technical data that it considered "sensitive." The DoD's implementation of this new authority included the ability to label documents under its control as containing export controlled technical data, effectively controlling the dissemination of those documents.

[21] Pub. L. No. 96–107, 93 Stat. 803 (1979); See H.R. Conf. Rep. No. 546, 96th Cong., 1st Sess. 1979.

[22] Dickson S. Academe Ponders Defense Curbs on Research, 11 SCI & GOV'T REP. 5, 5. March 1981.

[23] Atomic Energy Act of 1954, 42 U.S.C. § 2011.

[24] Invention Secrecy Act of 1951, 35 U.S.C. §§ 181–188.

[25] U.S. Congressional Research Service, The Export Administration Act: Evolution, Provisions, and Debate, (RL31832) May 5, 2005. See p. 18, "Deemed Exports are not expressly mentioned in the 1979 EAA. House versions of the EAA in the 107th Congress sought to explicitly define deemed export as exports falling under the jurisdiction of the act." [The language ultimately was not included.]

[26] Section 12 of the 1979 EAA: "It is the policy of the United States to sustain vigorous scientific enterprise. To do so involves sustaining the ability of scientists and other scholars freely to communicate research findings, in accordance with the applicable provisions of law, by means of publication, teaching, conferences, and other forms of scholarly exchange."

[27] 61 Fed. Reg. 58. See Sec. 730.5 "Coverage of more than exports." March 25, 1996.

[28] *United States v. John Reece Roth*, 628 F.3d 827 (6th Cir. 2011).

[29] [Online]. Available from: http://www.bis.doc.gov/index.php/compliance-a-training/export-administration-regulations-training/online-training-room?id=289.

[30] [Online]. Available from: http://www.bis.doc.gov/index.php/forms-documents/doc_view/412-part-734-scope-of-the-export-administration-regulations.

[31] [Online]. Available from: http://www.bis.doc.gov/index.php/enforcement/oee.

[32] [Online]. Available from: http://www.cbp.gov/.

[33] [Online]. Available from: http://www.ice.gov/eecc.

[34] 31 C.F.R. §§; 500–599.

[35] [Online]. Available from: http://www.pmddtc.state.gov/regulations_laws/itar.html.

[36] National Security Decision Directive 189 National Policy on the Transfer of Scientific, Technical and Engineering Information; 1985.

[37] 22 C.F.R. § 120.9.

[38] 22 C.F.R. § 120.10.

[39] 22 C.F.R. § 120.11.

[40] 76 Fed. Reg. 20592. April 13, 2011.

[41] [Online]. Available from: http://www.treasury.gov/about/organizational-structure/offices/Pages/Office-of-Foreign-Assets-Control.aspx.

[42] [Online]. Available from: http://www.treasury.gov/resource-center/.

[43] [Online]. Available from: http://www.treasury.gov/resource-center/sanctions/SDN-List/.

[44] [Online]. Available from: http://www.bis.doc.gov/Enforcement/UnverifiedList/unverified_parties.html.

[45] [Online]. Available from: http://www.bis.doc.gov/Entities/Default.htm.

[46] [Online]. Available from: http://www.pmddtc.state.gov/compliance/debar_intro.html.

[47] 15 C.F.R. Part 760.

[48] 26 U.S.C. § 999.

[49] 15 C.F.R. § 744.6(a)(2).

[50] [Online]. Available from: http://www.bis.doc.gov/index.php/enforcement/oac.

[51] [Online]. Available from: http://www.irs.gov/pub/irs-pdf/i5713.pdf.

[52] Export Controls: Agencies Should Assess Vulnerabilities and Improve Guidance for Protecting Export-Controlled Information at Universities, Government Accountability Office. 2006.

[53] 22 C.F.R. § 120.25.

[54] [Online]. Available from: http://efoia.bis.doc.gov/exportcontrolviolations/E2306.PDF.

[55] [Online]. Available from: http://www.uscis.gov/i-129.

[56] Anthony Decrappeo D.K.J.T.T.L.S. Reforming Regulation of Research Universities. Issues in Science and Technology. 2011.

[57] 15 C.F.R. § 734.8.

[58] 15 C.F.R. § 744 Supplement 2, FAQ D(8).

[59] As of publication these countries include Cuba, Iran, North Korea, Sudan, and Syria.

[60] For EAR violations, see 15 C.F.R. § 764.5; For ITAR violations, see 22 C.F.R. § 127.12(c).

[61] 22 C.F.R. § 127.12.

[62] [Online]. Available from: http://www.treasury.gov/resource-center/faqs/Sanctions/Pages/answer.aspx.

# Data Management and Research Integrity

*Shannon Wapole, David A. Stone*
**Northern Illinois University, DeKalb, IL, USA**

## 1. INTRODUCTION

Data management has always been central to the entire scientific research enterprise. Scientific progress depends on the ability to reproduce, extend, and challenge scientific findings. These activities all require that research, whether experiments or field studies, be properly documented in their procedures, processes, and findings. The scientific community further requires that these documents and other artifacts of scientific discovery be properly stored and managed to maintain their propriety, and that they be functionally accessible. In these ways, data management is understood to be central to the responsible conduct of research (RCR).

But over the past decade, the need for data management has taken on a new character and with it a new urgency. The capacity to produce and reduce scientific data to digital form has ushered in a completely new scientific era from the standpoint of data management. The dawning of this era was recognized in the United States by the National Science Foundation (NSF) at the turn of the new century and heralded by the release of two reports in 2003 that recognized the urgency of addressing the growing need for what was termed "cyberinfrastructure" for the collection, storage, archiving, and sharing of the vast quantities of digital data that science was producing and expected to produce in the future [1]. A decade later, the White House issued an executive order calling on all of the major federal research funding agencies to put forward more robust plans that allow for the retention and sharing of research data and the public availability of federally funded research findings [2]. It is therefore important for researchers, research office personnel, and library and information technology staff to understand the general rules of data management, the roles of researchers in regard to data management, the need to develop and implement data management plans, and how to ensure compliance with data management regulations.

In 2003, the National Institutes of Health (NIH) also responded to the need to address calls for data management, data sharing, and increased access to research results by issuing a data sharing policy and requiring applicants for large grants to submit data management plans with their applications [3]. Since then, the regulatory environment for data management is undergoing constant change. As big data and collaboration become scientific watchwords, regulations directly addressing data management are evolving, and are expected to become more comprehensive with time. Most federal agencies that fund the creation and use of data already have data management regulations, but as the nature of technology and the ways we use data change, these requirements can be expected to change to keep pace.

This chapter will provide researchers and research office personnel with a basis for understanding the current regulatory environment and its likely trajectory following the latest executive orders on data management of open access. In addition, because data management is now a research compliance matter, the chapter will also provide information on common compliance challenges and the role data management practices play in issues related to research integrity and scientific misconduct. As such, this chapter does not address other matters, such as the development of national and international data management tools, repositories, and other infrastructure supports, issues related to resources for implementation of data management plans, the need for training in the area of data management, or other issues that are important to addressing data management.

## 2. HISTORICAL PERSPECTIVES

### 2.1 Current Changes in Federal Agencies

#### 2.1.1 National Institutes of Health

The federal focus on issues related to data management arose as a confluence of matters relating to the safeguarding of the collection of unique and costly data; the need for data sharing to promote replication, extension, and innovation; and the desire to ensure that results of scientific research be made as widely available as possible to both the research community and the public at large. The NIH was the first institution to respond to these calls with regulations regarding data sharing [3]. According to NIH regulations, applications to NIH for funds exceeding $500,000 were required to include a management plan to promote the sharing of research data. Additionally, recipients of NIH funding were required to submit their papers to PubMed Central, a data repository where all publications are free to the public. A statement of this regulation promulgated in 2008 states: The Director of the NIH shall require that all investigators funded by the NIH submit or have submitted for them to the National Library of Medicine's PubMed Central an electronic version of their final, peer-reviewed manuscripts upon acceptance for publication, to be made publicly available no later than 12 months after the official date of publication: Provided that the NIH shall implement the public access policy in a manner consistent with copyright law [4].

#### 2.1.2 Multiagency Task Force

In January 2009, The Working Group on Digital Data issued a report, Harnessing the Power of Digital Data for Science and Society, calling for the promotion of data management plans [5]. This task force was represented by 22 federal agencies. The report contains a vision, calling for "a digital scientific data universe in which data creation, collection, documentation, analysis, preservation, and dissemination can be appropriately, reliably, and readily managed" [5]. The report also called for agencies to stress the importance of making data readily available to the public. Specific suggestions for data management plans were also outlined. In the wake of this report, federal agencies have already made changes regarding their data management policies.

### 2.1.3 National Science Foundation

In 2010, the NSF changed its requirements for all grant applications submitted after January 17, 2011 [6]. Under the change in regulations, all proposals must include a data management plan. This plan must include information on how the applicant will conform to NSF's data dissemination and sharing policy, which states: "Investigators are expected to share with other researchers, at no more than incremental cost and within a reasonable time, the primary data, samples, physical collections, and other supporting materials created or gathered in the course of work under NSF grants. Grantees are expected to encourage and facilitate such sharing" [6].

### 2.1.4 Office of Science and Technology Policy

In February 2013, the White House issued a new directive under the Office of Science and Technology Policy [7]. A memo accompanied the update regarding increasing access to the results of federal funded scientific research. Funding agencies with an annual research and development budget greater than $100 million dollars must develop a public access plan for distributing the results of their research [8].

Part of this requirement involves data management plans. "Ensure that all extramural researchers receiving Federal grants and contracts for scientific research and intramural researchers develop data management plans and, as appropriate, describing how they will provide for long-term preservation of, and access to, scientific data in digital formats resulting from federally funded research, or explaining why long-term preservation and access cannot be justified" [8].

It is expected that other federal agencies will develop policies requiring grant applications to include information regarding the collection, storage, protection, retention, analysis, sharing, and reporting of scientific data. These regulations will evolve with time and it is important that researchers become familiar with creating and implementing data management plans.

## 2.2 Data Management Defined

Historically, data management has referred to data ownership and sharing. However, data management has a much more expansive definition and contains many facets. Following is a brief outline of the different types of data management.

### 2.2.1 Data Collection

Data collection refers to what information will be recorded, how it will be recorded, and the design of any particular research project. Data collection should be planned beforehand and used consistently throughout the project. This is the best way to ensure the integrity of the data [9].

### 2.2.2 Data Analysis

Determining what raw data should be analyzed and how the data will be analyzed is data analysis. This is an important aspect of data management for researchers to consider because analyzing the wrong data could lead to false results [10].

### 2.2.3 Data Storage

It is necessary for the research to determine what, how, and where the data should be stored. Certain projects can yield a large amount of data, not all of which is valuable. Also, some data may need to be stored in specific conditions. When dealing with electronic data storage backup files should be created [9].

### 2.2.4 Data Retention

Many funding organizations have time requirements for retaining data. Institutions may also have restrictions on timelines for retaining data. Researchers should be aware of the timeframe prior to beginning research [11]. Data retention also includes proper destruction of data, such as making sure that all confidentiality laws are being followed [9].

### 2.2.5 Data Ownership

Data ownership concerns who owns the data. This can extend to laboratory notebooks, notations, and hard data. Data ownership questions extend beyond the researchers tenure with the institution where the research was performed [12].

### 2.2.6 Data Protection

It is necessary that the written and electronic data are protected from physical damage, tampering, or theft [11]. This may include encrypting digital data.

### 2.2.7 Data Sharing

Data sharing is one of the most commonly discussed issues regarding data management. This pertains to how the project data and research results are made available to the general public [10].

### 2.2.8 Data Reporting

After the research project is done, the results of the data should be published. This is not limited to positive results and is likely the final step in data management [9].

## 3. RELEVANT REGULATORY/OVERSIGHT AGENCIES, REGULATIONS, AND GUIDANCE DOCUMENTS

Following the changes in NSF in regulations, researchers at Cornell University conducted a study that reviewed the top 10 federal funding agencies and their data management regulations [13]. The study addressed specific criteria regarding data management plans and analyzed the current data management policies at the funding agencies. A key finding of the study is that there is no uniformity in the regulations across agencies. The remainder of this section briefly outlines the existing data management requirements for the major federal funding agencies, as well as select foundations and provides references for the specific policies.

## 3.1 National Science Foundation

### 3.1.1 Data Management Plan Requirement

A two-page data management plan must be submitted with all grant applications to the NSF. This plan must detail how the applicant will adhere to the NSF data management and sharing policy. The plan may include the types of data, the standards to be used for data format and content, the policies for access and sharing the data, the policies for reuse and redistribution of the data, and the plans for archiving data [6].

### 3.1.2 Data Sharing Requirement

Investigators are expected to prepare all significant findings from research done with NSF grants and submit them for publication. This should be at no more than incremental costs and within a reasonable time. The publication should include primary data, samples, physical collections, and other supporting material collected during an NSF-funded project [14].

Steps should be taken to avoid releasing protected or confidential information.

It is the opinion of the NSF that grantees share software and inventions created with NSF funds, though grantees may retain their legal rights to intellectual property. This does not reduce the researcher's responsibility to the scientific community regarding data sharing [14].

Collaborative projects that have subawards are considered one proposal and should only have one combined stat management plan [6]. Proposals for supplementary funding do not require a new data management plan. If an applicant feels a data management plan is not necessary, he or she must include justification in the application [6].

### 3.1.3 Specific Program Guidance

#### 3.1.3.1 BIOLOGICAL SCIENCES DIRECTORATE

With the increase in the amount of collaboration between the sciences, the Biological Sciences Directorate (BIO) recognizes that the biological subdisciplines may have their own data management standards. Consequently, BIO states that the data management plan should reflect the standards of the area of research being proposed [15].

It is requested that the data management plan be organized according to the guidelines. This includes leading with a description of the data that will be collected along with the standards. Next, a description of what physical and/or cyber resources and facilities will be used to store the data until the end of the project. Third, a description of the media and dissemination methods that will be used to make the data available after the project concludes. Next, the policies for data sharing and public access should be included. Finally, a description of the roles and responsibilities of the parties involved in the grant to the management of the data after the project is completed.

#### 3.1.3.2 ENGINEERING DIRECTORATE

The Engineering Directorate of the NSF also offers additional guidance on creating data management plans. The guidance document is available through the NSF Website and it provides a solid template for researchers to follow [16].

### 3.1.3.3 EDUCATION AND HUMAN RESOURCES DIRECTORATE

The Education and Human Resources Directorate stresses data on projects involving human subjects [17]. These data should be made available to the public, though subject to constraints imposed by institutional review board (IRB) decisions. The Education and Human Resources Directorate also outlines specific examples for investigators to follow. The examples include a proposal for a workshop that will result in a workshop report, a proposal for developing a new undergraduate course, and a proposal in an education program that requires all projects to report on the graduation rate of participants [17].

### 3.1.3.4 COMPUTER AND INFORMATION SCIENCES AND ENGINEERING

The Computer and Information Sciences and Engineering (CISE) Directorate is aware of the need to provide flexibility in assessment of data management plans [18]. Each community within CISE has its own definition of data. This will be taken into consideration when reviewing the data management plans submitted by these communities.

### 3.1.3.5 DIRECTORATE FOR GEOSCIENCES

The Geosciences Directorate recognizes that data management plans are complex. A task force has been created to determine the issues and answers surrounding data management [19]. The Geosciences Directorate has made a request for feedback from the community regarding the new requirements [19].

### 3.1.3.6 SOCIAL, BEHAVIORAL, AND ECONOMIC SCIENCE DIRECTORATE

This area of the NSF has outlined data management plan requirements [20]. It provides a thorough study on the background of data management plans and describes the required content. The content should include the types of data, how data will be managed, factors that might impinge on the investigator's ability to manage data, the lowest level of data that investigators might share with the scientific community, the mechanism for sharing data, and other types of information that should be maintained regarding the data.

### 3.1.3.7 MATHEMATICAL AND PHYSICAL SCIENCES DIRECTORATE

The Mathematical and Physical Sciences Directorate division of the NSF gives guidance on creating a data management plan created to each of its disciplines [21]. The areas of astronomical sciences, chemistry, material research, mathematical sciences, and physics all have guidance documentation for investigators to follow when creating their data management plans.

1. Physics states that there is no recommendation of a specific archiving approach [22].
2. Mathematics states that the statement of no data management plan is necessary will suffice for most proposals, provided that the justification is present [23].
3. The Division of Materials Research does not have a recommendation of a specific repository [24].
4. Chemistry recommends the use of a public database. Examples that are provided include The Protein Data Bank, Cambridge Crystallographic Data Centre, PubChem, and the National Institute of Standards and Technology Chemistry WebBook, to name a few [25].
5. Astronomical sciences does not suggest any specific repositories, but requests that these details be provided in all data management plans [26].

## 3.2 National Institute of Health

### 3.2.1 Public Access Policy

The goal of the NIH Public Access Policy is to make sure that the public has access to all data generated with NIH funds [27]. The NIH Public Access Policy requires researchers to submit final peer-reviewed journal manuscripts that arise from NIH funds to the digital archive PubMed Central immediately upon acceptance for publication.

The policy applies to any paper that is peer-reviewed, accepted for publication in a journal, and arises from one of the following four circumstances: direct funding from an NIH grant or cooperative agreement active in the fiscal year 2008 or beyond; any direct funding from an NIH contract sign on or after April 7, 2008; any direct funding from the NIH Intramural Program; or an NIH employee.

It is important for an investigator to take this policy into account when publishing a paper. The copyright agreement must ensure that the paper is able to be published in PubMed Central. There are no exceptions [27].

### 3.2.2 Data Sharing Policy

The NIH policy on data sharing requires the sharing of final research data. It is applicable to applications seeking $500,000 or more in direct costs in any single year of the project period or as a special requirement of a Funding Opportunity Announcement [28].

Applicants must include a data sharing plan with their application. The data sharing plan describes what data will be shared. This should include both final research data and metadata with descriptors. Information on who will have access to the data should also be provided. The data should be shared broadly, and only be limited by laws, regulations, rules, and policies that prohibit the release of specific data. If the data sharing is limited, a rationale must be included in the plan. The location of the shared data should also be included. The ideal place to share data is a data repository with common standards and an established infrastructure.

Data should be made available as soon as possible and for as long as possible. A schedule should be provided including whether any data will be made available prior to publication. The applicant must also include information relating to how the data will be located and accessed. Other researchers must be able to identify the location of any relevant data with ease. It is also necessary that accessing the data is a simple process.

## 3.3 US Department of Energy

### 3.3.1 Chief Information Officer

Previously, the chief information officer of the Department of Energy was responsible for ensuring that data was acquired and managed consistent with the policies of the department. This was a broad statement that provided some guidance to researchers with Department of Energy funding. As of October 2013, the Department of Energy's stance on data management became more specific [29].

### 3.3.2 Office of Science

As of October 2013, all proposals submitted to the Department of Energy Office of Science must include a data management plan. This modification responded to the White House

Office of Science and Technology's revised policy on expanding public access to the results of federally funded research.

The Office of Science has a Statement on Digital Data Management. The focus of the plan is on digital research data and stresses the need for sharing and preservation.

All applications must include a data management plan. It should be no more than two pages and should detail how the data will be shared and preserved. If the data cannot be shared or preserved a rationale must be presented.

The data management plan must describe the method the primary investigator (PI) intends to use to ensure that all data used in published research is available to the public by the time of publication. If any data are used in charts, figures, images, etc., they must be made available to the public. This can be done by including the data as a supplement to the article or by providing it in a repository. The published article must tell the reader where the data can be accessed [30].

If the researcher is planning to work at an Office of Science User Facility, he or she must consult the published data policy of that facility and reference the policy in her data management plan.

### 3.3.3 Climate and Environmental Sciences Division

The Department of Energy requests that data of potentially broad use in climate change research be archived [31]. This is intended to promote networking among the members of the global climate-change community and inform preparation of technical and informational reports, and sponsorship of scientific conferences.

### 3.3.4 North American Research Strategy for Tropospheric Ozone Projects

If a researcher is applying for a grant under the North American Research Strategy for Tropospheric Ozone (NARSTO) initiative of the Department of Energy, a data management plan must be submitted [32]. A guidance document is available instructing an applicant how to tailor their plan in the NARSTO context. More than 20 sample data management plans are provided depending on the type of funding one is applying for. The samples range from organization focus, data and metadata reporting, data documentation and archiving, and data systems management.

## 3.4 US Department of Education

### 3.4.1 Institute of Education Sciences

Researchers with funding provided through the National Center for Education Research and the National Center for Special Education Research, the two research centers of the Institute for Education Science (IES), are required to include data sharing plans [33]. The institute believes that sharing data will lead to more rigorous peer review, and so the production of more robust findings.

This requirement was instituted for 2013 grants and continues. All plans must describe the data to be shared, the method of sharing, the documentation that will accompany the data, the plan for keeping personally identifiable data confidential, the projected timeline for sharing data, the roles of the staff in the management and retention of the data, and the cost for sharing the data. The two methods of sharing described are through the Principal Investigator (PI) directly or a data archive/repository.

Data are expected to be made available upon publication of the attendant findings. The IES recognizes that this may not occur until the research is complete. The IES permits budgeting of data sharing costs. These costs may include preparing the data to be archived, as well as the data documentation. A guideline with further information is provided at the IES Website [33].

## 3.5 US Environmental Protection Agency

The US Environmental Protection Agency (USEPA) does not have an official data management and sharing policy. However, it does supply several documents describing the importance of data management that should be taken into consideration by researchers with USEPA funding.

### 3.5.1 *Open Government Data Quality Plan*

The Open Government Data Quality Plan is an internal policy of the USEPA [34]. It outlines the implementation of data quality framework stressing open communication and monitoring between the government and funded teams. It also discusses steps for reporting data and access to budgets regarding funding.

### 3.5.2 *Survey of the Environmental Protection Agency and Other Federal Agency Scientific Data Management Policies and Guidance*

In 2010, the USEPA released a report of its data management practices in comparison to other funding agencies [35]. The report is very detailed and covers data management plans in relation to assets or liabilities, the full data lifecycle, ability to identify metadata, and other data management related topics. The report concludes that there is yet to be a comprehensive data management policy among federal agencies, demonstrating that Data Management requirements continue to evolve.

## 3.6 US Agency for International Development

### 3.6.1 *Data Quality Assessment*

The five data quality standards the US Agency for International Development (USAID) holds key are validity, reliability, precision, integrity, and timeliness. The USAID encourages data quality assessment to ensure that data generated from USAID-funded research is up to their standards. There is no specific way to conduct a data quality assessment, stating a memo in the file or a formal report may be necessary, but the USAID suggests one be done at least every three years [36].

### 3.6.2 *American Schools and Hospitals Abroad*

The USAID provides funding under a number of different grant instruments. The award under the American Schools and Hospitals Abroad program requires a monitoring and evaluation plan [37]. Applicant must specifically outline how, when, and by whom data will be gathered, analyzed, and used. Although this plan may be brief in the application stage, it could lead to a larger plan.

## 3.7 National Oceanographic and Atmospheric Administration

### 3.7.1 Data Sharing Policy

Data sharing is one of the many facets of data management. The National Oceanographic and Atmospheric Administration (NOAA) has separate requirements for data sharing [38]. The NOAA is concerned with making the data visible, accessible, and understandable. Data sharing is limited by privacy concerns and any other superseding laws or regulations.

Under the NOAA data sharing policy, all data using NOAA funding must be shared in a timely manner. Typically, this is interpreted to mean no later than two years after the data are collected or created. A two-page data sharing plan is required as part of the project narrative. The information supplied should include the types of environmental data created, the standards to be used to format the data, policies accessing data preservation, previous data sharing experience, and procedures for providing access, sharing, and security. Data sharing plan templates are provided by the NOAA along with case examples.

When deciding on where to share the data, a researcher should first consider NOAA facilities that archive data. The NOAA Procedure for Scientific Records Appraisal and Archive Approval describes the process of contacting an NOAA archive [39]. It should be noted that failure to publish the data may result in diminished awards and denial of any future awards.

### 3.7.2 Oceanographic Data

When oceanographic data and related information are acquired with federal funds, the data must be submitted to the National Oceanographic Data Center [38]. This is a national repository that holds some international data as well. The National Oceanographic Data Center has acquisition specialists that will assist researchers with storing their data.

## 3.8 National Aeronautics and Space Administration

### 3.8.1 Data Rights and Related Issues

The National Aeronautics and Space Administration (NASA) details its data management requirements in its Data Rights and Related Issues policy [40]. NASA promotes the full and open sharing of all data. It lists the organizations with which data should be shared, such as academia and the general public. Archived mission project data management plans are available to the public. Although its official Data Management stance is general, specific areas of NASA funding require more information.

### 3.8.2 Earth Science Missions

Data management plans are required under the Earth Sciences division of NASA [41]. Guidance for creating a plan is provided by the agency. The Data management plan must include information on the development, maintenance, and management responsibility, the change control (plans for modification and updates to this document over time), all relevant documents, the project objectives, science objectives, mission summary, instrument overview, mission operations, science operations, post-mission stewardship and access, science data product summary, associated archive products, special considerations, and a section on acronyms.

### 3.8.3 *Heliophysics*

Heliophysics research provides its own requirements for Data management plans [42]. Guidelines are available for creating Data management plans, which must include preparing, accessing, using, and archiving heliophysics data. This policy stresses NASA's overall open access data policy mentioned above.

## 3.9 National Endowment for the Humanities

### 3.9.1 *Office of Digital Humanities*

All applicants must submit a data management plan supplementing their grant application [43]. The plan should be no more than two pages and answer two questions: What data are generated by your research and what is your plan for managing the data? The plan should articulate, in a clear and concise manner, how sharing of the primary data will be accomplished. The rights and responsibilities of the parties involved in relation to management and retention of data must also be outlined. Any costs of data sharing should be included in the budget. The matters that should be addressed are the type of data, how they will be managed and maintained until sharing is possible, factors that will impede sharing of data, the lowest level of data that can be shared, the mechanism for sharing data, and analytical and procedural information regarding the data. The data are expected to have a timely and rapid distribution; however, no minimum time requirements are provided.

## 3.10 Institute of Museum and Library Services

### 3.10.1 *Open Government*

The Institute of Museum and Library Services (IMLS) does not have specific data management requirements. It does stress open access government. It is a goal of IMLS to make the agencies work more transparent and encourage public participation. Meeting this goal may fall under data sharing guidelines.

## 3.11 American Heart Association

### 3.11.1 *Guide for Affiliate Research Awards*

The American Heart Association provides little guidance on data management. However, in its guide for affiliate research awards, it specifically mentions research misconduct including data falsification [44]. Implementing a strong data management plan can help a researcher defend against claims of scientific misconduct. In general, researchers should become familiar with creating data management plans regardless of the requirements because it is likely more and more agencies will look for them in the future.

## 3.12 Alfred P. Sloan Foundation

The Alfred P. Sloan Foundation offers only general guidance on the necessity of data management [45]. It makes reference to the importance of handling a wide variety of digital data and encourages researchers to make data publicly accessible. As the trend from general guidelines to specific requirements continues, researchers should create data management plans that follow these objectives.

### 3.13 Centers for Disease Control and Prevention

#### 3.13.1 *Data Sharing and Release Policy*

The Centers for Disease Control and Prevention (CDC) policy on data sharing includes all data collected for the CDC by institutions. The policy specifically mentions data generated through grants, contracts, and cooperative agreements. The policy requires that all data are released or shared as soon as possible without disregarding privacy and confidentiality concerns or other applicable laws [46]. The policy is vague and does not require a specific data management plan, but every researcher funded by the CDC should expect to release and share data in a reasonable timeframe.

### 3.14 Department of Defense

#### 3.14.1 *Department of Defense Directive 3200.12*

Similar to the CDC, the Department of Defense (DoD) only gives vague instructions regarding data management. It requests that researchers "establish and maintain a coordinated and comprehensive program to document the results and outcome of DoD-sponsored and/or performed research and engineering and studies efforts and provide access to those efforts in an effective manner consistent with the DoD Mission."

There is no requirement to submit a data management plan with grant proposals; however, it is expected the researcher have one. Many DoD grants come with stipulations and confidentiality agreements. Researchers must take these clauses into account before sharing any data to make sure they are in compliance.

### 3.15 National Institute of Justice

A brief data archiving strategy must be included in any application for National Institute of Justice (NIJ) research grants [47]. This should describe how the data will be prepared and documented. The NIJ gives details on its requirements and requires that the data archiving strategy includes information regarding the data formats, which software will be used to archive the data, a description of the procedures for data collection, and confidentiality details in the research involves human subjects.

Most NIJ-funded research must have its data sets archived with the National Archive of Criminal Justice. The data must be submitted 90 days before the end of the project period.

### 3.16 National Institute of Standards and Technology

The National Institute of Standards and Technology does not have requirements directed solely toward data management. In its document addressing information quality standards and administrative mechanism, data release is mentioned. It is required that data from

National Institute of Standards and Technology grants is disseminated for public use or made available through an ad hoc request that results in the steward no longer controlling the data [48].

## 3.17 US Department of Agriculture

The US Department of Agriculture Cooperative State Research, Education, and Service require all funded research be submitted into the public domain without restriction. There are few additional instructions provided to researchers. When there is a patent application, exceptions are sometimes allowed [49].

## 3.18 Office of Research Integrity

The Office of Research Integrity (ORI) is not a grant awarding body. It serves as a regulatory committee regarding misconduct and provides information and training regarding the RCR, among other things. Data management is one of the main areas of focus within RCR and the ORI offers a variety of information on the subject [11].

### 3.18.1 Guidelines for Responsible Data Management in Scientific Research

A course regarding data management is offered through ORI entitled Guidelines for Responsible Data Management in Scientific Research [50]. A 35-page course outline covers general data management, data ownership and retention, data collection and record keeping, data storage and protection, data sharing and publication, human subjects research, animal research, and research team leadership and communication. Case studies and real-world examples are also provided in this training. It is highly recommended every researcher take the time to review this document.

### 3.18.2 Data Acquisition and Management

ORI also offers training in data acquisition and management [50]. This exercise is intended for individuals with some knowledge of data management. The focus is on two separate case studies, what to look for, and the outcomes. It is the responsibility of the PI to offer continuous training in RCR to the research team and students. This training is a good way to keep data management issues present in researchers' minds.

### 3.18.3 Educating Clinical Research Staff in Clinical Data Collection and Data Management

This is an interactive tutorial provided by the ORI in conjunction with Saint Jude's Children's Research Hospitals and Cure4Kids [50]. The focus of this training is intended to address the needs of clinical staff members and covers issues regarding patient collection and recording. Data management plans are not limited to clinical research.

### 3.18.4 Interactive Data Management Module

ORI provides a link to Northern Illinois University's data management module [50]. This is an interactive training geared toward researchers with a very basic familiarity with data management. All areas of data management are covered in this tutorial and it can take up to 4 h to complete. One does not need to finish the entire course in one session. Although a PI can benefit from taking this module, it is a good practice for the PI to require training similar to this for his or her research staff.

## 4. KEY REGULATORY MANDATES

To date, the key regulatory mandates regarding data management are those promulgated by the NSF and NIH and subsequently modified and adopted in whole or in part by other federal agencies and private funding sources. The pillars of these mandates are: (1) that data be collected and stored in a manner that permits the scientific community and interested others to access, review, and make further use of that data. This mandate recognizes both the value (intrinsic and extrinsic) of that data collected and the need to safeguard that data for future use and the dramatic increase in problem spaces that require that data and scientific information be made easily and cheaply available to scientists from their own and other disciplines. (2) That the findings of scientific research, especially those resulting from publicly funded research projects, be made publicly available as widely and as quickly as practicable. Again, this mandate arises from the recognition of the need for scientists across distances and disciplines to have access to the latest scientific information in a timely manner to foster the cross-pollination of scientific thought and to ensure that scientific findings are further tested through replication and extension in order to solidify their basis as reliable knowledge.

The NSF data management policy simply states that "[I]nvestigators are expected to share with other researchers, at no more than incremental cost and within a reasonable time, the primary data, samples, physical collections and other supporting materials created or gathered in the course of work under NSF grants."

The NIH simply stipulates that: "Investigators seeking $500,000 or more in direct costs in any year should include a description of how final research data will be shared, or explain why data sharing is not possible" [51]. It then goes on to provide the following detail regarding the contents of the plan and opportunities for covering the costs of the plan within the budget justification:

> Applicants who are planning to share data may wish to describe briefly the expected schedule for data sharing, the format of the final dataset, the documentation to be provided, whether or not any analytic tools also will be provided, whether or not a data-sharing agreement will be required and, if so, a brief description of such an agreement (including the criteria for deciding who can receive the data and whether or not any conditions will be placed on their use), and the mode of data sharing (e.g., under their own auspices by mailing a disk or posting data on their institutional or personal website, through a data archive or enclave). Investigators choosing to share under their own auspices may wish to enter into a data-sharing agreement…
>
> Investigators working with archives can get help with data preparation and cost estimation. Investigators who are concerned about paying for data-sharing costs at the end of their grant can make prior arrangements with archives. Investigators facing considerable delays in the preparation of the final dataset for sharing should consult with the NIH program about how to manage this situation, such as requesting a no-cost extension.

These mandates, and similar language provided by other federal funding sources, address data management simply by requiring plans to be included in requests for funding.

However, to date, the plans do not play a significant role in the peer review process. In this sense, they function as an institutional assurance and no more. A regimen of stronger mandates would require not only explicit attention during peer review, but also more explicit recognition of the need to fund data management activities and, eventually, the need for the time and effort required to develop, populate, and monitor data management systems within the context of a research project to be recognized by investigator's departments as activity worthy of measurement for the purposes of tenure, promotion, and merit pay increases.

However, this picture may change as agencies respond to a White House executive order on increasing access to federally funded scientific research. The order requires agencies that fund in excess of $100 million in research to develop concrete plans for data management and open access.

In terms of digital scientific data and publications, the agency plans must contain the following elements:

1. a strategy for leveraging existing archives, where appropriate, and fostering public–private partnerships with scientific journals relevant to the agency's research;
2. a strategy for improving the public's ability to locate and access digital data resulting from federally funded scientific research;
3. an approach for optimizing search, archival, and dissemination features that encourages innovation in accessibility and interoperability, while ensuring long-term stewardship of the results of federally funded research;
4. a plan for notifying awardees and other federally funded scientific researchers of their obligations (e.g., through guidance, conditions of awards, regulatory changes);
5. an agency strategy for measuring and, as necessary, enforcing compliance with its plan;
6. identification of resources within the existing agency budget to implement the plan;
7. a timeline for implementation; and
8. identification of any special circumstances that prevent the agency from meeting any of the objectives set out in this memorandum, in whole or in part.

With respect to public access to scientific publications, the order requires that each agency shall:

1. Ensure that the public can read, download, and analyze in digital form final peer-reviewed manuscripts or final published documents within a timeframe that is appropriate for each type of research conducted or sponsored by the agency. Specifically, each agency:
   a. shall use a 12-month postpublication embargo period as a guideline for making research papers publicly available; however, an agency may tailor its plan as necessary to address the objectives articulated in this memorandum as well as the challenges and public interests that are unique to each field and mission combination, and
   b. shall also provide a mechanism for stakeholders to petition for changing the embargo period for a specific field by presenting evidence demonstrating that the plan would be inconsistent with the objectives articulated in this memorandum.
2. Facilitate easy public search, analysis of, and access to peer-reviewed scholarly publications directly arising from research funded by the federal government;
3. Ensure full public access to publications' metadata without charge upon first publication in a data format that ensures interoperability with current and future search technology.

Where possible, the metadata should provide a link to the location where the full text and associated supplemental materials will be made available after the embargo period;
4. Encourage public–private collaboration to:
   a. maximize the potential for interoperability between public and private platforms and creative reuse to enhance value to all stakeholders,
   b. avoid unnecessary duplication of existing mechanisms,
   c. maximize the impact of the federal research investment, and
   d. otherwise assist with implementation of the agency plan.
5. Ensure that attribution to authors, journals, and original publishers is maintained; and
6. Ensure that publications and metadata are stored in an archival solution that:
   a. provides for long-term preservation and access to the content without charge,
   b. uses standards, widely available and, to the extent possible, nonproprietary archival formats for text and associated content (e.g., images, video, supporting data),
   c. provides access for persons with disabilities consistent with Section 508 of the Rehabilitation Act of 1973, and
   d. enables integration and interoperability with other federal public access archival solutions and other appropriate archives.

Regarding agencies' plans to provide public access to scientific data in digital formats, the order stipulates that each agency will:

1. Maximize access, by the general public and without charge, to digitally formatted scientific data created with federal funds, while:
   a. protecting confidentiality and personal privacy,
   b. recognizing proprietary interests, business confidential information, and intellectual property rights and avoiding significant negative impact on intellectual property rights, innovation, and US competitiveness, and
   c. preserving the balance between the relative value of long-term preservation and access and the associated cost and administrative burden.
2. Ensure that all extramural researchers receiving federal grants and contracts for scientific research and intramural researchers develop data management plans, as appropriate, describing how they will provide for long-term preservation of, and access to, scientific data in digital formats resulting from federally funded research, or explaining why long-term preservation and access cannot be justified;
3. Allow the inclusion of appropriate costs for data management and access in proposals for federal funding for scientific research;
4. Ensure appropriate evaluation of the merits of submitted data management plans;
5. Include mechanisms to ensure that intramural and extramural researchers comply with data management plans and policies;
6. Promote the deposit of data in publicly accessible databases, wherever appropriate and available;
7. Encourage cooperation with the private sector to improve data access and compatibility, including through the formation of public–private partnerships with foundations and other research funding organizations;
8. Develop approaches for identifying and providing appropriate attribution to scientific data sets that are made available under the plan;

9. In coordination with other agencies and the private sector, support training, education, and workforce development related to scientific data management, analysis, storage, preservation, and stewardship; and

10. Provide for the assessment of long-term needs for the preservation of scientific data in fields that the agency supports and outline options for developing and sustaining repositories for scientific data in digital formats, taking into account the efforts of public and private sector entities.

Agency responses to this order will address some of the concerns raised here, for example, they will at least indicate that data management and public access plans must be made part of the peer review process, but motivation and incentive for faculty and research institutions to change their practices and their culture in this regard remain distant prospects.

# 5. KEY PERSONNEL AND UNIVERSITY COMMITTEES DESIGNATED TO IMPLEMENT REGULATORY MANDATES

Universities address the wide range of issues related to data management from a number of organizational directions. Libraries commonly have staff members, departments, and committees intended to support faculty, staff members, and students meet data management requirements and access library-based data management services. They often also cover issues related to copyright, rules for metadata use, connection with international and discipline-based repositories, and requirements related to data sharing and open access publishing. Research and Sponsored Programs offices may have staff members who can assist faculty in developing appropriate data management plans or accessing tools and templates for completing their plans (e.g., DMPTools [52]). Information Technology Services departments often have staff members and committees that address issues of data storage and transfer. Issues related to data management are also often addressed by legal counsel, Provost's Office committees, research committees, and arise as matters addressed by faculty senates. Data management is also one of the core elements of what has come to be termed RCR and so the development of policies and procedures often falls to RCR committees. Not all institutions use all of these institutional options or use them in the same ways; nor are all of them necessarily charged with ensuring compliance with regulatory mandates, but their goals are generally aligned around ensuring that legal, ethical, regulatory mandates are met in ways that support access to and the sharing of research data and information. Generally, the university units and committees charged with ensuring regulatory compliance for data management include the following.

## 5.1 Principal Investigators

In terms of project implementation and the ways in which specific agency requirements regarding data management and publication of finding are met and managed, the responsibility falls to the PIs as the leaders of the research project and the signatory on the grant award. They set the tone and assign the responsibilities to their staff and collaborators. They will plan out the project and have the final decision on all matters regarding how data are collected, stored, managed, and shared. The publication of the final results is a central responsibility of the PI as well, and so they are responsible for meeting all requirements regarding publication and access to results. The PI is also required to meet any university requirements regarding data management and sharing and to abide by university policies as they relate to data security, confidentiality, data ownership, intellectual property, and copyright.

## 5.2 Research Office

The Research Office generally houses a number of units that play important roles in developing and implementing data management policies and in ensuring adherence to regulatory mandates.

## 5.3 Research Compliance

Research compliance often promulgates general university policy as it relates to the ownership and use of research-related data, and to the requirements for meeting federal mandates (see Section 6). The Research Compliance Office is often also the home of the unit that addresses research misconduct, which may also involve issues related to data management and reporting as required by federal agencies (see Section 6).

## 5.4 Responsible Conduct of Research Committee

In response to NIH and NSF requirements that students participating on grants funded by those institutions receive training in the RCR, many institutions have RCR committees, which are usually housed within the university research office and generally made up of faculty and administrative staff representing those departments most commonly affected by the NIH and NSF mandates. Generally, these committees are responsible for a number of items, including design and implementation of core RCR programs and coordination with department-specific RCR training programs. Data management is one of the core elements of RCR training. Therefore, although RCR committees may develop RCR standards and implement policies that affect RCR, they are unlikely to make policy specific to data management, but simply ensure that students and faculty are properly apprised on issues related to data management through RCR training.

## 5.5 Sponsored Projects

This is the office that will assist researchers with applying for funding. In this capacity, it often assists investigators in developing appropriate data management plans based on the guidance provided by the funding agency or by directing them to specific data management tools. It is also responsible for reviewing proposals before they are submitted to ensure that all federal, state, and institutional requirement are met. For proposals to federal funding agencies, this includes a long list of assurances and, where mandated, inclusion of the required data management plan.

## 5.6 Institutional Review Board

The IRB is a committee responsible for approving, monitoring, and reviewing biomedical and behavioral research involving human subjects. Often these proposals come with confidentiality restrictions regarding information provided by or related to the human subjects. The IRB can be instrumental in determining the confidentiality concerns and offering guidance and regulations on how various types of data can be held and for how long.

## 5.7 University Libraries

University librarians, staff members, and committees are often experts in the regulations, technologies, services, and discipline-specific requirements related to data management and providing access to published material. They may be usefully consulted on matters relating to storage, archiving, curation, transfer, and the appropriate use of metadata. Libraries often house the university data repository, which is often available free of charge to investigators on campus. Storing data in a repository is often a safe way to ensure the integrity of the data and fulfill funding agency requirements.

## 5.8 Outside Parties

### 5.8.1 Journals

At present, journal involvement with research data most often arises in connection with disputes over findings or cases involving potential misconduct. In this role, many journals have become significant players in areas of data management related to data integrity. However, it is becoming more common for journals to request that data be made available along with the publication of findings. As this practice becomes more common, journals will play an ever larger role in data management. Discussions of open access writ large are beyond the purview of this chapter; however, as federal mandates stressing access evolve, the role of journals in this area will become ever more central.

### 5.8.2 Professional Societies

Professional societies often provide disciplinary standards and best practices guidance to their communities. They may also provide specific guidance on how to prepare appropriate data management plans. In some cases, they may also recommend data archives.

## 6. COMMON COMPLIANCE CHALLENGES

Every project will have unique situations that arise and must be dealt with on a case-by-case basis. However, the ORI in the Department of Health and Human Services (HHS) has recognized frequent issues that arise involving data management. These are summarized here and can be found in more detail at the ORI Introduction to the RCR Guide and the ORI Data Management Guidelines.

## 6.1 Creating Internal Policies

Many universities lack formal policies and tend to rely on "industry standards." Although a large number of funding agencies require some form of data management and record keeping, it is still beneficial for the university to have its own internal policies. In the event an ownership or access issue arises, universities without policies could find themselves in very difficult places. Because data management is a pillar of the RCR, any data management policy should supplement existing RCR and research misconduct policies and not contradict them.

### 6.1.1 University-Wide Policy

Different disciplines or departments may have their own particular policies, but it is important to have a university-wide policy regarding data management practices and procedures. These policies should protect the university and the researcher. It is difficult to regulate all the aspects of data management, but data usage, ownership, retention, and access should be addressed.

### 6.1.2 Data Usage

Internal policies should cover data usage. It may be helpful to identify a global standard, such as the ORI language, because this policy may cover a wide variety of disciplines. Any policy should grant the Investigators appropriate use of the data. The policy should stipulate that all data usage must be in accordance with contractual commitments by the university. The policy may also encourage investigators to create written plans regarding ownership, rights, access, and permissions for data use at the outset of projects.

### 6.1.3 Custody of Research Data

Because research awards from funding sources are usually granted to the institution, the university is generally the owner of any research data collected under the auspices of the university (i.e., by faculty in the normal course of their duties). The custody and stewardship of the research data are usually in the hands of the PI. In some cases, research participants or governments with jurisdiction of property from which samples are taken may seek to retain forms of ownership or rights to data collected from their samples. In such cases, it is important to document or address the apportionment of those rights in an informed consent document or some other form of written agreement.

Some university policies further expand upon this, explaining the chain of custody of the data if the PI becomes unavailable. This should include what will happen to the data in the event of research misconduct proceedings. The research misconduct policy and the data management policy should not contradict each other and ensure the university has access to the data.

As custodian of the data, the PI should also be charged with maintaining the integrity of the data. This could include responsibilities toward data collection, analysis, or storage among others.

### 6.1.4 Data Retention

Although many funding agencies have their own data retention policies, it may be in the interests of the university to implement their own standards. In some cases, there may be benefits to retaining data, because as the owner of the data, the university can set time limits the custodian must abide by. However, there are also cases where sensitive or personal data, such as video or audio need to be retained. In such cases, it is important to balance the needs of the investigators, and often the policies of the journals to which they submit articles, and the research participants, whose interest is in seeing that the data are destroyed as soon as is practicable. Whatever limits are set, the clock usually starts after submission of the final research data.

It is advised that alternative retention requirements are given if the work belongs to a student. These may include retaining the data until the student graduates or it is clear that the work has been abandoned.

Data retention policies need not limit themselves to funded projects. It is important to define who the policy applies to and possibly include provisions that exclude unfunded work for certain sections.

### 6.1.5 Data Access

Internal university data management policies should state that the university has access to all research data. Universities should not limit themselves to data regarding research preformed at the university and should include any research supported by university administered funds.

It is important that researchers not feel alienated by these clauses and be given ample warning before the university requests the data absent an emergency.

### 6.1.6 Confidentiality

Data management policies should ensure that all confidentiality agreements and requirements put forth in human subjects protocols and informed consent documents regarding the confidentiality of data be honored. Federal funding often requires that specific procedures be followed in order to safeguard confidential or otherwise sensitive data. Policies should specify adherence to such procedures.

### 6.1.7 Data Sharing

As mentioned previously data sharing is seen as a tenet of the scientific community. More and more organizations encourage data sharing. Striving for data sharing is something a university must consider, but with the demand for sharing increasing including a data sharing clause can be expected from faculty and administration alike.

It is important that confidentiality concerns are taken into consideration with data sharing. When a patent or other copyrighted material is involved researchers may be reluctant to share their data. Researchers should be made aware of any exceptions to data sharing requirements.

### 6.1.8 Data Transfer

If an investigator separates from his or her institution, he or she may wish to take the research to the new organization. The university is the owner of the data and has the right to deny that request; however, most organizations allow for some form of agreement. Mentioning this in the policy and even putting a blanket statement this will be handled on a case-by-case basis can make the transition easier for separating investigators. Make sure that there are people in place to handle the transfer.

Some of the transfer arrangements may include the university keeping the originals, whereas the investigator takes copies or vice versa. There can also be steps put into place where the investigator can take the research, but the university retains the rights to access all the data.

### 6.1.9 Data Ownership

Prevailing higher education practice indicates that the university is the owner of all the research data. This should be made clear throughout the policy. This statement should take preference over any other policy that mentions this topic, whether they be intellectual property policies or human resource issues.

### 6.1.10 Disputes

The policy should include a reference to where to handle disputed issues. This could be handled by going to the vice president for research or the RCR Committee for example. The details do not have to be written out, but just some basic direction where the individual should go if they have any issues regarding the internal data management policy.

## 6.2 Project-Based Data Management Plans

Many funding agencies require data management plans with their grant applications. Several of these plans are limited to two pages. Some organizations, such as NASA, provide sample data management plans for applicants. It is a good idea for researchers to examine these plans before creating their own.

Universities will normally have an administrator who will be able to assist researchers with drafting their project-based data management plans; there are also a number of resources available online. The California Digital Library has a free data management plan tool for investigators at https://dmp.cdlib.org/. This module is tailored for each funding agency. This can be a great help to ensure all the requirements of the funding agency have been met.

Even if the specific funding agency does not require a data management plan it is advised that the PI create one for the team. Data management plans organize the research, guide the team, and streamline the process. The following should be considered when the PI creates the data management plan.

## 6.3 Project Needs

To avoid confusion and make the project run smoothly, the PI should outline the needs of the research project. These should cover all the areas of data management from data collection to data reporting. Breaking them down step by step will give a clearer picture of what needs to be done regarding the data.

### 6.3.1 Team Member's Skills

As researchers work together longer, they will become aware of new or increasing skills, as well as areas where individuals need improvement. Most universities offer a variety of training options and the PI should be aware of what the people on the team can handle and where they can get more assistance.

### 6.3.2 Roles and Responsibilities

If each member of the team knows what is expected of them, the research can run smoothly. This not only benefits the PI because it save the project time, but it will also ensure the integrity of the project because the team will be aware of expectations and what to perform.

### 6.3.3 *Potential Problems*

If the researcher is aware of potential problems before they arise, he or she will also be aware of potential solutions. It is best to evaluate the options available, especially if a data ownership or confidentiality issue may arise. That way the PI will know what steps to take next.

### 6.3.4 *Timespan*

Data management plans can keep the project moving forward. The PI should look at the finished plan and set goals, including specific dates, and make sure that the team is aware of these aims. The goals should also include any mandatory deadlines set by the funding agency. Progress should be checked against the timeline to ensure that the project will be finished in a timely manner.

It is recommended that the timeline extends beyond the date of publication, especially if there is a data sharing requirement. Many organizations give the PI a time limit before the team must share its data. This should be noted and honored or else the PI risks violating the grant agreement.

## 6.4 Types of Data

Most data management requirements are less than a decade old. This is a changing landscape and some researchers may be reluctant to change. In 2012, the journal article "Prepared to Plan? A Snapshot of Researcher Readiness to Address Data Management Planning Requirements" was published. The authors surveyed current and prospective NSF PIs from Cornell regarding data management plans. The responses to the survey indicated that 62% would be interested in guidance for writing a data management plan.

The results of the study showed two challenges when offering support for data management plans. The first challenge was that researchers were confused regarding the definition of what is considered data. Universities must be prepared to provide guidance on this issue. It is important that a set definition for data is provided and that researchers understand it. This can be accomplished with training or through guidance provided by data management plan servicers.

The second issue was the vast array of digital content. As technology continues to advance, it is important that the people giving guidance on data management plans are aware of what storage and analytical tools are available to address the specific needs generated by various kinds of content and the ways in which that content is most effectively accessed.

## 6.5 Standards for Data and Metadata

### 6.5.1 *Understandings*

Metadata is a set of data that gives information about other data. Standards vary among disciplines. Any persons giving data management advice must know what field they are working with before attempting to answer questions dealing with standards. The same study mentioned previously [53] showed not all researchers are aware of whether their data or metadata conforms to the standards of their discipline.

There was also an apparent lack of understanding regarding the definition of metadata, along with a reluctance to use metadata in one's research.

### 6.5.2 Recommendations

NSF's recommendation that researchers specify "standard to be used for data and metadata" should be interpreted to mean formally, or de facto, standards of the discipline, not within a single laboratory.

The same confusion appears to exist among data management plan servicers. This should be seen as an opportunity to create and implement training programs. These could consist of online or face to face trainings and explain data standards and how one creates metadata.

## 6.6 Data Sharing

The dilemmas a research may face when sharing data are the necessity of protecting the privacy of all research participants, maintaining the confidentiality of sensitive information, monitoring and preventing inappropriate use of the data shared [54].

### 6.6.1 What to Share

When sharing data, two challenges researchers face. The first is determining what the investigator should share. Research can generate a large amount of data, but not all if it may be relevant to the research. This is a difficult question for researchers to answer. They should look at their final discoveries and make sure that the data shared can recreate their research. They should also look to their peers for guidance and see what has worked best for other researchers in the past.

### 6.6.2 Confidentiality

There is a concern regarding confidentiality and data sharing. A significant amount of research experiments contain confidential information, especially those involving human subjects. Institutions should make sure their research infrastructures are up to date and in place. Educating investigators on confidentiality laws will also ease issues they have with sharing their data.

### 6.6.3 Where to Share

NIH has internal systems for sharing data, but not every funding institute is the same. Certain publications may also offer a data repository if the article is to appear in one of their editions. Some institutions offer internal repositories that are open to the public for researchers to share their data. These services are generally free and it is recommended they are used by investigators. Some disciplinary repositories exist as well. These repositories include the Inter-University Consortium for Political and Social Research, GenBank, and ArXiv. There are many other options available as well. Finally, a researcher may use public services such as Good Docs or Dropbox.

## 6.7 Financial Requirements

Many of the data management requirements make mention of costs. They promote data management initiatives at the lowest cost possible to investigators. Even with this caveat, there are some concerns regarding the costs of implementing data management plans.

### 6.7.1 Storage and Retention

When dealing with large amounts of hard data, the cost of storing the items can add up. Some biological specimens can require refrigeration, which may be more costly than storing laboratory notebooks. The length of retention should be noted as well. Even if the funding agency has a specific requirement, this should be checked against internal university policies. Whichever one is longer will be the one the investigator needs to follow. Costs should be examined before the start of the research and extend through the retention period. If these financial concerns are addressed early, they should not be a problem for the investigator later on.

### 6.7.2 Digital Data

Research can generate large amount of digital data. The larger amount of data, the more the researcher has to work with—but also the higher the costs. Sometimes analyzing large amounts of digital data will require a third party. The fees these companies charge can vary. It is important the PI knows upfront their plan for analyzing large electronic files.

### 6.7.3 Protection

Certain data come with confidentiality restrictions or can be sensitive to public knowledge. Regardless of whether the data are physical or digital, protecting these data can come with some costs. If the data are physical, a safe, a locked room, or even video monitoring may be required.

Digital security comes with a variety of options. This can include encrypting files, creating secure logins, monitoring who accesses the files, and using a private server. Many universities have internal technology departments who will be able to assist the PI in protecting the digital data, but in some cases a third party may need to be used. It is good planning to make sure the researcher is aware of these costs.

### 6.7.4 Destroying Data

The cost of destroying the hard data should also be calculated before beginning the project. This could include shredding services or hard drive wipes. It is difficult to predict the cost of the destruction of data because some retention periods are as far as five years after the project completion, but an estimate for these services should be recognized.

## 6.8 Communication

Even if the PI has a very detailed data management plan, he or she cannot expect everything to run smoothly for the duration of the project with engaging in communication. The PI needs to communicate well with the team. He or she should personally educate the members regarding RCR issues, encourage team members to engage in open discussion regarding the data, and promote open communication regarding any issues or problems the team might face. Encouraging open communication among the team will make sure that everyone is aware of details involving the grant and helps strengthen the integrity of the data.

### 6.8.1 Communication Plan

By the time the project commences, the PI should implement a communications plan. It is best if this plan is in writing and available to all members, whether in hand out form, e-mail, or available on a Website. Copies may even be posted in the laboratory.

It is important that the communications plan establish a chain of command. It should also outline who is able to make decisions regarding the research and data. The team members must be aware of what information is to be communicated, who will be told, and how they will be informed. The plan should also let the team know what forms of communications should be in writing, electronic, or oral.

It is a good idea to integrate a communications plan with data collections issues. The approach for collecting data and who to inform about that steps have been taken can be integrated. This should outline the way data collection will be recorded as well and serve as a benchmark among the project's timeline.

A sample idea would be requiring team members to send an e-mail every time they leave the laboratory. The communication should include how much data was collected, who collected the data, in what format was the data collected, and so on. This would create an easy paper trail promoting the integrity of the data.

The communication does not have to be limited to internal dialogs. The plan can include communication within the institution, including updates with the Office of Sponsored Projects. They may also mention communications directly with the funding agency as well as set time to speak with peers working in different laboratories or institutions.

## 6.9 Leadership

It is necessary that the PI be the leader of the research as well as the research team. To be an effective leader, the PI should conduct himself or herself in a manner that provides the project's goals. The PI needs to set the vision of the project and control the way it is heading. If the PI is able to involve every team member in the goal-setting process, it will unify the team, and the work will demonstrate the care put into the research. Creating goals will also provide the PI with a way to self-check the project and note who is accountable for which parts of the research.

It is necessary that the PI remains a figure of authority but does not alienate team members or appear unapproachable. Open communication should be encouraged or problems may arise that the PI is unaware of, which could affect the data. Fostering trust among the team members will allow the PI to be more aware of what is happening on the project.

An effective leader strengthens the integrity of the data. The PI should make sure he or she is creating a healthy environment for the team and leading by example with specific goals and open communication.

## 6.10 Managing Conflicts

It is a safe assumption that conflicts will present themselves over the course of a project. These issues may be between team members or a team member and the PI. As the leader, it is the PI's responsibility to recognize and deal with the conflicts. Failure to act quickly can endanger the integrity of the research.

Some issues that could arise include conflicting outlooks between team members, lack of recognition, authorship disputes, feeling over- or underworked, a belief that not all of the resources are being used to their full potential, refusal to follow protocols, frustration with the project, unhappiness over the goals of the project, or refusal to accept negative outcomes.

If the PI has created an environment in which the team members feel like they can openly communicate among each other and express themselves, these issues will be brought to the PI's attention before they get out of control and cause a major issue within the laboratory.

The PI should provide constructive feedback and address the problems as soon as they arise.

One of the best ways to deal with an issue is to simply listen. Active listening, which is done with body language, attentiveness, and awareness of the issues, will let the offended party know he or she is being taken seriously. The PI should never interrupt, react to, or correct the team member. Once the person is finished expressing the initial concerns, the PI should continue in a calm and open manner.

The PI should not show judgment or pick sides, but rather talk softly and explain his or her views on the issues. This might include emphasizing contributions the team has made or reiterating the initial goals of the project. It is important the PI continue to stress his or her approachability and not shut down open communications.

Although the PI cannot predict every conflict that will arise, he or she should address them in a calm and consistent manner. The PI should focus the discussion on the conflict itself and not let any member of the team feel attacked. If a strong communication plan is in place and the PI has demonstrated leadership skills, then the team will come to the PI with any issues. By handling these issues in a quick and consistent manner, the PI is preserving the integrity of the research.

## 7. ADDRESSING NONCOMPLIANCE

### 7.1 Research Integrity

Data management policies and regulations are put into place to ensure the integrity of the research. A violation of data management practices and procedures will normally amount to research misconduct.

In 2005, processes were put into place by the Public Health Service (PHS) regarding allegations of research misconduct [55]. These regulations only apply to projects funded by a PHS organization. Universities who receive funding from a PHS organization must have internal policies that reflect the requirements of these regulations. In many cases, the internal policies expand to all research and are not limited to PHS funded projects.

The ORI is the agency that enforces research misconduct rules. It provides a sample policy that gives great detail and guidance when creating a research misconduct policy. Following is a detail of the requirements the internal policies should contain.

### 7.2 Research Misconduct

When an accusation of research misconduct arises, it is normally a unique case. There is no way to predict exactly what the issue may be. The parties and the university itself may be very affected by an accusation. A finding of research misconduct can lead to suspension of one's career as well as distress of reputation. It is important that all of these cases are treated carefully and follow the orders of procedure outlined by any policy [56].

Many issues may arise regarding research, but not all of them will constitute research misconduct. The ORI defines research misconduct as fabrication, falsification, and plagiarism. Fabrication is making up data or result and recording or reporting them. Falsification is manipulating research materials, equipment, or processes, or changing or omitting data or results such that the research is not accurately represented in the research record. Plagiarism is the appropriation of another person's ideals, processes, results, or works without giving appropriate credit [57]. The key to defining research misconduct is intent. Research misconduct does not include honest error or differences of opinion. Research misconduct must consist of intentional fabrication, falsification, or plagiarism.

## 7.3 Parties

When following the guidelines of the ORI, it is easiest to become familiar with its terminology and incorporate the mechanism into internal policies. These are the generally accepted terms used across PHS-funded institutions.

### 7.3.1 Research Integrity Officer

The Research Integrity Officer is often referred to as the RIO. The RIO is an institutional official who is responsible to the initial assessment of research misconduct allegations [58]. His or her assessment will determine whether the allegations warrants further review. If an accusation moves forward, the RIO will oversee the entire investigation and inquiry. A committee will be formed by the RIO, who will take the lead in assessing the information. The RIO will collect and securely store all evidence gathered and serve as the key point throughout the entire proceeding. Institutions vary in regards to who serves the role of RIO. The individual is often a member of the Division of Research or similar office. In smaller institutions, the RIO may also be a faculty member, but this is not always the case. The RIO's identity should not be kept secret. It is important that the entire university, including undergraduates, is easily able to ascertain who the RIO is.

#### 7.3.1.1 RESEARCH INTEGRITY BOOT CAMP

The ORI offers a boot camp for RIOs. Many different aspects of the RIO position are covered in great detail. It is extremely helpful for new RIOs. The boot camps are not regularly scheduled. If someone is interested in attending they should contact the ORI for further details.

#### 7.3.1.2 ASSOCIATION OF RESEARCH INTEGRITY OFFICERS

In 2013 the first Association of Research Integrity Officers meeting was held. This is designed to be an organization separate from ORI, where RIOs can stay up-to-date on issues affecting research misconduct. The organization is in early stages of development, but as membership grows it is expected to have a large impact on the RIO community and strengthen the resources available to RIOs.

### 7.3.2 Deciding Official

The deciding official (DO) is an institutional official who is responsible for final determinations of research misconduct [58]. Generally, they are removed from the inquiry and investigation phases. They are informed of the findings of the investigation and will make the final call based on the information provided. In certain institutions, they are responsible for listening to any appeals regarding research misconduct findings. The DO will decide what administrative actions should be taken and ensuring they are enforced. This often may be detailed as other university policies and procedures will come into play, such as any union agreements, tenure policies, and human resource requirements. The DO and the RIO must never be the same person; however, in many cases, the DO has the right to appoint individuals to serve on a committee.

### 7.3.3 Complainant

Researchers do not draw attention to their own instances of misconduct. The complainant, sometimes referred to as the whistleblower, is the person who notifies the institution of the potential misconduct [59]. Organizations should encourage complainants to come forward and make the process as easy as possible. Some organizations allow for anonymous complainants. If this is the case, then the RIO will act as the complainant for purposes of record.

The first person the complainant should speak with is the RIO. Often potential complainants will go to a dean or department chair. These individuals should immediately refer the complainant to the RIO instead of trying to handle this issue themselves. It is in the best interests of the complainant to study any internal policies before making an accusation. The policy should let them know who the RIO is, where the allegation should be reported, what they can expect from the process, and what protections they are provided. After misconduct proceedings start, the complainant does not carry any additional responsibilities. They may be called to investigations in the role of witness, but they will not be considered a party to the proceedings [58].

#### 7.3.3.1 RETALIATION

In accordance with 42 CFR 93, organizations must "take all reasonable and practical steps to protect the positions and reputations of good faith complainants, witnesses and committee members and protect them from retaliation by respondents and other institutional members."

It is important that the allegation is made in good faith for this provision to come into play. The complainant must have an honest belief that there is an instance of research misconduct. When there is an allegation made with reckless disregard or willful ignorance of facts, these protections are not awarded to the complainant.

If the accusation is in good faith it is the responsibility of the university to ensure that there is no retaliation taken against the complainant (ORI, http://ori.hhs.gov/guidelines-whistleblowers [accessed 12.17.14]).

### 7.3.4 Respondent

The Respondent is the party accused of research misconduct [60]. All allegations should be taken seriously as even an allegation can damage a researcher's reputation and career. The majority of allegations of research misconduct will not stop after initial review by the RIO, but once the respondent is informed of the accusation, he or she should start by reviewing all policies, both internal and external.

It is recommended that the respondent start to identify witnesses, gather documentation, decide whether or not an expert should be consulted, make sure that no retaliation is taken against whoever he or she believes the complainant to be, and try to maintain confidentiality of the proceedings.

The respondent should receive a fair and objective investigation. They should also be given an opportunity to admit to research misconduct and avoid the procedure. They must be given an opportunity to comment on the findings, a copy of any reports, access to the evidence, and be notified throughout the stages of the proceedings (42 CFR 93).

If there is no finding of research misconduct the University should take all steps possible to restore the reputation of the respondent (ORI, Survey of Accused but Exonerated Individuals in Research Misconduct Cases [accessed 12.17.14]). If the respondent leaves the institution before the proceedings are over, the proceedings will continue. Resigning or transferring will not stop any research misconduct cases.

## 7.4 Initial Allegations

The institution's policy should outline methods that initial allegation may be made [61]. This should include whether anonymous allegations are accepted and what form the allegations must take, whether it be oral or written. Individuals may make complaints directly to ORI or the PHS funding institutions.

## 7.5 Initial Assessment

The initial assessment phase is where most accusation of research misconduct cease [58]. The RIO will meet with the complainant, whether face-to-face or by electronic means. After hearing the allegation, the RIO may conduct interviews, analyze documents, and any other investigation activities deemed necessary.

The RIO will decide whether or not the allegation falls within the scope of research misconduct. He or she will also determine how credible the accusation is and whether or not there is potential evidence. If the RIO believes the allegation is credible and fits the definition of research misconduct, the case will move forward to the inquiry phase.

## 7.6 Inquiry Phase

The inquiry phase is not designed to determine guilt, rather to make an evaluation of the available evidence, including witnesses, and determining whether there is evidence to move forward to the investigation phase [58].

### 7.6.1 Inquiry Committee

At this point, the RIO will establish the inquiry committee. The internal university policy should reflect how many members serve on the committee, usually ranging from three to six. They may be institutional officials, experts in the field under inquiry, or faculty members. It is normally at the discretion of the RIO who forms the inquiry committee.

#### 7.6.1.1 SEQUESTRATION

The respondent must be notified that the accusation is moving toward an inquiry. It is normally in the RIO's best interests that any sequestration of computers, notebooks, and any other possible evidence be sequestered at this time. Evidence that is valuable to the inquiry and investigation should be sequestered as efficiently and speedily as possible.

It is important that procedures are in place for securing the original documentation and any other records that are relating to the research. Items can be lost or destroyed that will greatly hinder the inquiry and further investigation phases. This process may be intrusive and stressful for the respondent and the university as well.

ORI is available to offer any technical assistance and a variety of forensic tools that may be used to evaluate the evidence [62].

### 7.6.2 Final Report

After the inquiry phase, a report should be generated detailing the findings. This should summarize the evidence, list the witnesses, and indicate whether or not an investigation is warranted. If an investigation is warranted, then justification should be provided.

PHS regulations mandate that the inquiry report be finished within 60 days from the commencement of the inquiry. The inquiry report must be submitted to ORI [63].

## 7.7 Investigation Phase

If the inquiry committee recommends the proceedings move forward, the investigation phase will take place next. The investigation will explore the details and examine all the evidence in depth. It is necessary that the investigation broaden the scope of the inquiry committee and determine whether there are any additional concerns regarding research misconduct [58].

The investigation will consist of a variety of activities. This can include, but are not limited to, reviewing the evidence, reviewing published materials, inspecting laboratories, interviewing parties, and pursuing all leads regarding the conduct in question.

### 7.7.1 Investigation Committee

In a similar manner to the inquiry phase, an investigation committee will be brought forward. It is at the discretion of the university policy whether the inquiry committee and investigation committee have the same makeup.

### 7.7.2 Investigation Report

The report must include the nature of the allegation, the documentation of all PHS support (if applicable), the specific allegation of research misconduct, the institutional policies and procedures under which the proceedings were conducted, a summary of the evidence, a list of the evidence taken into custody, and a statement of the findings for each allegation.

The DO will review the investigation report and has the final decision on whether or not to accept the findings. If the research is PHS funded, the investigation report must be submitted to ORI for review as well as the PHS funding agency [58].

If the research is PHS-funded and if the investigation cannot be completed in 120 calendar days, then the RIO will submit a written request to the ORI for an extension. If the request is granted, the university will file periodic progress reports as requested by the ORI.

## 7.8 Institutional Decision

Once the decision has been made on whether or not research misconduct occurred, the institution must inform the respondent and the complainant of the final determination in writing [57].

The DO must also determine what other organizations must be notified. This could include publications, licensing boards, professional societies, or law enforcement.

## 7.9 ORI Oversight

Both the inquiry and investigation reports must be sent to ORI for final review. ORI will examine both documents carefully and request any subsequent data or information necessary to complete their overview.

Once the overview is completed, ORI will draft an oversight report. If the allegation of research misconduct was supported, then ORI will try to work with the respondent to create a Voluntary Exclusion Agreement in which the respondent accepts impositions based on the misconduct. If an agreement cannot be reached, ORI will recommend impositions of administrative actions to the Assistant Secretary for Health or submit a charge letter to the HHS Departmental Appeals Board.

## 7.10 Appeals

### 7.10.1 *Institutional Level*

It is up to the institution whether or not an internal appeal process will be created. There is no requirement for an appeal to exist from the ORI [58]. If an appeal option exists, the institution must include this information in its policy. This includes the grounds and procedures for filing an appeal and who may file the appeal.

### 7.10.2 *ORI*

A respondent may request a hearing on the PHS finding or administrative action before the HHS Department Appeals Board within 30 days of receipt of the final report from the ORI. This is conducted by an administrative law judge.

## 7.11 Case Summaries

ORI offers case summaries of research misconduct proceedings on its Website. The case summaries can be very informative for RIOs and others interested in research misconduct processes [64].

## References

[1] Atkins Daniel, Droegemeier Kelvin, Feldman Stuart, Garcia-Molina Hector, Klein Michael, Messerschmitt David, et al. Revolutionizing science and engineering through cyberinfrastructure: report of the national science foundation blue-ribbon advisory panel on cyberinfrastructure. National Science Foundation; 2003.
[2] H.R, 708 – 113th Congress (2013-2014). http://beta.congress.gov/bill/113th-congress/house-bill/708 [accessed 02.02.14].
[3] NOT-OD-03-032, National Institute of Health. http://grants.nih.gov/grants/guide/notice-files/NOT-OD-03-032.html [accessed 12.12.13].
[4] PL 110–161, Section 218. http://publicaccess.nih.gov/policy.htm [accessed 12.12.13].
[5] Interagency Working Group on Digital Data. Harnessing the power of digital data for science and society. Executive summary. Committee on Science of the National Science and Technology Council; 2009.

[6] Chapter II.C.2.j. Grant proposal guide. National Science Foundation; 2011.

[7] http://www.whitehouse.gov/administration/eop/ostp/initiatives#Openness [accessed 27.11.13].

[8] Holdren John P. Section 4b Increasing access to the results of federally funded scientific research. Office of Science and Technology Policy; 2013.

[9] Clinical Tools Inc. Guidelines for responsible data management in scientific research. 2006.

[10] Kalichman Michael. Data management. In: Kulakowski EC, Chronoister LU, editors. Research administration and management. 2006. Sudbury, Massachusetts.

[11] Stenech Nicholas H. Introduction to the responsible conduct of research. Office of Research Integrity; 2000.

[12] http://ori.hhs.gov/education/products/n_illinois_u/datamanagement/dotopic.html [accessed 02.12.13].

[13] Dietrich Dianne, Adamus Trisha, Miner Alison, Steinhart Gail. De-mystifying the data management requirements of research funders. ISTL Summer 2012. http://www.istl.org/12-summer/refereed1.html. [accessed 17.12.14].

[14] Chapter VI.D.4. Awards and administration guide (AAG). National Science Foundation; 2013.

[15] Updated information about the data management plan required for all proposals. http://www.nsf.gov/bio/pubs/BIODMP061511.pdf [accessed 14.12.13].

[16] Data management for NSF engineering directorate proposals and awards. http://nsf.gov/eng/general/ENG_DMP_Policy.pdf [accessed 14.12.13].

[17] Data management for NSF EHR directorate. National Science Foundation; March 2011.

[18] Data management guidance for CISE proposals and awards. http://www.nsf.gov/cise/cise_dmp.jsp [accessed 14.12.13].

[19] Directorate for Geosciences—Data policies. http://www.nsf.gov/geo/geo-data-policies/index.jsp [accessed 14.12.13].

[20] Data management for NSF SBE directorate proposals and awards. October 2010.

[21] Dissemination and sharing of research results. http://www.nsf.gov/bfa/dias/policy/dmp.jsp [accessed 14.12.13].

[22] Directorate of Mathematical and Physical Sciences Division of Physics Advice to PIs on Data Management Plans. http://www.nsf.gov/bfa/dias/policy/dmpdocs/phy.pdf [accessed 14.12.13].

[23] Directorate of Mathematical and Physical Sciences Division of Mathematical Sciences Advice to PIs on Data Management Plans. http://www.nsf.gov/bfa/dias/policy/dmpdocs/dms.pdf [accessed 14.12.13].

[24] Directorate of Mathematical and Physical Sciences Division of Materials Research Advice to PIs on Data Management Plans. http://www.nsf.gov/bfa/dias/policy/dmpdocs/dmr.pdf [accessed 14.12.13].

[25] Directorate of Mathematical and Physical Sciences Division of Chemistry Advice to PIs on Data Management Plans. http://www.nsf.gov/bfa/dias/policy/dmpdocs/che.pdf [accessed 14.12.13].

[26] Directorate of Mathematical and Physical Sciences Division of Astronomical Sciences Advice to PIs on Data Management Plans. http://www.nsf.gov/bfa/dias/policy/dmpdocs/ast.pdf [accessed 14.12.13].

[27] PL 110-161, Div G, Title II, Section 218. http://publicaccess.nih.gov/policy.htm.

[28] NOT-OD-03-032. Final NIH statement of sharing research data. February 2003.

[29] Office of the Chief Information Officer. http://energy.gov/cio/office-chief-information-officer [accessed 14.12.13].

[30] Biven Laura. Office of Science Statement on Digital Data Management. United States Department of Energy; March 2013.

[31] Climate and Environmental Sciences Division. http://science.energy.gov/ber/research/cesd/data-management/ [accessed 17.12.13].

[32] Hook, L.A., Christensen, S.W. Developing data management policy and guidance documents for your NARSTO program or project. http://cdiac.ornl.gov/programs/NARSTO/DM_develop_guide.pdf [accessed 17.12.13].

[33] Policy statement on data sharing in IES research centers. http://ies.ed.gov/funding/datasharing_policy.asp [accessed 17.12.13].

[34] U.S. Environmental Protection Agency. Open government data quality plan 1.0. May 2010.

[35] U.S. Environmental Protection Agency, Office of Research and Development, Office of Science Information Management. Survey of EPA and other federal agency scientific data management policies and guidance. April 2010.

[36] Meeker Sherwin. ADS chapter 203 assessing and learning. Sections 203.3.1.8; 203.3.2–203.3-17. November 2012.

[37] USAID/DCHA/ASHA Annual Program Statement. II 3.6. Monitoring and evaluation plan. November 2013.

[38] National Oceanographic Data Center. Long version of the data submission guidelines. http://www.nodc.noaa.gov/General/NODC-Submit/submit-guide.html#polguide [accessed 17.12.13].

[39] Guch Ingrid. It's time to share: proposed NOAA data policy. September 2011.

[40] Data rights and related issues. http://science.nasa.gov/earth-science/earth-science-data/data-information-policy/data-rights-related-issues/ [accessed 18.12.13].

[41] Earth Science Division, NASA Science Mission Directorate. Guidelines for development of a data management plan. Version 1.0. January 2011.

[42] Fisher Richard R. NASA heliophysics science data management policy. Version 1. April 2009.

[43] Data management plans for NEH office of digital Humanities proposals and awards. http://www.neh.gov/files/grants/data_management_plans_2013.pdf [accessed 18.12.13].

[44] American Heart Association. Guide for affiliate research awards. December 2011.

[45] Alfred P. Sloan Foundation. Digital information technology. http://www.sloan.org/major-program-areas/digital-information-technology/data-and-computational-research/ [accessed 18.12.13].

[46] CDC-GA-2005-14. CDC/ATSDR policy of releasing and sharing data. September 2005.

[47] National Institute of Justice, Data archiving plans for NIJ funding applicants. http://www.nij.gov/funding/data-resources-program/applying/Pages/data-archiving-strategies.aspx [accessed 19.12.13].

[48] National Institute of standards and technology guidelines, information quality Standards, and administrative mechanism. http://www.nist.gov/director/quality_standards.cfm [accessed 19.12.13].

[49] United States Department of Agriculture, Grants. http://www.csrees.usda.gov/funding/electronic.html [accessed 19.12.13].

[50] ORI. https://ori.hhs.gov/data-management-0 [accessed 01.12.13].

[51] NOT-OD-03-032, National Institute of Health. http://grants.nih.gov/grants/guide/notice-files/NOT-OD-03-032.html [accessed 12.12.13].

[52] University of California. https://dmp.cdlib.org/ [accessed 17.12.14].

[53] Dietrich D, Adamus T, Miner A, Steinhart G. De-mystifying the data management requirements of research funders. 2012.

[54] Jahnke LM, Asher A. Dilemma of digital stewardship a: research ethics and the problems of data sharing. In: Research data management. Council on Library and Information Resources; 2013.

[55] Responsibility of PHS Awardee and Applicant Institutions for dealing With and Reporting Possible Misconduct in Science, 42 CFR 50, 93. 2005.

[56] ORI. http://ori.hhs.gov/handling-misconduct [accessed 12.01.14].

[57] Responsibility of PHS Awardee and Applicant Institutions for dealing With and Reporting Possible Misconduct in Science, 42 CFR 93. 2005.

[58] ORI, Sample policy and procedures. http://ori.hhs.gov/sites/default/files/SamplePolicyandProcedures-5-07.pdf [accessed 12.01.14].

[59] ORI. http://ori.hhs.gov/complainant [accessed 12.01.14].

[60] ORI. http://ori.hhs.gov/respondent [accessed 12.01.14].

[61] ORI. http://ori.hhs.gov/handling-allegations [accessed 12.01.14].

[62] ORI. http://ori.hhs.gov/forensic-tools [accessed 12.01.14].

[63] ORI. http://ori.hhs.gov/sites/default/files/SamplePolicyandProcedures-5-07.pdf. The inquiry report [accessed 12.01.14].

[64] ORI. http://ori.hhs.gov/case_summary [accessed 12.01.14].

# Intellectual Property

*James H. Bratton*

Office of Technology Development, University of Oklahoma, Norman, OK, USA

## 1. SUMMARY

Commercial institutions often rely on innovation as a means to achieve success and will vigorously protect their inventions through legal and strategic means as a way to ensure that competitive advantage is maintained and exploited for the benefit of shareholders. Research universities produce scientific discoveries that not only inform our understanding of the world, but in some cases generate revenue that support the activities of the institution. As a result, such institutions find it essential to maintain an intellectual property (IP) policy to regulate the process for disclosure and protection of IP. Such a policy typically outlines the governance of IP ownership, its use, and the allocation of compensation resulting from commercialization. Employees typically agree to the terms of the policy when signing their employment agreement.

## 2. KEY PERSONNEL AND UNIVERSITY COMMITTEES DESIGNATED TO IMPLEMENT REGULATORY MANDATES

The administrative structure for the management of IP at a given university will vary according to each university's historical experience and precedence, as well as the priorities the university has set for itself regarding commercialization of research, entrepreneurship, and economic development. Regardless of these conditions, there are several core functions that are replicated widely and coordinate regularly inside and outside the university to ensure the proper implementation of IP regulation and each university's own IP policy. Relevant offices and committees may consist of employees from different departments across campus and may coordinate vertically throughout the institution, involving both academic and administrative personnel as well as representatives from outside the university hierarchy, in decision-making and operating activities. The key personnel responsible for compliance with IP regulation at universities typically include someone who functions as the executive director of the technology transfer office (TTO) or equivalent, the vice president (or vice chancellor) for research (VPR), and university general counsel. Other personnel who may be involved at various times include college deans, the provost, outside advisors, faculty or staff appointed to oversight committees, and members of the university's board of regents or trustees.

Although the practice of implementing an IP policy for a university may be coordinated through these key personnel and their offices, it is important to understand that the responsibility of adherence to the policy rests with every employee. Typically, faculty (and staff) hired by research institutions consent to the provisions of policies established for faculty (and/or staff) as a condition of their employment. Often such policies are indicated within a handbook of institutional guidelines and policies. The handbook will outline the employees' responsibilities and document their consent to the university's IP policies, including those the university implements as a recipient of external funding. As an example, the University of Oklahoma's Faculty Handbook [1] states:

> Section 3.3 Faculty Accountability "Persons who accept full-time employment at the University owe their first duty to the University."
> Section 3.29.1 Intellectual Property Policy: "It is the responsibility of University employees to disclose intellectual property and to foster an entrepreneurial attitude within the work force by involving students in the creation of intellectual property."

These principles are important to remember because innovation and the creation of IP are, at most universities, the result of a collaborative effort between and among faculty and students, as well as colleagues at other institutions, both academic and industrial. A university's IP policy is designed to enable the protection of IP for the benefit of the institution's mission, which includes teaching, continued research, and commercial exploitation of innovation. Therefore, researchers and students must be aware of, and adhere to, self-policing practices to ensure the integrity of the university's policies and the protection of IP.

## 2.1 Technology Transfer Office

While the form and content of the IP policy for any given university may originate from the university's board of regents, the basis of virtually every IP policy is to ensure that (1) all university faculty and staff disclose and assign to the university inventions made in the ordinary course and scope of their employment; and (2) the process of managing IP is compliant with the university's mission, for the benefit of the academic process, and is consistent across all aspects of the university. The central, coordinating entity for the IP policy is typically the TTO. Occasionally, this office may have a different name, such as office of technology development or office of licensing and commercialization, but the central responsibilities of this function are consistent: implementation and enforcement of the university's IP policy and compliance with federal or other contracted IP regulation. This office may be a centrally organized, independent, administrative function [2], integrated as a part of research services [3] unit, or integrated into a university academic entity (e.g., college of business) [4]. Alternatively, the functions may be decentralized across a university system through a distributed network of semiindependent campus-based technology transfer programs.

Depending on the size and scale of a university's commercialization and entrepreneurship activities, the TTO is often staffed by a diverse team of people with scientific, legal, commercialization, and administrative experience and run by an executive director who oversees operations of the office and may report to the university president or university vice president. The executive director usually has a background from either academia or industry and is tasked with authorizing the business decisions for patenting and licensing technology. In addition, the executive director will be responsible for ensuring that the IP policy is followed and adhered to by all university employees and for coordinating with other university individuals, departments, and/or committees to do so. In addition, the TTO may liaise with corporate or federal funding counterparts to negotiate or coordinate IP management before, during, and after a research project.

Upon the creation of IP, the implementation of IP regulation typically begins with an invention disclosure to the TTO. Someone who functions as a technology manager, within the TTO, typically will evaluate (or coordinate the evaluation of) the disclosure for IP protection and commercialization via licensing. During this process, the technology manager may interact with the university inventors, external sponsors of research, the university office that coordinates research service, including export controls, the internal office of legal counsel, and outside patent counsel to establish patentability, inventorship, assignability, and ownership of the invention depending on how many inventors and different institutions are involved. In addition, the technology manager may consult with entrepreneurs and operating companies who might be potential licensees and/or commercialization partners in an effort to assist with the commercialization strategy.

Regardless of the structure or composition of the TTO at any given university, management of IP assets and decisions about treatment of IP generation and rights may involve other offices at the university.

## 2.2 Office of Research Services

Most universities coordinate research administration activities through an office of research services (ORS) or some similar entity. Such an office is frequently involved in decisions related to IP at a university. ORS typically provides pre- and post-grant services to researchers regarding funding and grant contract administration. This office is usually managed under the purview of the university VPR. It is sometimes led by an associate vice president for research or an executive director who has strong administrative and contract management skills and is familiar with university and government funding agency research and regulations.

Ordinarily, during contract negotiations for grant funding, ORS will use standard IP language crafted by the TTO or university office of legal counsel that is based on, and consistent with, the university's IP policy. However, in some instances, circumstances unique to the sponsor or type of research will invoke a waiver by the university of IP rights that would typically inure to the university in favor of the research sponsor. This situation is most commonly experienced when universities participate in clinical trial studies sponsored on site by a pharmaceutical or medical device company seeking US Food and Drug Administration regulatory approval for a drug compound or medical device. In such circumstances, the executive director of the TTO may consult the VPR, the principal investigator(s), the college dean(s), the provost, and/or the university chief financial officer, because relinquishing such rights may place deleterious restrictions on the research (e.g., those which are contrary to the university's mission and may trigger unrelated business taxable income for the university).

These limitations might include, but may not be limited to, inhibited academic freedoms (e.g., publication, teaching, or further research) (see Section 3.2).

## 2.3 Financial Services

The commercialization of IP generally results in licensing agreements with companies that develop, manufacture, and sell the products and services that result from IP created at a university. Licensing terms often include upfront fees, royalties, milestone payments, and reimbursement of patent expenses, all of which must be accounted for and distributed to the appropriate parties as dictated by the university's IP policy.

The sharing of royalties, fees, and other receipts related to licensing activities between inventors and their institutions varies greatly among universities (Table 1). Some universities recover specific costs before allocating monies to inventors and university departments, while others allow inventors to share directly in the first dollars received as a way to reinforce and encourage commercialization activities among researchers.

In addition, many universities encourage the formation of startup and spinout companies to foster economic development within their community, region, or state. As a result, the university may take an equity position in the nascent company in lieu of any upfront payment of licensing fees to help the management team preserve cash for operations. Consequently, offices responsible for university financial services (e.g., the bursars office) may be involved from time to time to receive cash payments; allocate receipts according to the IP policy; hold and exchange stock certificates as needed for the continued capitalization activities of the portfolio companies; and receive and act on K-1 and other tax forms received from licensees in which the university holds an equity stake.

TABLE 1    Sample Waterfall Comparison of Licensing Revenue Distribution Policies

|  | University of Oklahoma | University of Kansas | University of Texas | University of Colorado |
|---|---|---|---|---|
| Amount to inventors | 35% of gross | 1/3 of net | 50% of net | 25% of net |
| Deductible costs | After distribution to inventors, unreimbursed patent expenses | Unreimbursed patent expenses | Tech transfer operating, expenses and unreimbursed patent expenses | Unreimbursed patent expenses |
| University allocations | 5% president<br>10% vice president of research<br>10% inventor college(s)<br>20% TTO<br>20% growth fund | 1/3 KU Research Center<br>1/3 inventor college(s) | 50% to the University of Texas system | 25% campus chancellor<br>25% inventor's lab<br>25% university use |
| Source | www.otd.ou.edu/forms.htm | https://documents.ku.edu/policies/research/technology transfer.htm | www.utsystem.edu/bor/rules/90000Series/90101.pdf | www.cu.edu/sites/default/files/1013.pdf |

While royalties, licensing fees, and patent reimbursements are not taxable receipts for tax-advantaged universities, distributions of profit and loss allocated to, or received by, a university as a result of an equity position it holds are considered by the Internal Revenue Service (IRS) to be unrelated business taxable income [5]. Therefore, universities with equity positions in startup companies who receive such allocations or member distributions must report these receipts to the IRS (both real and "in kind"): document revenue, costs, and any income; and pay tax on the income [6].

## 2.4 Office of Legal Counsel

Because IP is a legal asset, legal resources should be devoted to the creation, protection, management, and commercialization of the asset. Patenting and licensing expertise are two obvious areas of legal proficiency required for successful compliance. However, other legal issues such as export controls, litigation, and employment may come into play regarding the creation, management, and/or disposition of IP.

Specifically regarding the protection of IP, the level of involvement of the office of legal counsel can vary widely across US universities. Given the technical and often nuanced nature of filing, prosecuting, and maintaining patents, access to strong patenting expertise across a variety of scientific domains is a must for universities. Some TTOs employ a staff of patent attorneys to file patent prosecutions on behalf of the university. Others hire outside counsel, but have a patent attorney and patent agent on staff to assist with the patent strategy and to oversee coordination of outside counsel activities. Others still rely exclusively on outside counsel. Much of the decision regarding in-house versus outsourced filing is driven by financial resources available to the TTO.

Aside from filing for IP protection, the office of legal counsel may become involved in other issues related to the management of IP, such as litigation with licensees and/or infringers; litigation between inventors and the university related to ownership and assignment of IP; and issues related to export controls and the establishment of technology control plans for handling export controlled technologies.

Because many researchers collaborate with peers at other institutions and may even change employment among universities or between universities and industry, the dates on which, and location(s) where, an inventive concept is derived and reduced to practice can become germane to the issues of assignment and ownership for the inventor and his or her employer. It is prudent for universities to obtain a day zero disclosure summary from any newly arriving faculty member and also a last day disclosure summary from any departing faculty to record the then-current state of that faculty member's research, especially if funding for research is being transferred from one institution to another.

## 2.5 Equity Management Committee

Oftentimes, universities will accept equity ownership in a startup company as a consideration for licensing to the company's IP developed at the university. Equity ownership may be in the form of stock, membership interest, options, warrants, convertible notes, debentures, or other financial instrument(s).

When a university takes equity in a startup, it does so with the intent of helping the company preserve cash by reducing or eliminating licensing payments in the early stages of the company's life cycle. This exchange enables a more efficient use of capital by the company for operations and commercial development, thereby reducing the risk and helping the company attract outside investors. As a stockholder (or member), a university obliges itself to act as a fiduciary for the company and the interests it represents. Sometimes these activities involve filling board seats, voting on actions of the company, and maintaining confidentiality of proprietary company information. Under these circumstances, university employees managing the equity positions are also fiduciaries to internal constituents (e.g., inventors, the university departments that benefit from equity realizations and tax payers at public universities).

Acceptance, management, and disposal of equity positions may be at the sole discretion of the TTO or the responsibility of an internal committee. Some universities have accelerated processes for taking equity in startups, with the goal of decreasing delay associated with decision-making. Others have established equity management committees [7] to provide objective assistance, perspective, and guidance to the university administrators about the risk, liability, and operational insight relative to the acquisition management and disposition of equity positions the university might seek to hold [8]. This committee might comprise alumni, trustees, and/or industry experts with experience in financial markets, entrepreneurship, venture capital, and/or private equity.

## 3. COMMON COMPLIANCE CHALLENGES

There are several common compliance issues related to the management of IP at research institutions. Some issues are the result of a researcher or an administrator not being aware of the institution's policies, while others are more intentional. Regardless of the motive(s), consequences for noncompliance can be severe.

### 3.1 Failure to Disclose the Creation of Intellectual Property

Most institutions, both academic and industrial, that emphasize research and innovation have an employment policy requiring all employees to disclose to their employer and further assign their rights to any inventions created during the course of employment. This practice is based on the logic that because the institution is paying the employee's salary, directing the employee's activities, and providing the resources for the employee to work, the employee's work product is "work made for hire" and therefore the property of the institution (employer). Occasionally, employees may not be aware of their company policy or may not be aware of the procedure for disclosure and therefore fail to disclose an invention. Other times (particularly at universities), researchers may wish to publish and explicitly not protect their work so that it may be used solely for teaching and further research. Sometimes, researchers from different institutions may collaborate on a project that produces joint IP, and disclosure of the invention is made to only one of the organizations. Sometimes, too, for whatever reason (e.g., lack of policy awareness, personal gain, etc.), researchers may try to seek protection for their work-related inventions on their own. Regardless of the cause, it is the responsibility of the executive director of the TTO to initiate corrective action to obtain assignment for inventions that should have been disclosed under the institution's policies for management of IP.

An appropriate process for handling policy violations may involve the university legal counsel, those responsible for university research administration and internal audit, and the representatives of the provost (because the researchers' actions could have academic ethics implications). A thorough due-diligence effort examining laboratory notebooks, interviews with students and colleagues, and IP protection searches is typically necessary to gather adequate evidence to determine whether or not a breach of duty has occurred.

## 3.2 Waiver or Assignment of Rights to Intellectual Property

Many research institutions conduct collaborative or sponsored research with, and for, industrial partners, in which a condition of the funding is the assignment or transfer of ownership of any foreground IP to the sponsor. Examples include clinical trial testing of new drugs and medical therapies developed and owned by a pharmaceutical company[1]; research based on proprietary products and processes patented or otherwise protected by the industry partner; and scientific analysis of materials for further research. Under these circumstances, it is not necessarily expected that the university researcher will invent anything new; to safeguard against that rare occurrence, corporate sponsors will require a waiver or assignment of the university's IP rights in favor of the sponsor.

While this practice of "work made for hire" is common among private sector collaborators, it is in direct violation of a university's mission to disseminate freely new knowledge (as per the standard tax definition of educational institution) and an objective "business use" test used by the IRS to monitor an institution's ongoing tax-advantaged status and ensure compliance with the use of funds generated from the issuance of tax-advantaged bonds. Other situations in which a university agrees in advance to license royalty rates for an as-yet uninvented technology are also considered "work made for hire" and violate the university's tax-advantaged mission. These tests apply not only to the type of revenue the institution receives, but also govern the terms of tax-advantaged bonds issued by the institution to underwrite the building in which the research is conducted.

Sponsored research that requires the waiver of IP rights in favor of the sponsor (e.g., work made for hire) may trigger business use issues for the university [9]. As a result, unrelated business taxable income (UBTI) may need to be accounted for and reported. Perhaps more problematic, however, is that when a tax-advantaged entity engages in nonmission-related activities, the tax-advantaged status may be challenged. Furthermore, the tax-advantaged nature of bonds used to underwrite the funding of buildings where "work made for hire" research is conducted may be called into jeopardy.

## 3.3 Conflicts of Interest

Many university researchers consult outside their regular university appointments—perhaps during summer months or during a sabbatical, or even during the school year. Usually, companies that rely on and pay for consultants from academia want clear title to IP generated by the consultant without additional compensation (i.e., "work made for hire," not a

---

[1] Many universities consider phase I and phase II US Food and Drug Administration clinical trial testing to be "for benefit" and therefore protected activities commensurate with their tax-advantaged status (see IRS PLR 8,230,002 April 30, 1982).

licensing arrangement). Because academic researchers are typically hired to consult specifically for their expertise in a given domain, their duty of assignment of invention is conflicted between the university and the corporation for which they consult.

Another form of conflict of interest often arises when a university researcher desires to form a start-up around his or her invention. In these situations, the researcher's duty of loyalty is conflicted on several levels. With respect to IP, the researcher takes on the dual roles of being both a university employee (obliged to disclose and assign interest in IP to the university) and a company employee (obliged to disclose and assign interest in IP to the company). Furthermore, the researcher is expected to aid in promoting the company's financial success whether as a spokesperson, leveraging their university affiliation, or by putting the company's financial interests above those of the university.

Resolving the conflict related to duty of assignment in both of these cases is often solved through discussions and negotiations with the company and the university researcher. Demarcating and documenting the topics, areas of research, scopes of work, and use of university and/or company facilities and resources used in the course of work of the researcher are usually the best ways to ensure compliance with the university's IP policy and communication of expectations related to employee performance.

However, the remaining issue of financial reward related to a researcher's private enterprise based on university's IP is more complicated, nuanced, and difficult to manage. Just as one example, establishing licensing terms between the university and the company for IP incentivizes the researcher as the company owner to negotiate for the most favorable financial terms. In addition, when inventing improvements, the researcher as the company employee has strong incentives to make sure the invention (and therefore ownership) occurred as a result of his or her company employment or use of company resources.

### 3.4 Inappropriate Sharing of Intellectual Property

It is common knowledge and practice that university faculty shares research. The foundation of universities throughout the history and throughout the world is the sharing of knowledge. But protection is the cornerstone of IP, and sometimes researchers share their invention publicly (e.g., at a conference or via a poster or publication), or they share it inadvertently with someone outside the university before patent or copyright filings protect the invention. Even a dissertation defense by a master's or doctoral candidate is considered a public disclosure and can result in forfeiture of protection rights. Faculty and advanced degree students who disclose inventions to their TTO prior to publication or theses defense often are able to protect their inventions while obtaining scholarly attribution for their innovation.

## 4. ADDRESSING NONCOMPLIANCE

While some noncompliance issues are complex and rife with challenges (e.g., conflicts of interest), most are resolved through a clear communication by the university of policies, practices, and expectations. Continuous communication and education may be necessary in some cases, particularly involving the hiring of new faculty who may be unfamiliar with the university's policies or with the protection of IP in general.

When instances of noncompliance arise, however, addressing them usually involves both administrative and academic input. Violations of IP regulation(s) often cross multiple institutional codes, as mentioned above, and rectifying the infringement may involve the TTO, university legal counsel, and representatives from the provost's office, the office overseeing export controls, internal audit, and the vice president for research.

# References

[1] University of Oklahoma Norman Campus Faculty Handbook. https://apps.hr.ou.edu/FacultyHandbook/ [accessed 04.03.15].

[2] Stanford University Office of Technology Licensing. http://otl.stanford.edu/ [accessed 12.05.14].

[3] Emory University Office of Technology Transfer. http://www.ott.emory.edu/ [accessed 12.05.14].

[4] University of Oklahoma Office of Technology Development. http://www.ou.edu/otd.html [accessed 12.05.14].

[5] 26 U.S.C. 512-Unrelated Business Taxable Income. http://www.gpo.gov/fdsys/granule/USCODE-2010-title26/USCODE-2010-title26-subtitleA-chap1-subchapF-partIII-sec512 [accessed 30.11.14].

[6] Harding Jr BM. The tax Law of Colleges and universities. 4th ed. Washington (DC): National Association of College and University Business Officers; 2012.

[7] University of Oklahoma Norman Campus Faculty Handbook, Intellectual property policy Section 3.27.1(C). https://apps.hr.ou.edu/FacultyHandbook/ [accessed 04.03.15].

[8] University of Oklahoma Norman Campus Faculty Handbook, Intellectual property policy Section 3.27.2(C). https://apps.hr.ou.edu/FacultyHandbook/ [accessed 04.03.15].

[9] US Internal Revenue Service. Revenue procedure 2007-46. July 16, 2007.

# Financial Conflicts of Interest in Research

## Julie D. Gottlieb

**Johns Hopkins University, Baltimore, MD, USA**

*It is difficult to get a man to understand something, when his salary depends on his not understanding it.* **Upton Sinclair [1]**

## 1. INTRODUCTION

Americans holds science and scientists in high regard. Yet more than 60% of the public say they worry that new medicines and health care treatments do not receive adequate testing before they reach the market [2]. It is hard to know whether this concern reflects media reports about ethical lapses in biomedical science or the inherent challenges of developing safe and effective drugs. But along with the growing role of industry in science, there has been a series of scandals, some involving harm to patients and research subjects, which have made the scientific community and some of the public wary of commercial relationships.

Industry involvement in the scientific research enterprise in universities, hospitals, and research institutes can be immensely valuable and is virtually the only way that ideas and inventions generated in the academy become commercially available products with the promise for improving human health and welfare. The involvement takes many forms. Companies sponsor research projects, conduct collaborative research, license inventions, hire consultants, acquire university startup companies, and provide grants and philanthropy. These relationships nearly always include the transfer of money or equity to researchers and research institutions.

Scientists are trained to seek the truth and follow the data wherever they lead. It is rare for a scientist to be accused of deliberately falsifying data, cutting corners, or slanting results because that investigator has money riding on the outcome, in part because it is difficult to prove causality. But there is a broad consensus in the biomedical research community that financial interests are a source of bias. A growing body of research shows that individuals with even small financial incentives make decisions designed to maximize personal gain [3].

Still other studies show that there are strong associations between industry-supported studies and those where researchers have financial interests and positive study conclusions [4].

Science and scientists are not about to pull back from relationships with industry that bring critical financing and expertise to bear on the increasingly complex and costly research enterprise. Instead, to address the risks of bias associated with economic interests, the scientific community and regulators have sought to devise structures for identifying financial interests, evaluating their risks, and "reducing, managing, or eliminating" conflicts of interest (COIs) that threaten research objectivity or the safety of research subjects. This chapter describes some of the key historical events and trends in COIs in research and discusses regulation, community standards, and the challenges for scientists and research administrators.

Financial interests that have potential to influence research come in many forms. The major currency in science is publication, and those with strong publication records are best positioned to win competitively awarded grants that most scientists depend on. Scientific and medical journals want to publish studies with interesting or positive results, not those that show inconclusive or negative results. Journals themselves have financial COIs because the best way to sell advertisements and reprints to companies is to publish studies with compelling results in fields of interest to them. So the enterprise of science is biased toward generating publishable data, often in the form of studies with positive results. In addition, research funding from industry, an increasingly important source of support, creates risks of bias because the studies often are designed to demonstrate the safety and effectiveness of the sponsor's products or technology. Even grant agreements that are structured carefully to protect academic independence cannot eliminate the appearance of company influence on the research. Research institutions' budgets also are increasingly dependent on the funds from grants, licenses, and collaborations with industry as well as philanthropy. Through these relationships research institutions accumulate financial interests (for example, stock and potential sales royalty) in companies involved in research on their campuses. To address these "institutional conflicts of interest," the research community has devised a set of standards that, while generally not binding, are being adopted by more and more institutions.

This chapter deals with the personal economic interests of researchers—consulting income, licensing payments, and equity interests—that are the subject of federal regulation. The focus is largely on biomedical research because of its direct impact on medical care and human health and because it is the setting for most of the problems and regulatory responses. However, COIs in economics, food and agriculture, education, and energy research are gaining more attention in the media [5,6].

The chapter begins with a discussion of the history and background to the current regulatory environment. The 2011 Public Health Service (PHS regulation), the one of most interest to leaders and administrators in research institutions, is discussed in detail, along with descriptions of the resources institutions should consider as they build a COI program. The chapter closes with a discussion of some of the major challenges posed by the regulation, and hypothetical cases are provided throughout to help illustrate approaches to addressing the challenges.

## 2. HISTORICAL PERSPECTIVES

### 2.1 The Growth of Academic–Industry Relationships

Financial COIs in research are largely a phenomenon of the late twentieth and early twenty-first centuries. Before this period, the academy and industry operated quite independently of one another. Large companies had in-house research and development operations; academic researchers published their findings without regard to intellectual property protection or potential economic value; and small life science companies were few in number because they had no access to novel technology and the investment it might attract.

The situation changed in 1980. The move toward large-scale commercialization of biomedical research universities started with Congressional passage of the University and Small Business Patent Procedures Act of 1980, commonly known as the Bayh-Dole Act. The act was designed to help end the economic stagnation of the 1970s by spurring commercial development of scientific discoveries made in university laboratories. For the first time, research institutions receiving federal funds were allowed to retain title to the inventions made in their laboratories with federal funding. They were expected to file for patent protection on intellectual property and to transfer it to firms for commercial development so that innovations resulting from the taxpayers' investment in research would lead to new diagnostic tests, medications, and other tools for advancing public health and welfare. The act directed institutions to give preference to small firms and required that the income from commercialization be shared with the inventors of the technology. So Bayh-Dole set the stage for universities and other research institutions to exploit their inventions and, in the process, generate financial interests for institutions and researchers [7].

In the early 1980s, universities established technology transfer offices. They hired patent attorneys to protect intellectual property, and licensing and business development specialists to make deals for commercial development of inventions. University leaders hoped that, in addition to generating wealth and incentivizing researchers to disclose novel ideas, income from commercial licenses would help support their research laboratories.

Another important outgrowth of the Bayh-Dole Act was an increase in the number of researchers consulting for industry. Companies that licensed technology from universities recognized the value of having regular access to the inventors as development continued in industry labs. Companies also knew that paying researchers for their advice helped cement relationships, particularly for small startup companies eager to have enthusiastic inventors on board as their champions when seeking investment capital.

Because established companies often are not interested in the early-stage inventions coming out of academic laboratories, faculty inventors and entrepreneurs founded startup companies, or spinoffs, to take advantage of licensing opportunities. In 2012, 17.1% of university technology licenses were awarded to startup companies [8]. Researchers who start companies that will license and develop their inventions often remain full-time faculty members but they acquire a variety of financial interests in the new company. They share in licensing payments (e.g., royalties) from their inventions, receive fees for consulting, and own stock in their startups. It is common for startups to compensate consultants at least partly with stock or stock options because they generally have little cash. Having multiple financial interests and relationships with a company whose business is to develop one's technology while conducting university-based research on that technology creates a complex web of interests. Entrepreneurial faculty members continue to do research, often with federal support, which is related to and may impact the value of their commercial interests.

Consulting arrangements became very common between both new and established companies and university researchers. A 2006 survey showed that 49.5% of academic scientists were consultants or served on scientific advisory boards for industry [9]. Firms sought advice from expert scientists and physicians, asking them to serve on scientific advisory boards and to brainstorm about product development strategies, the design of research studies, and how to meet the demands of the health care market. Large pharmaceutical companies and medical device companies engaged physician "thought leaders" in their marketing strategies. It became common for academic physician investigators, reputed to be the best in their fields, to give scripted dinner talks to health care practitioners. Whether the objectives of these engagements were commercial or scientific, the result was to generate a steady and in some cases large stream of income for those researchers willing to work with industry. Academic institutions supported consulting activity for various reasons. It was another way to disseminate knowledge. They expected that consulting relationships would lead to research support for the university or medical school. And the outside income supplemented academic salaries, helping institutions retain talented scientists and physicians who could earn higher salaries elsewhere.

Another source of personal gain, involving mainly physicians and physician researchers, came in the form of gifts from industry. Pharmaceutical firms in particular have long doled out modest gifts to doctors and other clinical staff in the form of pens, coffee mugs, bagel breakfasts, and pizza lunches. It was common practice to give physicians samples of the newest—and usually most expensive—drugs so patients could try them out. Thought leaders and others were taken on trips to expensive resorts, often with their families, given theater and sporting event tickets, and lavished with other gifts, sometimes in connection with consulting and sometimes simply to buy influence. Although many academic institutions have banned personal gifts and entertainment, there are still physician researchers who accept them, so they need to be considered a possible source of bias, whether in prescribing medications or conducting research involving a company's product.

## 2.2 Emergence of Regulation and Guidance on Individual COI in Research

As the relationships between industry and research institutions proliferated, concern grew that personal financial interests in companies with closely related businesses would either consciously or unconsciously bias scientists in favor of a company's products. In particular, there was a risk that taxpayer dollars would be misused if research supported by federal agencies such as the National Institutes of Health (NIH) were rife with bias.

The government responded to worry about COIs in research by promulgating a regulation titled "Responsibility of Applicants for Promoting Objectivity in Research" (1995 PHS regulation). The 1995 PHS regulation required that institutions receiving federal research grants establish policies and procedures to identify and manage investigators' financial interests to protect the objectivity of federally funded research. The regulation specified that investigators must disclose to the institution those personal financial interests that, in their view, were related to research projects. (Under the 1995 regulation, income exceeding $10,000 per year had to be reported, a threshold that was lowered in the 2011 revised regulation.) The grantee institution was responsible for judging whether the interests represented a risk to the objectivity of the research and, if so, managing the COI and reporting its existence to the awarding agency. The regulation was widely misunderstood and inconsistently implemented by grantee organizations. One its many weaknesses was allowing investigators themselves to judge which of their financial interests was related to research projects.

In 1995 the National Science Foundation (NSF) issued a grants management policy on COI that largely mirrored the PHS regulation. The NSF rule is far less detailed and specific than the 1995 or revised 2011 PHS regulations [10].

The Food and Drug Administration (FDA), which regulates drugs, medical devices, and biologics, followed suit and instituted a financial COI policy regulation in 1998. The FDA required that organizations or individuals submitting requests for marketing approval collect financial interest disclosures from clinical investigators in "covered studies" and submit the information to the FDA. The financial interest disclosure thresholds differ from those of the PHS regulation and reporting is not required until studies are completed. So although the FDA's collection of disclosures allows the agency to disregard data from studies with unacceptable investigator financial interests, the regulation does not prospectively address the risks of investigators' financial interests for data objectivity or the safety of research subjects [11].

## 2.3 A Focus on COIs in Human Subject Research: The Gelsinger Case and Protocol 126

In 1999, Jesse Gelsinger, an 18-year-old with a mild form of the often-fatal nitrogen metabolism disorder known as ornithine transcarbamylase deficiency, volunteered to participate in a clinical study at the University of Pennsylvania. The investigational therapy was invented by the University of Pennsylvania researcher, James Wilson, and the university licensed it to a startup company, Genovo. Genovo's technology had attracted significant investment from large biotech companies. Dr. Wilson, some of his colleagues, and the University of Pennsylvania owned stock in the company and the university's Institute for Human Gene Therapy, led by Dr. Wilson, was funded substantially by the company. The university was aware of the COI and put in place some measures to protect the research from COIs.

Gelsinger died within a few days of receiving the study drug. In the ensuing lawsuit, his family charged that Wilson and Penn failed to fully disclose the FCOI. The study consent form included a general disclosure of financial interests [12] but it did not specifically state what the interests were. Whatever the causes of Jesse Gelsinger's death, public reporting of the financial interests of Dr. Wilson and the University of Pennsylvania set off a firestorm of criticism and calls for action [13].

Another major scandal unfolded in 2001 when the *Seattle Times* published its investigation of "Protocol 126," a clinical trial conducted at the Fred Hutchinson Cancer Research Center (FHCRC) between 1981 and 1993 [14]. The study, which lasted 12 years, tested whether using monoclonal antibodies to kill T cells would prevent the immune system reaction graft-versus-host disease in bone marrow transplant patients. There was a far higher rate of death among patients in the study than was to be expected with standard care. The *Seattle Times* series revealed that FHCRC had licensed some of the monoclonal antibodies used in the study to Genetic Systems, Inc., and that the Protocol 126 investigators owned stock in and received consulting fees from the company. Although FHCRC adopted a COI policy at one point during the study, the financial interests were not reported to the institution or reviewed for COI.

## 2.4 Responses by Government, Institutions, Scientific and Professional Societies, and Journals

Eleven months after Gelsinger's death, on August 15–16, 2000, the Department of Health and Human Services (DHHS) convened the first-ever conference on human subject protection and financial COI. Soon thereafter, in response to the issues highlighted at the conference, the major associations representing academic medical institutions crafted standards to limit financial interests in the high-risk setting of clinical research. A series of reports and recommendations focused on individual investigators' financial interests and on those associated with research institutions' own financial interests (institutional conflict of interest or ICOI).

In 2001, the Association of American Medical Colleges (AAMC) issued guidelines setting a "presumptive" limit of $10,000 per year in a researcher's income (and similar limits for equity and other financial interests) from the sponsor or another financially interested company when conducting clinical research [15]. In 2002, the AAMC published recommendations for limiting the financial interests of institutions in clinical research conducted under their auspices [16]. Institutional interests were defined as those of the organization itself and of the "institutional officials" with supervisory responsibility for the research. The Association of American Universities (AAU) issued guidelines on individual and institutional COIs in 2001, focusing on accountability in university research [17].

The AAMC and AAU guidelines and recommendations are not binding, but many in the academic research community and others came to view them as the gold standard. In a survey of its member medical schools conducted in 2003–2004, the AAMC found that, in response to its recommendations, 52% of institutions had modified their policies to increase protection for human subjects in studies involving individual COIs.

In 2004, the DHHS issued guidance on how institutions that receive PHS grants should manage financial conflicts [18]. The guidance was an outgrowth of the DHHS-sponsored conference on financial COI and human subject protection in August 2000 and reflected many of the recommendations in the AAMC and AAU reports. It called on institutions, investigators, and institutional review boards (IRBs) to take steps to ensure that conflicting financial interests would not compromise the protection of research subjects. Although the guidance does not suggest specific limits on investigators' financial interests in human research, it sets forth points to consider in evaluating the risks of those interests for research safety and objectivity.

The Association for the Accreditation of Human Research Protection Programs, a new and important actor in the clinical research community, added COI and ICOI, respectively, in 2004 and 2009 to its list of standards for accrediting human subject research organizations.

In 2003, senior administrators from several leading medical schools and teaching hospitals who were responsible for handling COI issues at their organizations met to discuss their common challenges. The meeting led to formation of the Forum on COI in Academe, a grass-roots working group to exchange ideas and share best practices. In 2006, the forum became part of the AAMC. The Forum on COI in Academe holds an annual national meeting and is the primary forum for discussion of regulation, standards, policy development, and administrative management of COI. It hosts discussions with regulators and members of the media, disseminates model practices, and offers those new to the field instruction on how to interpret standards and regulations.

Many scientific and medical professional societies, journals, and conference organizers followed suit and introduced or strengthened standards for disclosure of financial interests and mitigation of COIs. Several barred conflicted investigators from authoring certain types of articles. Others required that members of their governing boards eliminate most or all personal financial interests that could be viewed as COIs.[2] Many professional societies tightened standards for accepting industry funds to support their meetings, and industry itself devised protections to minimize the appearance of undue influence in its support of fellowships, travel grants for trainees, and other forms of support for education and research.

## 2.5 Scandals of the 2000s

Notwithstanding the federal regulations and the many organizational policies adopted in the 1990s and early 2000s, during the first decade of the 2000s there was a series of high-profile scandals involving researchers' and physicians' financial interests. The scandals raised concern among members of the public, media, and regulators about the effectiveness of existing standards and the impact of researchers' financial interests on the practice of medicine. The visibility and wide scope of the scandals motivated a second wave of regulations beginning toward the end of that decade.

Reports of perhaps the most pervasive practice—pharmaceutical company payments to physicians—highlighted the close ties between industry and clinical providers, triggering additional worries about the integrity of research and undue influence on doctors' clinical decision-making. Media reports revealed that well-known investigators at major research institutions received large speaking and consulting fees from the manufacturers of drugs that they were studying with federal funds. Dr. Charles Nemeroff, head of the psychiatry department at Emory University Medical School, earned $2.7 million between 2000 and 2007 in consulting arrangements with pharmaceutical companies. The *New York Times* cited Congressional documents stating that Dr. Nemeroff earned more than $960,000 from GlaxoSmith-Kline between 2000 and 2006 but listed earnings of less than $35,000 for the period on his university disclosure forms. At the same time, he was conducting NIH-sponsored research on the company's drugs [19]. NIH suspended his grant in 2008. In Boston, Dr. Joseph Beiderman, an influential child psychiatrist at Harvard and researcher at the Massachusetts General Hospital, was mired in a similar scandal. In 2011, the *Spine Journal* devoted an entire issue to repudiating several studies it had published about Medtronic's bone cement, declaring that as a result of the authors' financial ties to the company, they had dramatically underreported serious complications experienced by study participants. The authors received millions of dollars in consulting and royalty payments from Medtronic.

In parallel, the US Department of Justice investigated orthopedic surgery device companies' payments to physicians, contending the payments were inducements to purchase their medical devices and that federal health insurance dollars (e.g., Medicare) were at risk. The investigations exposed sham consulting agreements, outsized advisory board and speaking payments, lavish trips and gifts, and illegal marketing practices. The government reached settlements with the major vendors in the industry requiring, among other things, that they publicly disclose their payments to physicians.

In 2004 the NIH, the predominant funder of biomedical research in the United States and an agency charged with receiving and evaluating COI reports from grantee institutions, faced its own scandal. The agency discovered that a number of its intramural investigators had failed to report their financial ties with the pharmaceutical and biomedical device industry. As a result, NIH director Dr. Elias Zerhouni imposed strict new financial COI rules, effectively preventing NIH's own scientists from consulting for industry.

As the scandals unfolded, Sen. Charles Grassley, a Republican senator from Iowa who served as either ranking member or chair of the Senate Finance Committee from 2001 to

2010, conducted investigations and held hearings on financial interests in research and clinical practice. He pushed NIH to tighten COI regulations and introduced the Sunshine Act provision of the Patient Protection and Affordable Care Act of 2010, which required public disclosure of drug and device industry payments to physicians.

## 2.6 More Stringent Federal Regulations on COI in Research

After a two-year rule-making process, in August 2011, the PHS promulgated revised regulations on FCOI. Many of the provisions of the revised regulation reflected the scandals of the preceding decade, which had exposed weakness and inconsistencies in organizations' standards for reporting of financial interests. The revised regulation greatly broadened the scope of information investigators need to report. Institutional responsibilities for review of financial interest disclosures are outlined in copious detail, and institutions must provide granular information on FCOIs and their management to the PHS awarding agency. In response to arguments that previously there was inadequate transparency of researchers' financial interests, the 2011 PHS regulation included a requirement that details of FCOIs to be made public, either on a Website or in response to any public inquiry.

Although the revised regulation imposes a much greater burden on investigators and research institutions, it does not dictate institutional responses to FCOIs. No limits are placed on the magnitude or types of financial interests that institutions can allow researchers to have, and the final rule does not prescribe any specific management measures to protect objectivity. So, in theory, for example, a researcher using federal funds to conduct a clinical study involving a novel cancer therapy can own substantial stock in and receive large consulting fees from the manufacturer of the therapy—if his or her institution believes that its management measures will successfully protect the objectivity of the research. The institution has to defend the rationale for allowing the arrangements and describe its management plan in detail, and the PHS awarding agency may question or challenge an institution's decision. The goal of the regulation is to compel institutions to carefully consider the facts and make well-informed judgments about the risks to research objectivity. In principle, the review process acts as an important brake on what might otherwise be unfettered risks to research from COIs. But ultimately, as with all regulated activity, the public must rely on institutions' and investigators' integrity.

## 2.7 Physician Payments Sunshine Act

Although regulations on COIs in research focus mainly on establishing frameworks (albeit burdensome) and objectives and leave many details up to institutions, the Physician Payments Sunshine Act is much more prescriptive. It has a different focus and a larger intended audience. The goal is to ensure that patients can obtain information about companies' payments to their physicians. The act, whose implementation began in 2013, requires that manufacturers of drugs, medical devices, and biologics report detailed data about their payments to doctors and teaching hospitals to the federal Centers for Medicare and Medicaid Services (CMS). CMS must make the information available to the public by posting it on a Website. Manufacturers have to report payments of more than $10 and for a wide range of purposes such as consulting, teaching, travel, gifts, and research. Because industry financial support for research at academic institutions is almost always the subject of institutional contracts and funds are provided to the institution rather than to individual physician researchers, CMS will report payments for research separately from payments to physicians, but the names of physician principal investigators will be listed. Although only a small minority of physicians conduct research, the biomedical research community is concerned that journalists, interest groups, politicians, and regulators will draw attention to the inevitable discrepancies between information about COIs in research disclosed publicly under the PHS regulation and data published in accordance with the Sunshine Act.

## 2.8 Institutional Conflict of Interest

An important part of the COI landscape is the role of institutions—universities, medical schools, teaching hospitals, and research institutes. They license laboratory inventions to commercial firms, seek philanthropy from companies with related businesses, and develop research collaborations and partnerships with industry. Institutions' financial relationships with industry are significant and they have the potential to lead to bias in research. Institutional leaders, such as deans, presidents, and department chairs can exert influence, often through allocation of resources, which may impact the success or failure of research. The argument goes that when there is research that could financially benefit the institution, directly or indirectly, it is important to exercise caution to avoid the appearance or risk that leaders will exercise influence to support or favor certain outcomes. In addition, when individuals with executive or senior leadership roles in an organization have personal financial interests in a technology that is being studied at their institutions, their interests should be viewed as potentially creating institutional COIs because their roles give them the authority to influence others' research.

A well-known case of ICOI in research is illustrative. In the late 1990s, Dr. Nancy Olivieri, a University of Toronto hematologist working at the Hospital for Sick Children in Toronto, was conducting a clinical trial of an experimental iron-chelating drug (deferiprone) for patients with thalassemia. Finding that the drug's efficacy was declining and that it was causing serious adverse events, Dr. Olivieri planned to inform the trial participants. The study sponsor and manufacturer of the drug, Apotex, disagreed, withdrew its support, and terminated the trial. Dr. Olivieri nevertheless presented her results and submitted them for publication. The university and hospital, fearful of losing a promised multimillion dollar donation from Apotex, failed to support Dr. Olivieri and instead allowed unsubstantiated misconduct allegations to be pursued against her [20]. This well-known story offers lessons for those concerned that institutions' financial interests can lead to institutional actions that violate research integrity and endanger research subjects and future patients [21]. During the 2000s, many academic medical centers, acknowledging that their industry ties were likely to remain important but recognizing the risks to the research enterprise voluntarily adopted ICOI policies.

The PHS federal conflict of interest (FCOI) regulations do not address ICOI. Although some expected that the 2011 revision of the PHS regulation would do so, government officials decided that there needed to be more discussion with members of the biomedical research community before they drafted regulation on ICOIs.

## 3. RELEVANT REGULATORY/OVERSIGHT AGENCIES, REGULATIONS, AND GUIDANCE DOCUMENTS

The chart that follows lists the major government agencies, regulations, and key documents related to COIs in research. There are many other organizations, professional societies, and journals that maintain policies and guidance on COIs in research.

| Agency/organization | Name of regulation/document | Date issued | Topic |
| --- | --- | --- | --- |
| US Public Health Service (includes NIH and other agencies) | Responsibility of applicants for promoting objectivity in research for which PHS funding is sought (42 C.F.R. Part 50, Subpart F) and responsible prospective contractors (45 C.F.R. Part 94) | 1995; revised 2011 | Objectivity in research; management of investigators' conflicts of interest. Compliance burden is on grantee institutions. |
| US National Science Foundation (NSF) | NSF Award and Administration Guide: Conflict of Interest Policies | 1995 | Objectivity in the design, conduct or reporting of NSF-funded research or educational activities; management of investigators' conflicts of interest. Compliance burden is on grantee institutions. |
| US Food and Drug Administration (FDA) | Financial Disclosures by Clinical Investigators | 1998 | Financial conflicts of interest of investigators in clinical studies of safety and efficacy being submitted to FDA for marketing approval of drugs, biological, and devices. Compliance burden is on companies and others applying for marketing approval. |
| Centers for Medicare and Medicaid Services | Physician Payments Sunshine Act | 2010 | Transparency of industry payments to physicians and teaching hospitals, including payments for research. Compliance burden is on manufacturers. |
| US Department of Health and Human Services | Financial Relationships and Interests in Research Involving Human Subjects: Guidance for Human Subject Protection | 2004 | Determining whether personal financial interests could affect the rights and welfare of human research subjects and how to protect those subjects |
| State regulations (Massachusetts, Vermont, Minnesota, District of Columbia) | Various | | Transparency and restrictions on physicians' payments from industry. |
| Association of American Universities (AAU) | Report on Individual and Institutional Conflicts of Interest | 2001 | Guidelines for addressing conflicts of interest to ensure accountability of university research. |
| Association of American Medical Colleges (AAMC) | Protecting Subjects, Preserving Trust, Promoting Progress—Policy and Guidelines for the Oversight of Individual Financial Interests in Human Subjects Research | 2001 | Recommended institutional policies limiting investigators' financial interest in human subjects research. |
| AAMC | Protecting Subjects, Preserving Trust, Promoting Progress II: Principles and Recommendations for Oversight of an Institution's Financial Interests in human Subjects Research | 2002 | Recommended approaches for addressing institutions' financial interest in human subjects research. |

—cont'd

| Agency/organization | Name of regulation/document | Date issued | Topic |
| --- | --- | --- | --- |
| AAMC and AAU | Protecting Patients, Preserving Integrity, Advancing Health: Accelerating the Implementation of COI Policies in Human Subjects Research | 2008 | Addresses individual and institutional conflict of interests and policy implementation. |
| Council on Government Relations | Recognizing and Managing Personal Financial Conflicts of Interest | 2002 | Individual conflicts of interest in research, mentoring, and procurement in academic institutions. |
| Institute of Medicine of the National Academies of Science | Conflict of Interest in Medical Research, Education, and Practice | 2009 | Conflicts of interest in medical research, education, practice, and practice guideline development; recommendations on policy design and implementation. |
| Association for the Accreditation of Human Research Protection Programs | AAHRPP Accreditation Standards | 2004, 2009 | Standards for accrediting human research protection programs that include addressing conflicts of interest in human subject research. |

A few foreign countries regulate FCOIs in research. In Japan, for example, there have been well-publicized scandals involving COIs in biomedical research, and the Ministry of Education, Culture, Sports, Science, and Technology and the Ministry of Health, Labor, and Welfare have issued COI regulations [22].

## 4. KEY REGULATORY MANDATES OF THE 2011 PUBLIC HEALTH SERVICE REGULATION

This section deals with the revised Public Health Service (PHS) regulation on COIs in research that was issued in 2011 and became effective in 2012 (2011 regulation) [23]. The stated purpose of the regulation is to "promote(s) objectivity in research by establishing standards that provide a reasonable expectation that the design, conduct, and reporting of research funded under PHS grants or cooperative agreements will be free from bias resulting from Investigator financial conflicts of interest" [42 CFR Part 50 §50.601].[3] It was the first major revision to the 1995 regulation, and it substantially increased the compliance burden for researchers and institutions.

### 4.1 Policies Must Be Publicly Available

Institutions must have up-to-date, written, enforced COI policies and must make them available on a publicly accessible Website. If an institution does not have a Web presence, the policy must be provided to any requestor within five business days of the request. Institutions also must make their investigators aware of the policy and of the investigators' obligations under the regulation and policy.

## 4.2 Determining Who is an Investigator

The regulation defines "investigator" as the "project director, principal investigator, or any other person regardless of title or position, who is responsible for the design, conduct, or reporting of research funded by the PHS, or proposed for such funding, which may include, for example, collaborators or consultants." It is a challenge for institutions to interpret the definition in a way that meets the intent of the regulation but is not so broad as to be impossible to administer. Because the definition is not congruent with "key personnel" or "study team," institutions must decide whether some individuals, such as senior research technicians or graduate students, should be considered investigators. In most cases, those listed as key personnel qualify as investigators. But what about, for example, laboratory technicians who are responsible for the "conduct" of the research by following scientific protocols, but do not have independent authority for any portion of the research? Should they be considered investigators?[4] The regulation specifies that "consultants" on research projects may be investigators, so institutions need to judge whether a consultant's contribution qualifies as design, conduct or reporting of research and, if so, whether a consultant from another institution should be made subject to a contract with the prime awardee.

## 4.3 Requirement to Disclose Significant Financial Interests

Institutions must solicit and investigators must disclose "significant financial interests" (SFIs) to the institutional official no later than the time of application for PHS funding. Disclosures have to be updated annually and within 30 days of acquiring or learning about a new SFI. SFIs are defined more broadly than in the 1995 regulation. The financial threshold for SFIs in the original regulation was defined, in part, as income of $10,000 per year. Under the 2011 regulation, SFIs include the following, whether on the part of the investigator or his or her spouse or dependent children:

1. Income from publicly traded entities (other than the applicant institution) that, when aggregated for the 12 months preceding the disclosure, exceeds $5000. This may include, for example, consulting fees, honoraria, and paid authorship, and may be in the form of cash, equity, or stock options, where the value of the equity is derived from public prices or other reasonable measures of fair market value.
2. Income from nonpublicly traded entities (other than the applicant institution) when the remuneration exceeds $5000 or where the investigator or his or her family members have *any* equity or ownership interest. For example, an investigator who owns 50% of the equity in a nonpublicly traded startup company must report the interest.
3. Intellectual property rights such as patents and copyrights upon receipt on income from such rights. This provision does not set a "floor" of more than $5000 in income from intellectual property rights. Some institutions have interpreted it to mean all income exceeding $0 or being named on a patent or copyright even if there is no license that entitles the individual to fees or royalty payments.

It is important to note that the regulation refers to SFIs in "entities," not only for-profit companies. So investigators have to disclose income from or ownership interests in not-for-profit organizations that are related to their institutional responsibilities. Examples include professional societies, patient advocacy or other community organizations, international advisory or regulatory bodies, and non-US universities. Regulators cast the net broadly to ensure that institutions capture and scrutinize information about payments from and ownership in bodies such as a foundations and nonprofit organizations that are supported solely or largely by companies in a particular industry. The effect is to require that investigators disclose a great deal of data about income and financial interests that are highly unlikely to affect research objectivity, and institutions must devote resources to processing the information.

4. Exceptions. There are some notable exceptions to the disclosure requirements. First, income from investment vehicles where the investigator does not directly control the investment decisions, such as mutual funds, is exempt. Second, the regulation exempts "income from seminars, lectures, or teaching engagements sponsored by a [U.S.] Federal, state, or local government agency, an Institution of higher education as defined at 20 U.S.C. 1001(a), an academic teaching hospital, a medical center, or a research institute that is affiliated with an Institution of higher education; or income from service on advisory committees or review panels for a Federal, state, or local government agency, an Institution of higher education as defined at 20 U.S.C. 1001(a), an academic teaching hospital, a medical center, or a research institute that is affiliated with an Institution of higher education."

These exemptions do not cover, for example, service as a consultant to a government agency if it involves work other than serving on an advisory committee or review panel. Also not exempted is income from non-US government agencies and non-US institutions of higher education.

## 4.4 Scope of Financial Interests to Be Disclosed

1. *Relationship to institutional responsibilities.* The 1995 regulation allowed investigators to decide which of their significant financial interests were related to PHS-funded research, so the institution's obligations for addressing and managing potential COIs were limited to those financial interests judged by the investigators themselves to be related. The 2011 regulation vastly expanded investigators' disclosure requirements by requiring that they disclose SFIs *related to their institutional responsibilities,* and it made institutions, rather than investigators, responsible for determining whether the disclosed SFIs are related to PHS-funded research.

SFIs are defined as those interests that "reasonably appear[s] to be related to the Investigator's *institutional responsibilities*" [italics added]. Institutional responsibilities include the investigator's professional responsibilities on behalf of the institution including, but not limited to, research, teaching, professional practice and service on committees such as IRBs.

Consider the example of researcher Dr. Smith, who serves on his institution's animal care and use committee (IACUC) and receives royalty income exceeding $5000 per year on sales of a book he published about the composition and operations of animal care and use committees. He is an investigator on an NIH-supported clinical trial and his role is to conduct a key assay of tissue samples derived from participants in the trial. Although the royalty income from his book bears no relationship to his work on the NIH-funded clinical study, Dr. Smith must disclose it because it is related to his role on the IACUC, which is an institutional responsibility. His institution has to determine whether the SFI, royalty from a book on IACUCs, is related to his role as investigator on a clinical study.

2. *Travel.* Although not defined as SFIs, investigators must disclose sponsored or reimbursed travel when entities other than the applicant institution or certain

government agencies or US educational institutions sponsor (i.e., directly pay for) or reimburse the individual. In a clarification issued in October 2012, the NIH notified the research community that institutions could opt to limit disclosure requirements for sponsored or reimbursed travel to instances where the value of the travel from a single entity exceeds $5000 in the 12 months before the disclosure. This modest reduction in institutional burden was welcomed by institutions whose staff members were reviewing disclosures of $100 train tickets for travel to professional society meetings.

## 4.5 Disclosure Review

Disclosure review comprises two main activities: determining relatedness and judging whether a related financial interest is an FCOI.

1. *Relatedness determination.* The institution must review an SFI and decide whether it is "related" to PHS-funded research. It is related if it "could be affected by the PHS funded research; or is in an entity whose financial interest could be affected by the research." Although institutions are ultimately responsible for determining relatedness, they may involve the investigator in making the assessment. This is very helpful because it is often difficult for administrators, and even scientists other than the investigator, to know whether the work scope of a federal grant, particularly for basic or animal research, could affect a company for which the investigator is a consultant or to which she has licensed intellectual property.

2. *FCOI determination.* Determining whether an SFI that is related to one's research represents an FCOI is at the core of the PHS regulation. Institutions must conduct a fact-based analysis of each SFI in light of the research to judge whether an FCOI exists. The regulation states, "A financial conflict of interest exists when the Institution, through its designate official(s), reasonably determines that the significant financial interest could directly and significantly affect the design, conduct, or reporting of the PHS-funded research." Making an FCOI determination involves having complete information about the investigator's relevant financial interests and relationships; understanding the research design or protocol and its specific aims; knowing the investigator's role in the study; and assessing whether those aspects of the study the investigator can influence could be affected by his financial interest. The "directly and significantly" standard can be difficult to apply in practice. It sets a high bar for finding an FCOI, but institutions sometimes make FCOI determinations in more ambiguous cases to ensure that financial arrangements are disclosed to funders and the scientific community.

Following are three hypothetical examples of COI cases that illustrate some of the most common arrangements and institutional reviews.

a. When the investigator has an SFI in a company whose drug or device is being directly tested in the research, making an FCOI determination is straightforward.

*Dr. Green and NuBiomarker, Inc.* Dr. Green, a professor in the Oakville University Medical School's oncology department, discovered a novel biomarker for colorectal cancer and demonstrated its utility in animal models. The biomarker was licensed to a nonpublicly traded startup company, NuBiomarker, Inc., in which Dr. Green owns stock and from which she receives $30,000 per year in consulting fees. In her NIH grant,

Dr. Green will study the utility of the biomarker in tests using human tissue samples. If the research shows that the biomarker can identify colorectal cancer earlier or more effectively than existing diagnostic markers, the results are likely to enhance the value of NuBiomarker and the value of Dr. Green's stock. Oakville University's conflict of interest committee concludes that her interest could have a direct and significant impact on the value of the startup company and that therefore it represents an FCOI.

**b.** Some institutions struggle to decide whether there is an FCOI when a study involves a product in which the investigator has an interest, but the study is not directly testing the product.

*Dr. Blue and InSite Behavioral Systems, Inc.* Dr. Blue, a senior researcher in Elmwood University's Department of Psychology, is the founder of InSite Behavioral Systems, a company that markets surveys, evaluation tools, and other behavioral science instruments to researchers, therapists, and corporate human resource departments. Originally a startup based on inventions licensed from Elmwood University, the company now has 120 employees and its stock is publicly traded. Dr. Blue owns 5% of the company's stock and earns $50,000 per year as chair of its scientific advisory board. Dr. Blue is submitting a grant application to NIH for a project in which his lab will compare how a control group and an intervention group perform on a series of tests designed to evaluate executive functioning skills. The intervention group will receive intensive counseling from an expert; the control group will receive no counseling. Eight of the ten tests that will be used to evaluate the intervention are owned and marketed by InSite. They are novel tests that, although "validated" by the company internally, are new to the market. The study's specific aims focus on the effectiveness of counseling in enhancing executive functioning skills. Most of the evaluation tools are owned and sold by InSite. Could Dr. Blue's financial interest have a direct and significant impact on the value of the instruments or the company?

Some institutions might conclude that the instruments themselves are not being evaluated in the study, so there is no potential FCOI. Others might judge that although efficacy of the tools is not a study endpoint, the decision to use primarily InSite instruments for a major research project—including several that are new to the market—could enhance their value. And since the study PI, Dr. Blue, has a large SFI, the design—if not the conduct or reporting—of the research may be directly affected.

**c.** In some cases, the product in which the investigator has a financial interest is being used in the study incidentally as a tool.

*Dr. Red and MRIs-R-US.* Dr. Red, a radiology researcher at Maple Leaf University Medical School, earns $20,000 per year as a consultant to MRIs-R-US, a large magnetic resonance imaging (MRI) manufacturer. In her federally funded research project, Dr. Red is using the MRIs-R-US machine purchased by the hospital in which she conducts research to study whether a new contrast agent is more effective than existing agents for visualizing certain brain lesions. Dr. Red has no financial interest in the contrast agent manufacturer. Maple Leaf University Medical School's institutional official decides that Dr. Red's consulting income from the MRI manufacturer does not have the potential to directly and significantly affect the objectivity of her research on the contrast agent because she is using, not studying, the MRI machine.

## 4.6 Managing FCOIs

When an institution identifies an FCOI with PHS-supported research, it must take measures to "manage" the FCOI or, in effect, minimize its impact on the objectivity of the design, conduct, and reporting of the research. The most extreme way to deal with an FCOI is to eliminate it—that is, require that the investigator eliminate the financial interest by ending a consulting relationship or selling his or her stock or, alternatively, by prohibiting the investigator from participating in the research project. Most institutions are eager to support their investigators' constructive engagement with industry, whether through scientific consulting, licenses of novel technology, or other appropriate arrangements. So it is reasonable to assume that in the majority of cases, institutions apply management tools other than elimination of FCOIs. Standard FCOI management tools include disclosure of financial interests in relevant publications, presentations and human subject consent forms; oversight of research to ensure it is conducted according to scientific protocol; modification of the research plan; changing the responsibilities of research team members to protect the study from bias due to the FCOI of a particular investigator; and reducing the magnitude of the financial interest.

The management plan must be in place and reported to the PHS awarding agency before the institution spends funds on the project.

## 4.7 Reporting to PHS Awarding Agency

The 2011 regulation substantially increased institutions' FCOI reporting obligations. Although reporting is done through an enhanced electronic portal, it still represents an additional administrative burden. The regulation sets forth a series of elements that must be included in the report. They include:

1. Name of the project director/principal investigator;
2. Name of the investigator with the FCOI;
3. Name of the entity with which the investigator has an FCOI;
4. Nature of the financial interest (e.g., equity, consulting fee, travel reimbursement, honorarium);
5. Value of the financial interest within a series of dollar ranges or a statement that value of the interest cannot be readily determined (for example, in the case of a nonpublicly traded startup company);
6. A description of how the financial interest relates to the PHS-funded research and the basis for the determination that the financial interest conflicts with such research; and
7. A description of the key elements of the institution's management plan, including:
    a. Role and principal duties of the conflicted investigator in the research project;
    b. Conditions of the management plan;
    c. How the management plan is designed to safeguard objectivity in the research project;
    d. Confirmation of the investigator's agreement to the management plan;
    e. How the management plan will be monitored to ensure investigator compliance; and
    f. Other information as needed.

## 4.8 Public Reporting of FCOIs

The 2011 PHS regulation responded to a call for more transparency in researchers' relationships with industry by instituting a public disclosure requirement. The scandals of the mid-2000s led to claims that the interests were obscured, making it impossible for the public to know whether research funded with taxpayer dollars was at risk for bias. The public disclosure requirement can be fulfilled in one of two ways. Institutions can post information about FCOIs on a publicly accessible Website, which must be kept up-to-date in accordance with regulatory provisions. Alternatively, institutions can respond to FCOI information requests from any member of the public within five business days. The vast majority of NIH grantee institutions have opted for the second approach. Anecdotally, as of this writing, there have been very few public information requests to institutions. The regulation prescribes the content of FCOI information to be provided to requestors. It is very similar to the information institutions must provide the PHS awarding agency.

### 4.9 Retrospective Review

A particularly vexing provision of the regulation is the requirement that institutions conduct a "retrospective review" if an investigator makes a disclosure late or the institution does not address the COI in the required time frame. In these circumstances, the institution must first determine whether the belatedly disclosed financial interest represents an FCOI. If so, it must impose "corrective actions" and institute a review of the research that was already undertaken to assess whether it was biased because of the undisclosed interest or absence of FCOI management. This requires guidance on how to recognize bias in the context of the research. And it means that the institution needs to engage disinterested, knowledgeable individuals to review the design, conduct, and collection, analysis, and reporting of data to judge whether bias affected objectivity.

## 5. KEY PERSONNEL AND UNIVERSITY COMMITTEES DESIGNATED TO IMPLEMENT REGULATORY MANDATES

### 5.1 Key Personnel

*Institutional officials.* Under the 2011 regulation, there must be a designated institutional official to solicit and review investigators' financial interest disclosures. This individual must be given guidelines for determining whether SFIs (1) are related to PHS-supported research and, if so, (2) present an FCOI with the individual's PHS-supported research. At larger institutions, the institutional official oversees staff members who may make initial assessments about whether a financial interest is related to an investigator's research, and the institutional official and staff work with a committee of senior researchers and other leaders who make official FCOI determinations and develop recommendations for management.

*Staff.* There is no mandatory training for institutional staff members who work on COI issues. However, they must be familiar with all relevant federal and state regulation, accreditation standards that address COI, and national organization standards. COI issues can be structurally complex, potentially involving one or more of the following: institutions and investigators with licensed technology, consulting arrangements, equity, basic research, clinical trials, and involvement of students and trainees. So it is important for COI staff members to have more than incidental familiarity with research and its administration, technology transfer, medical, and scientific graduate and postgraduate education, and clinical (or other professional) practice. Many COI staff members have law degrees, some have scientific backgrounds, and others have experience in academic research administration. Although not unique to COI work, the most valuable "soft skills" include the ability to synthesize and clearly communicate complex information, critical thinking skills, an ability to work effectively in a complex organization, and awareness that one is providing a service and also acting in a compliance role.

*COI committee.* Institutions, especially larger ones, appoint COI committee (sometimes called a "disclosure review committee") to review and render judgment or make recommendations regarding the permissibility and management of research and other activities where an investigator or the institution has financial interest. One advantage of assigning this role to a COI committee instead of an individual is that decisions benefit from many individuals' judgment and expertise. In addition, decisions made by a respected group, particularly if it is a group of one's peers, are less prone to be viewed as arbitrary or influenced by personal bias. Ideally, an institution's COI committee will include several senior faculty researchers who have a sophisticated understanding of science, the research process, and implications for the relevant field (e.g., medical care, health care, engineering, environmental science, nursing); a balance between members who themselves are involved with industry (and have COIs) and those who are not; and reasonable representation of the institution's departments, schools, or divisions. There is an important role for nonfaculty participants. These may include:

1. senior COI staff members who understand all the relevant relationships and have up-to-date knowledge of the status of the conflicted investigator's research and financial interests;
2. technology licensing professionals, who are familiar with the status of licensing arrangements and associated financial terms;
3. staff from the IRB and sponsored research offices, who bring knowledge of human subject research protocols and research grants and contracts;
4. institutional counsel, who can advise on legal other risks;
5. institutional media relations staff, who can advise on the potential public relations impacts of COI situations and decisions; and
6. the institutional official, who will gain insight into the thinking of the committee members.

## 5.2 Related Committees and Offices

*IRBs.* With one exception, the PHS regulation does not direct institutions to set any particular policy or follow any guidelines with respect to the permissibility or management of COIs in human subject research as compared with basic research.[5] Since the Gelsinger case, however, major research institutions, accreditation groups, and important interest groups have taken the position that COIs in human subject research should be treated as creating greater risk than nonhuman subject research. The presence of an investigator's financial interest in a human research project could, in theory, cause investigators to enroll participants who do not meet study criteria, to overstate a study's benefits and understate its risks, to underreport serious adverse events, and to overrepresent the benefits of a study drug or device in publications that impact the medical care of whole populations. So many institutions, following AAMC and AAU guidelines, set specific limits on investigators' (and in some cases, institutions') allowable financial interests in human subject research projects or clinical trials. Many institutions' IRBs do not approve study protocols until all COI issues are fully addressed.

Close coordination between the COI office and the IRB administration is therefore extremely important.

*Sponsored project office.* The sponsored projects (or grants and contracts) office administers research funding applications and, in the case of grants from PHS agencies, certifies the institution's commitment to comply with the FCOI regulation. The flow of grant applications and awards must be well coordinated with the COI review process so the institution can effectively solicit, review, manage, and report on disclosures related to PHS-supported projects effectively and within regulatory time frames.

*Technology transfer office.* At most research institutions, income from licenses of patented and copyrighted inventions (intellectual property)—fees, royalty, etc.—is paid to the institution that, in turn, shares specified portions of the income with the inventors. The PHS FCOI regulation requires that investigators disclose their income from intellectual property, but not the income that is received from the institution. Some institutions have concluded that because of this exemption, they do not need to review institutionally derived intellectual property income for COI. Others take the position that the exemption exists simply because institutions are expected to know of the income they share with their inventors, and that intellectual property income from the institution has the same potential to generate risks of bias in research as does income from other sources. So they require investigators who receive invention income from their employers to disclose it for purposes of COI review. In that context, a good working relationship between the technology licensing and COI offices is very valuable.

Consider the following example.

> Pineview University is licensing Professor Black's invention, a noninvasive test to screen for macular degeneration, to MacuScreen, a startup company. The proposed terms of the license agreement include postmarketing royalties and milestone payments that are tied to research events such as enrollment of clinical trial subjects at Pineview University Medical School. As an inventor, Dr. Black is entitled to a share of the fees, including milestone payments, and royalty income that MacuScreen pays Pineview University. The University's COI policy requires disclosure of financial interests investigators have through the university, including future licensing income.
>
> Dr. Black would like to conduct a first-in-human proof of principle study of the noninvasive screening test to further develop the technology and provide preliminary data on its efficacy. He has a financial interest in the royalty payments, but they will not flow until the research is completed, definitive studies have demonstrated efficacy, the test receives FDA approval, and it is on the market. The university's COI committee balances the potential for bias as a result of Dr. Black's interest in potential sales royalty with the low risk of the study to research subjects, his academic interest in conducting translational research, and the institution's goal of advancing contributions to public health through technology transfer. It concludes that the risks of bias due to future royalty income are acceptable and can be managed.
>
> However, Dr. Black's interest in a share of research milestone fees troubles the committee. It believes that payments triggered by events such as enrolling subjects in a clinical study are likely to jeopardize objectivity and potentially the participants' safety and welfare. Because there is a close working relationship between the COI and technology transfer offices, COI staff members advise the technology transfer office not to include milestone payments in the license agreement with MacuScreen. If the financial interests are limited to postmarketing royalty, Dr. Black will be able to participate in the early-stage clinical study. The licensing staff negotiates with MacuScreen for a somewhat higher royalty interest in lieu of milestone payments. Making this adjustment, which balances the institution's interests with those of the researcher, is possible because there is close communication between the two offices.

*Legal office.* As with all areas of regulatory compliance, institutional counsel can help interpret regulation, advise on risks to the institution and investigators, and help ensure that the institution's policies and procedures are structured to support compliance with regulations, standards, and institutional principles.

*Media relations.* Financial COIs in medicine and science, widely reported on since the 1990s, have captured the public's attention. Stories of financial interests in environmental, energy, and food science research also appear regularly in the media. Society expects research to be objective. And it traditionally holds those in the health care professions in high esteem. So revelations that a physician researcher pocketed hundreds of thousands, or even millions of dollars, for speaking favorably about a company's new drug, can destroy the individual's reputation and wreak havoc at his institution. Public reporting of industry payments to physicians as required under the Sunshine Act—and comparisons between that information and financial interest reports associated with PHS research—is likely to generate media attention. It is important for institutions' media relations staff to understand the facts and public perception issues associated with COIs so they can protect or at least minimize harm to the reputations of the organization and its researchers.

## 6. COMMON COMPLIANCE CHALLENGES

*Educating investigators.* The PHS regulation requires that institutions train investigators about COI every four years and on other triggering events. The form and content of training are not specified, and institutions take many different approaches. Some employ online training courses. These are available from the Collaborative Institutional Training Initiative and other sources, or can be developed in-house. Other institutions require investigators to attend didactic sessions. Much depends on the size and structure of the organization. In a large, decentralized institution, it is difficult to reach all investigators with didactic training, so online modules guarantee that there is at least minimal exposure to the topic. Didactic sessions, with an emphasis on case examples and interaction between teachers and learners, are most effective in engaging investigators' attention.

*Soliciting and receiving full and timely disclosure.* Obtaining timely and accurate financial interest disclosures from investigators is an ongoing challenge. Investigators are weighed down by myriad regulatory requirements including biosafety, animal welfare, export controls, human subject research, and effort reporting. Those who are physicians also contend with billing requirements, electronic medical records, privacy, patient safety, and others. Financial interest disclosure can get lost in the mix. So it is important for institutions to find the right "signal-to-noise" ratio in reminding investigators to make and update disclosures. Many institutions have instituted electronic disclosure processes to make the process as straightforward as possible.

*Coordination of complex systems and offices in large institutional bureaucracies.* In most organizations, one office, with responsibility for dealing with COIs, receives information about financial interests and another office manages research grants and contracts. Other offices are in charge of human subject research and technology transfer. Each has custody of information that needs to be collected and reviewed in a coordinated way to identify or rule out financial COIs in research. In very complex organizations, such as large university campuses or systems, there may be more than one office that manages disclosures or grants and contracts.

Although imperfect, interactive electronic systems that can draw from each administrative unit's database are immensely helpful.

*Role of information technology systems.* Addressing COI is an administratively complex undertaking, and the value of a robust information technology (IT) system cannot be overstated. Ideally, an IT system will support three major sets of activities. First, an online system, especially the one that is interactive and not simply a warehouse for forms, allows investigators to submit, update, revise, and terminate financial interest disclosures easily and from anywhere there is internet access. Making disclosure easy greatly supports compliance. Second, an effective system will integrate some or all of the following types of information: investigators' financial interest disclosures, grants and contracts, IRB projects, technology licensing, and purchasing. Finally, the COI disclosure lifecycle should be managed within the IT system so that disclosures, reviews for COIs, data about reporting to PHS, COI management plans, and interactions with investigators and other institutional offices are all managed in a single location. Instituting and maintaining an effective IT system is costly, but it is a wise investment for most medium-sized and large institutions.

*Monitoring investigator compliance.* Institutions must "monitor investigator compliance with the management plan on an ongoing basis until the completion of the PHS-funded research project." Some management measures can be monitored with straightforward, administrative practices. For example, the IRB can be engaged to monitor a requirement that FCOIs be disclosed to research subjects in consent forms (and even to monitor disclosure in the consent process). Investigators can be directed to submit all their publications and presentations to ensure that there is appropriate disclosure of FCOIs to the research community. The IRB and sponsored projects office also can be enlisted to ensure that an investigator with an FCOI fulfills a requirement that he or she step down as principal investigator or adjust his or her role on a project. The COI office can require an investigator to document changes in his or her financial interest, such as selling stock or reducing consulting income, as required under a management plan. Other measures are more difficult to implement. When a management plan calls for independent monitoring or oversight of research, it is often necessary to engage other senior disinterested researchers to review and report on the conduct of the project. Oversight can take significant time and energy, and supporting this process usually falls to the COI office staff. Some institutions even pay a small stipend to the individuals who conduct the oversight in recognition of their contributions.

*Subrecipients.* Identifying and addressing COIs of investigators at subrecipient institutions is a daunting task. Subrecipient institutions range from large academic and research organizations to domestic clinical practices and small businesses, and universities, clinics, and other organizations located overseas. The PHS regulation specifies that if a subrecipient certifies it has a COI policy that complies with the regulation, the "sub" can identify and manage FCOIs itself and simply needs to report FCOIs to the prime awardee. The "prime" in turn submits FCOI reports to the awarding agency. If, however, the sub does not have a compliant policy, the prime awardee must assume more responsibility. (Some institutions direct subs to adopt template COI policies. This may be effective in some settings. In others, there is a risk that a policy will be adopted but not effectively implemented.) Specifically, it must require the sub to collect disclosures of investigators' SFIs *related to the project* (a narrower range of disclosures than the requirement for the prime's investigators, i.e., SFIs related to one's institutional responsibilities) and submit them to the prime for review under the prime's COI policy. The sub must agree to comply with any COI management plan adopted by the prime to manage the COI. One of the many difficulties with this arrangement is that the prime has no way of knowing whether the sub has effectively implemented or monitored a management plan.

*Clinical trial networks.* NIH has established several networks of institutions and investigators to participate in trials in a particular area such as diabetic retinopathy or AIDS. Each network is structured differently. Funds may flow from NIH to a coordinating center and from the coordinating center to participating sites. Or there may be direct flows of money from NIH to the coordinating center, a statistical analysis center, and participating sites. These varied arrangements require the prime and subawardee institutions to understand the flow of funds and comply with COI regulation accordingly. In addition, many NIH institutes require that network steering committees establish and implement their own COI policies. Some network policies are more stringent than institutional policies, and other networks have little or no experience with COI. The combination of varied administrative structures with sometimes multiple prime and subawardee institutions and network-specific COI policies makes it difficult for institutions and investigators to sort out multiple disclosures, standards, and management plans.

*More stringent standards.* The PHS regulation stipulates that if an institution's COI policy is more stringent than the regulation, it must adhere to its own policy, provide the awarding agency reports of FCOIs identified under its policy, and do so within regulatory time frames. Research institutions' COI policies reflect their cultures as well as regulatory requirements. Some institutions require that investigators disclose financial interests of any value, not just those set by the regulation. Others require investigators to disclose royalty payments received from the institution and they review those interests for FCOI. The "more stringent standard" provision adds to the institution's reporting burden.

## 7. ADDRESSING NONCOMPLIANCE

*PHS regulation requires policies to cite disciplinary procedures.* Institutional policies must provide for sanctions or administrative actions in the event an investigator fails to comply with the policy. Although institutions maintain umbrella policies that trigger disciplinary review if an investigator violates institutional policies or research regulations, the COI policy itself needs to incorporate this type of provision.

*Determining deliberate versus unintentional noncompliance.* Given the complexity of the regulation, institutional COI policies, and in many cases the administrative procedures needed to stay in compliance, it is not uncommon for investigators to under-disclose or disclose their financial interests belatedly. Even at institutions that do a good job of educating investigators and providing them tools to comply with COI policies, disclosures are sometimes late or incomplete. The COI staff members need to judge when an investigator has made an honest or unintentional error and to provide ongoing guidance and education. Of course, there are cases of knowing and intentional failures to disclose financial interests or comply with management plans. It is incumbent on institutions to address those situations promptly under their disciplinary procedures, not only to be in compliance with regulation but also to signal that the institution takes its policies, particularly those related to ethical conduct of research, seriously.

## 8. END-OF-CHAPTER NOTES

1. The term "COI" is used throughout this chapter to refer to all financial COIs in research. The term "FCOI" is used to refer to financial COIs in the context of the PHS regulation on financial COIs in research.
2. For example, the American Academy of Orthopaedic Surgeons adopted a policy banning members of its senior governing boards and executive management from consulting or speaking for orthopedic device companies.
3. Contractors are covered under a parallel regulation [42 CFR Part 94]. Small Business Innovation Research Program Phase I applications are exempt from the regulation.
4. The Johns Hopkins University School of Medicine adopted the following interpretation. "The phrase 'responsible for the design, conduct, or reporting of research' should be interpreted to mean any individual involved in the research who works independently enough to affect the objectivity of the design, collection, or analysis of research data or reporting of research results. In addition to faculty members, this may include graduate and post-doctoral trainees, research staff, consultants, or other collaborators. The ultimate determination as to who is considered an investigator in PHS-supported research is the decision of the PI of the project."
5. The regulation requires that if a conflicted investigator in a PHS-supported clinical study testing a drug, device, or treatment fails to disclose a financial interest or the institution fails to manage it, upon disclosure or management the institution must require notification of the interest in all public presentations about the study, and there must be addendums to previously published presentations. This is the only provision of the PHS regulation that is specific to human subject research.

## References

[1] Sinclair U. I, candidate for governor: and how i got licked. University of California Press; 1994.
[2] Scientific achievements less prominent than a decade ago: public praises science; scientists fault public, media. http://www.people-press.org/2009/07/09/section-1-public-views-of-science-and-scientists/ [published 09.07.07].
[3] The scientific basis of influence and reciprocity: a symposium. https://members.aamc.org/eweb/upload/The %20Scientific%20Basis%20of%20Influence.pdf [published 12.06.07].
[4] Yank V, Rennie D, Bero L. Financial ties and concordance between results and conclusions in meta-analyses: retrospective cohort study. Br Med J 2007;335:1202–5.
[5] Efstathiou J, Drajem M. Texas energy head quits amid fracking study conflicts. http://www.bloomberg.com/news/2012-12-06/texas-energy-institute-head-quits-amid-fracking-study-conflicts.html [published 06.12.12].
[6] Dismal ethics: an intensifying debate about the case for a professional code of ethics for economists. http://www.economist.com/node/17849319 [published 06.01.11].
[7] 35 U.S.C, pp. 200–212. http://www.gpo.gov/fdsys/pkg/USCODE-2011-title35/pdf/USCODE-2011-title35-partII-chap18.pdf.
[8] Association of University Technology Managers (AUTM) U.S. licensing activity survey: FY2012, p. 30.
[9] Zinner DE, Clarridge B, Blumenthal D, Campbell EG. Participation of academic scientists in relationships with industry. Health Aff (Millwood) 2009;28(6):1814–25.

[10] NSF 05-131 July 2005, Chapter V—Grantee Standards. http://www.nsf.gov/pubs/manuals/gpm05_131/gpm 5.jsp#510.

[11] 21CFR54,p.54.1–54.6.http://www.accessdata.fda.gov/scripts/cdrh/cfdocs/cfcfr/CFRSearch.cfm?CFRPart=54 &showFR=1 [revised 01.04.13].

[12] Steinbrook R. The Gelsinger case. In: Emanuel EJ, editor. The Oxford textbook of clinical research ethics. New York: Oxford University Press; 2008.

[13] Nelson D, Weiss R. Hasty decisions in the race to a cure? Gene therapy study proceeded despite safety, ethics concern. The Washington Post November 21, 1999:A01. http://www.washingtonpost.com/wp-srv/WPcap/ 1999-11/21/101r-112199-idx.html.

[14] Wilson D, Heath D. Uninformed consent. Seattle Times; March 11–15, 2001. http://seattletimes.com/uninform ed_consent/.

[15] Task force on financial conflicts of interest in clinical research. December 2001. https://www.aamc.org/download /75302/data/firstreport.pdf.

[16] Protecting subjects, preserving trust, promoting progress II: principles and recommendations for oversight of an institution's financial interests in human subjects research. https://members.aamc.org/eweb/upload/Prot ecting%20Subjects,%20Preserving%20Trust,%20Promoting%20Progress%20II.pdf; October 2002

[17] U.S. medical school policies on individual financial conflicts of interest: results of an AAMC Survey. https:// www.aamc.org/download/75296/data/coiresults2003.pdf; September 2004

[18] Financial relationships and interests in research involving human subjects: guidance for human subject protection. http://www.hhs.gov/ohrp/archive/humansubjects/finreltn/fguid.pdf; May 5, 2004

[19] Harris G. Top psychiatrist didn't report drug makers' pay. N Y Times. http://www.nytimes.com/2008/10/04/ health/policy/04drug.html?pagewanted=1; October 3, 2008

[20] Report of the committee of inquiry on the case involving Dr. Nancy Olivieri, the hospital for sick children, the University of Toronto, and Apotex Inc, p. 29–32. http://www.caut.ca/docs/academic-freedom/summary-of-the-olivieri-report.pdf

[21] Nathan DG, Weatherall DJ. Academic freedom in clinical research. N Engl J Med 2002;347:1368–71.

[22] Minaguchi M. Conflicts of interest in drug evaluation. http://www.yakugai.gr.jp/topics/file/en/Minaguchi abstract(English).pdf.

[23] 42 CFR Part 50 and 42 CFR Part 94. http://www.gpo.gov/fdsys/pkg/FR-2011-08-25/pdf/2011-21633.pdf; 2011.

# Good Laboratory Practices (GLPs)

*Anne M. Brooks[1], Michael A. Koch[2], Asheley B. Wathen[2],*
*Tim Valley[2]*

[1]WuXi AppTec, Inc., Shanghai, China; [2]Covance, Inc., NJ, USA

## 1. INTRODUCTION

Pharmaceutical companies in the United States develop new drugs through a time-honored process that involves several phases from discovery of the drug through marketing of the drug to patients through physicians [1] (Figure 1). Those phases include early discovery research, preclinical (also known as nonclinical) toxicology studies, human clinical trials, and postmarketing studies. The US Food and Drug Administration (FDA) regulates the development process through so-called good laboratory practices (GLPs), good clinical practices, and good manufacturing practices codified in Part 21 of the code of federal regulations (CFR). These regulations are relatively complex and intended to ensure efficacy and safety of new pharmaceutical products. The pharmaceutical industry and its supporting contract research organizations must navigate these myriad regulations and secure FDA approval as the new products move through the phases mentioned above.

Discovery research is the earliest phase of drug development and the least regulated of the phases. Laboratory studies generally establish whether a new drug candidate is efficacious and safe enough to move along the development pathway. Lead optimization and pharmacology studies explore the safety of new drug candidates and set the stage for rigorous preclinical toxicology studies. The discovery research studies may or may not be done in the "spirit" of the GLPs.

Relatively short-term (e.g., 14–28 days) preclinical toxicology studies using animals are performed to determine if the drug candidate is safe enough to enter the human clinical trial phases of drug development. The FDA generally requires that these studies be run in a rodent species and a large animal species (e.g., dogs, macaques), and that they are done under rigorous conditions and according to the GLPs. The package of information generated by discovery and early toxicology work can then be presented to the FDA in an Investigational New Drug (IND) application. The FDA reviews the data and determines if drug development can proceed to the human clinical trial phases. Longer term (e.g., 13–104 weeks) preclinical

*Research Regulatory Compliance*
http://dx.doi.org/10.1016/B978-0-12-420058-6.00011-3

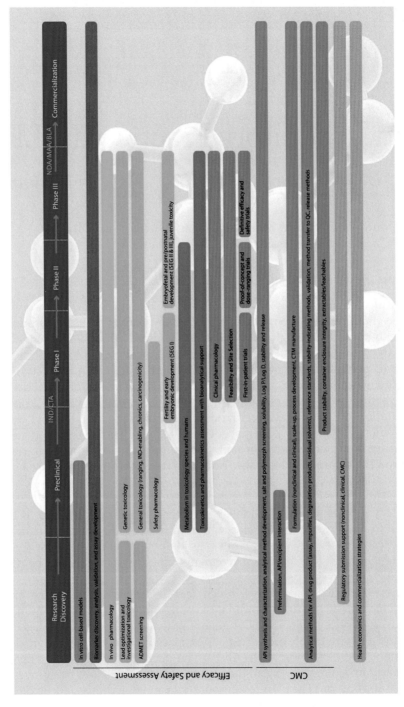

FIGURE 1    Drug development process map. *Reproduced with permission from Covance, Inc.*

toxicology studies using animals will commence and run concurrently with early clinical trials after submission of the IND. A "clinical hold," which is an order from the FDA to the sponsor to delay or suspend a clinical investigation, could be placed on the program if the FDA finds problems in the data at any point.

Clinical trials are done in human research subjects to determine if the new drug candidate is effective for its intended purpose and the side effects associated with its use (if any). There are four clinical trial phases in which the new drug candidate is initially tested in healthy human volunteers and then introduced into larger populations with the clinical problem the drug is intended to treat (Figure 1). The data from the clinical trials are then submitted by the pharmaceutical sponsor to the FDA through a New Drug Application (NDA). The FDA reviews all pertinent data and determines if the drug can be marketed for use in the human patient population. Patent law is often used by sponsors to protect their investment by ensuring that they have the sole right to market the drug during the life of the patent.

This chapter will provide information on historical perspectives, relevant regulations, agencies and guidance documents, key personnel, common compliance challenges, and addressing noncompliance as these items relate to the GLPs. The long history of drug development in the United States has led to a complex, modern-day regulatory environment that will be described in the following pages.

## 2. HISTORICAL PERSPECTIVES

### 2.1 Origins of the Food and Drug Administration

The path toward the current, large, complex FDA began during the mid-nineteenth century. The origin of the FDA can be traced back to around 1848 when the US Patent Office appointed Lewis Caleb Beck to run chemical analyses of agricultural products [2]. President Lincoln established the Bureau of Chemistry, the predecessor of the FDA, in the new Department of Agriculture in 1862 by appointing Charles Wetherill as chemist. A significant concern about food adulteration developed in the late 1800s, which led to calls for passage of a national food and drug law. More than 100 such bills were introduced in the US Congress during the late 1800s and the early 1900s before a food and drug law was enacted.

The modern era of food and drug regulatory oversight began with the passage of the original Pure Food and Drugs Act of 1906 [3]. The law prohibited sales of food and drugs with fraudulent label claims or that were adulterated. The law was challenged in the US court system, and the Supreme Court eventually ruled in 1911 that it did not prohibit false therapeutic claims. Congress passed the Sherley Amendment in 1912 to overcome the Supreme Court's ruling. The new law established that sellers could not intentionally defraud customers with false claims. This standard was difficult to prove and set the stage for calamitous events later in the twentieth century that led to a complete revision of the 1906 law and increased regulation of food and drugs. By 1930, the Bureau of Chemistry had been reorganized and the FDA was established as a separate regulatory entity.

## 2.2 Mid-Twentieth Century Events

Congress passed the Federal Food, Drug, and Cosmetic Act of 1938 after one of the most calamitous and tragic events related to drug development [3,4]. In 1937, elixir of sulfanilamide, which contained the poison diethylene glycol, killed more than 100 people. This episode demonstrated the clear need to establish drug safety before marketing and led directly to consideration and passage of the 1938 law. The law defined "new drugs" as those not generally recognized as safe, established the NDA and authorized the FDA to review new drugs to ensure that they were safe prior to marketing.

Regulatory oversight of drug development increased further in 1962 in the wake of the famous thalidomide episode. This new drug, intended to treat sleep problems, caused birth defects in thousands of babies in western Europe [3]. Public support for stronger regulation of drug development grew substantially in the wake of this tragedy and led to the Kefauver-Harris amendments to the 1938 Federal Food, Drug, and Cosmetic Act. These amendments required drug makers for the first time to demonstrate to the FDA that new compounds were safe and effective [4]. Safety and effectiveness were to be determined through controlled investigations by appropriately qualified scientific experts. The previously described system of preclinical investigations and clinical trials, in its earliest form, was born as a result of these amendments. Finally, through this system it was required that the FDA review all NDAs to ensure that new drugs were effective for their intended use.

As this system of drug development regulatory oversight progressed during the 1960s and 1970s, concerns with the validity of preclinical studies developed [5,6]. FDA inspections revealed instances of inadequate planning and execution of studies, lack of appropriate documentation of study methods and results, and even fraudulent activities. These issues were made public during the Kennedy hearings in Congress and led the FDA to propose regulations on GLPs in 1976 and a final rule (published in 21 CFR 58) in 1979. The GLP regulations were established to ensure that preclinical data submitted to the FDA as part of IND and NDA submissions would accurately reflect the scientific work carried out to determine the effectiveness and safety of new drugs. The US Environmental Protection Agency also promulgated GLP regulations in the late 1970s because of similar concerns in the chemical and pesticide field. Internationally, the Organization for Economic Cooperation and Development (OECD) and some member countries followed the US lead and recognized the GLPs in the early 1980s and 1990s as best practice for generating preclinical safety data. Much of the rest of this chapter will focus on important aspects of the GLPs.

## 2.3 Late Twentieth Century and Twenty-first Century Events

Globalization of drug development processes accelerated during the 1990s and into the twenty-first century. Drug makers currently have significant interest in marketing products internationally and mutual acceptance of safety test data across international boundaries is important to this globalization process. Compliance with GLP principles is a prerequisite to mutual acceptance of data [5,6]. As a consequence, OECD member countries developed procedures for monitoring GLP compliance that include laboratory inspections and study audits. Expert foreign inspectors may conduct inspections and audits in developing countries that currently lack national compliance programs. Thus, the principles of GLP have spread across the globe as a necessary component of the international drug development industry.

The GLP standards, within the United States and internationally, have also been revised substantially in more recent times because of several factors [6]. Those standards, as originally written, reflected the way studies were conducted at the time. Most data were recorded by hand, so the standards emphasized clarity of the handwritten record, appropriate footnoting, and other related items. Laboratory automation and computerized records have become commonplace, so GLP standards and associated guidance documents were updated in the 1990s and 2000s to address these emerging issues. GLP was also revised during this time because of ongoing recognition of inconsistencies in data such as detection of a test article in control samples as part of toxicokinetic evaluations [6]. GLPs will likely continue to evolve as the science of toxicology evolves and the trend toward globalization continues.

# 3. RELEVANT REGULATORY/OVERSIGHT AGENCIES

## 3.1 Food and Drug Administration

### 3.1.1 *Place in the US Government*

Formed in 1906, the FDA is an agency within the US Department of Health and Human Services, consisting of the office of the Commissioner and four directorates overseeing the core functions of the agency including Medical Products and Tobacco, Foods, Global Regulatory Operations and Policy, and Operations [7]. Responsibilities of the FDA include protecting and promoting public health through the regulation and supervision of these elements. The Food, Drug, and Cosmetic Act was first passed in 1938 and includes most federal laws concerning the FDA, which are codified in Title 21, Chapter 9, of the US Code. The FDA also enforces laws including Section 361 of the Public Health Service Act and associated regulations, parts of the Controlled Substances Act, and the Federal Anti-Tampering Act, among others.

### 3.1.2 *Responsibilities Related to Drug Safety*

Prescription, over-the-counter (OTC), and generic drugs are regulated by FDA's Center for Drug Evaluation and Research. Drug companies seeking FDA approval of a new prescription drug in the United States must test the drug first in laboratory and animal tests followed by tests in humans. These levels of testing evaluate if the drug is safe and effective when used to treat or diagnose a disease. After testing, the company sends the FDA an NDA. If made out of biologic materials, a Biologics License Application is used for approval. OTC drugs are most often marketed without an NDA by following a regulation called an OTC drug monograph, which tells what kind of ingredients may be used to treat certain diseases or conditions without a prescription, appropriate dose, and instructions for use. If an OTC product meets a monograph's requirement, it may be marketed without FDA review. Otherwise, an application such as those used for prescription products must be used for approval. Generic drugs do not need additional testing for safety and effectiveness as long as the generic drug is shown to be the same as an already approved drug. Generic drugs are approved under abbreviated NDA.

### 3.1.3 *Laws and Regulations Related to Drug Development Oversight*

#### 3.1.3.1 THE FEDERAL FOOD, DRUG, AND COSMETIC ACT

Passed by Congress in 1938, this set of laws gives authority to the FDA to oversee the safety of food, drugs, and cosmetics. The introduction of this act was spurred on by the elixir sulfanilamide disaster during which more than 100 patients died from a sulfanilamide medication that was dissolved into liquid form using diethylene glycol [7].

#### 3.1.3.2 21 CODE OF FEDERAL REGULATIONS AND SUBPARTS

Title 21 of the CFR governs food and drugs within the United States for the FDA (Chapter I), the Drug Enforcement Administration (Chapter II), and the Office of National Drug Control Policy (Chapter III). Chapter I, Part 58, details GLP for nonclinical studies.

## 3.2 Good Laboratory Practice Regulations (21 Code of Federal Regulations Part 58) [8]

### 3.2.1 *General Provisions*

The scope of the GLP regulations includes conduct of nonclinical laboratory studies that support or are intended to support applications for products regulated by the FDA. Subpart 58.3(d) defines a nonclinical laboratory study as follows:

> *Nonclinical laboratory study* means in vivo or in vitro experiments in which test articles are studied prospectively in test systems under laboratory conditions to determine their safety. The term does not include studies utilizing human subjects or clinical studies or field trials in animals. The term does not include basic exploratory studies carried out to determine whether a test article has any potential utility or to determine physical or chemical characteristics of a test article.

The FDA regulates food and color additives, animal food additives, human and animal drugs, medical devices for human use, biological products, and electronic products. Compliance with GLP regulations is to assure quality and integrity of the safety data filed as it relates to the Federal Food, Drug, and Cosmetic Act and relevant sections of the Public Health Service Act. Consulting laboratories, contractors, and grantees performing services for a sponsor in efforts to conduct a nonclinical laboratory study must conduct work in compliance with GLP regulations. During such conduct, a testing facility must permit an authorized employee of the FDA to inspect the facility, including all records and specimens. Refusal of inspection will result in the FDA not considering a nonclinical laboratory study in support of an application for a research or marketing permit. Definitions are a critical part of any regulatory document and are key to understanding and interpreting statements and recommendations given in the document [6].

### 3.2.2 *Organization and Personnel*

Every individual involved in conduct of or supervision of a nonclinical laboratory study will have adequate education, training, and experience (or combination thereof) to adequately perform their assigned functions. Personnel qualifications will be maintained by the testing facility, and a sufficient number of personnel will be ensured to provide timely and proper conduct of the study according to the protocol. Personnel will use appropriate personal sanitation and health precautions to avoid contamination, appropriate clothing for duties they perform and be excluded from duties if found to have an illness that may adversely affect study quality or integrity.

Management has specific responsibilities to provide an optimal environment for GLP compliance of the test facility and all GLP-compliant studies conducted within the test facility [8]. A study director is designated by management before study initiation and is replaced promptly if necessary during the conduct of a study. Management must assure that there is a quality assurance unit (QAU); that test and control articles have been tested appropriately before use; that personnel clearly understand functions they are to perform; and that appropriate resources are available including personnel, facilities, equipment, and materials. Last, management must report any deviation from these regulations, that are reported by the QAU, to the study director and corrective actions taken and documented.

The study director is typically a scientist or other professional of appropriate education, training, and experience who has the overall responsibility for the technical conduct of the study. Responsibilities of the study director also include interpretation, analysis, documentation, and reporting of results. Therefore, the study director represents the single point of study control. The study director must assure that the protocol and any changes are approved and followed; that all experimental data are accurately recorded and verified; that unforeseen circumstances that may affect quality or integrity of the study are noted and corrective action taken and documented; that all applicable GLP regulations are followed; and that all raw data, documentation, protocols, specimens, and final reports are transferred to the archives during or at the close of the study.

A QAU is responsible for monitoring each study to ensure that the facilities, equipment, personnel, methods, practices, records, and controls are in compliance with the GLP regulations. The QAU must be entirely separate from, and independent of, the personnel engaged in the direction or conduct of the study, meaning separate reporting lines within the organizational structure. QAU responsibilities include maintaining a copy of a master schedule sheet of all nonclinical laboratory studies at the testing facility; maintaining copies of all protocols; inspecting each study to ensure integrity of the study with records of any noted findings or problems and recommended actions; providing management with periodic status reports on each study; reviewing final study reports for accuracy; and preparing and signing a statement to be included with the final study report to management and the study director. Upon inspection of the testing facility, the FDA representative must have access to inspections performed by the QAU.

### 3.2.3 Facilities

Testing facilities must be of suitable size such that there is a degree of separation that will prevent any function or activity from having an adverse effect on the study. Sufficient numbers of animal rooms are necessary to ensure proper separation of species or test systems, isolation of projects, quarantine of animals, and routine or specialized housing of animals. Studies with test or control articles known to be biohazardous, including volatile substances, aerosols, radioactive materials, and infectious agents, must be appropriately isolated through a sufficient number of animal rooms or areas. Collection and disposal of all animal waste and refuse or safe sanitary storage of such waste before removal must be facilitated through appropriate means such that vermin infestation, odors, disease hazards, and environmental contamination are minimized. Storage areas must be provided for feed, bedding, supplies, and equipment with feed and bedding storage separated from areas housing the test systems and protected against infestation or contamination.

Separation of certain areas must be provided to prevent contamination or mix-ups. As necessary, separate areas should be provided for receipt and storage of test and control articles, mixing of the test and control articles with a carrier, and storage of test and control articles. Additionally, storage areas for test and control articles should be separate from areas housing the test systems and adequate to maintain the identity, strength, purity, and stability of the articles and mixtures. Separate laboratory space is needed for performing routine and specialized procedures required by nonclinical studies. Limited access to authorized personnel only should be maintained for space dedicated to archive and retrieval of all raw data and specimens from completed studies.

### 3.2.4 Equipment

Equipment must be of appropriate design and adequate capacity to function according to the protocol while being suitably located for operation, inspection, cleaning, and maintenance. Written standard operating procedures (SOPs) will describe methods, materials, and schedules to be used in routine inspection, cleaning, maintenance, testing, calibration, and/or standardization of equipment. SOPs also designate the person responsible for performance of each operation. Written records must be maintained of all inspection, maintenance, testing, calibrating, and/or standardizing operations. Any nonroutine repairs performed as a result of failure or malfunction of equipment must be documented, including the nature of the defect, how and when it was discovered, and any remedial action taken in response to the defect.

### 3.2.5 Testing Facilities Operation

Management must ensure adequate SOPs in writing to set forth methods. All deviations in a study from SOPs must be authorized by the study director and also documented in the raw data. SOPs detailing a variety of testing facility operations should exist to ensure quality and integrity of the data generated. Laboratory manuals and SOPs need to be immediately available in or near the room where the activities occur. Maintenance of a historical file of SOPs and all revisions, including dates implemented, is also necessary.

Upon arrival, animal health status should be determined through isolation and evaluation. Animals need to be free of any disease or condition that might interfere with the purpose or conduct of the study. Treatment for disease or suspected disease should not interfere with the study. Diagnosis, authorization of treatment, description of treatment, and date of treatment should be documented and retained.

Unique animal identification is required for all warm-blooded animals, including suckling rodents requiring removal from their home cages for any reason. The cage card is an acceptable method of identification if the animal is never taken from and returned to the cage during the course of the study. Best practice is to maintain only one species from a single vendor per study room, although if mixed housing is necessary, differentiation of space and identification must be made. Feed and water must be analyzed periodically to ensure that contaminants are not present above those levels specified in the protocol and included in documentation as raw data.

### 3.2.6 Test and Control Articles

Identity, strength, purity, and composition must be determined for each batch and documented as well as methods of synthesis, fabrication, or derivation of the test and control articles. Stability of each test or control article must be determined by the testing facility or sponsor either before study initiation or in parallel according to SOPs. Storage containers should be labeled by name, chemical abstract number or code number, batch number, and expiration date. For studies longer than 4 weeks' duration, reserve samples from each batch of test and control articles must be retained. Established procedures must be in place to ensure proper storage, distribution without contamination, deterioration or damage, and proper maintenance of identification, and receipt and distribution of each batch must be documented. When test or control article is mixed with a carrier, uniformity of the mixture and stability of the test and control articles within the mixture must be determined either before study initiation or in parallel, according to SOPs.

### 3.2.7 Protocol for and Conduct of a Nonclinical Laboratory Study

Each study must have an approved written protocol that clearly indicates the objectives and all methods for study conduct. Appropriate items in the protocol include: descriptive title and statement of study purpose; identification of test and control articles; name of the sponsor and name/address of the testing facility; test system specifics; procedure for test system identification; description of experimental design; dosage level and method and frequency of administration; type and frequency of tests/analyses/measurements; records; approval date of protocol by sponsor and dated signature of study director; statistical methods. Note that the "testing facility" and "sponsor" may be the same entity in certain circumstances such as in an academic setting. All data generated during study must be recorded directly, promptly, and legibly in ink with all dated entries dated on the date of entry with signature or initial of person entering the data. Any changes in entries will be made so as not to obscure the original entry (e.g., single line-out) indicating reasons for change with date and signature at time of the change.

### 3.2.8 Records and Reports

A final report should be prepared for each study including detailed information similar to that of the protocol. The study completion date is that time at which the final report is signed and dated by the study director. Any corrections or additions to the final report must be in the form of an amendment by the study director. All raw data, documentation, protocols, final reports, and specimens must be retained with the exception of those specimens obtained from mutagenicity tests and wet specimens (blood, urine, feces, and biological fluids). Archives must be employed for orderly storage and retrieval of all study-related information with storage conditions to minimize deterioration of documents or specimens. An identified individual must be responsible for the archives and only authorized personnel shall enter the archives. Specific requirements for retention of records are specified by GLP regulations dependent on the type of submission to the FDA and other factors. The shortest time frame prevails for record retention. In general, records must be maintained for 5 years after the date on which the results of the studies are submitted to the FDA in support of an application of a research or marketing permit (i.e., 5 years after application for an IND or NDA). Most companies retain documents, paraffin blocks, microscope slides, and digital images indefinitely, however. If a facility goes out of business, all raw data, documentation, and other material is transferred to the archives of the sponsor of the study with the FDA notified in writing of such transfer.

### 3.2.9 Disqualification of Testing Facilities

Disqualification exists to allow for exclusion from consideration completed studies that were conducted by testing facilities that fail to comply with requirements of GLPs until it can be determined that noncompliance did not affect the validity of data generated by a study. Also, this is done to exclude from consideration all studies completed after the date of disqualification until the testing facility can satisfy the Commissioner that it will conduct studies in compliance with GLP regulations. The applicant for a research or marketing permit must still submit results to FDA despite disqualification of a testing facility. Disqualification may occur by the Commissioner upon finding: failure of the testing facility to comply with one or more of the regulations; noncompliance that adversely affected the validity of the nonclinical laboratory studies; and when other lesser regulatory actions have not been or will probably not be adequate to achieve compliance with the GLPs. The Commissioner may issue a written notice proposing that the testing facility be disqualified and a hearing will be conducted. Determination that a testing facility has been disqualified and administrative records are disclosable to the public.

Once a testing facility has been disqualified, each application for a research or marketing permit may be examined to determine whether the study was or would be essential to a decision. If a study is determined to be essential, the FDA will also determine whether the study is acceptable, notwithstanding the disqualification of the facility. Persons relying on the study may be required to establish that the study was not affected by the circumstances that led to the testing facility disqualification. No nonclinical laboratory study initiated by a testing facility after the date of the facility's disqualification will be considered in support of any application for a research or marketing permit unless the facility has been reinstated.

Reinstatement of a disqualified testing facility may occur if the Commissioner determines that the facility can adequately ensure that it will conduct future studies in compliance with GLPs and that any ongoing studies being conducted have not been compromised in regard to quality and integrity. The testing facility may present in writing to the Commissioner why it should be reinstated with detailed description of the corrective actions it has taken or intends to take to ensure that the acts or omissions which led to its disqualification will not recur. If reinstated, the Commissioner will notify the testing facility and all others who were notified at the time of disqualification. Determination of reinstatement is also disclosable to the public.

### 3.2.10 Guidance Documents

Refer to Table 1 for some applicable guidance documents.

TABLE 1    Relevant Guidance Documents

| Guideline | Reference |
| --- | --- |
| ICH guidelines | http://www.ich.org/products/guidelines.html |
| OECD guidelines for the testing of chemicals | http://oberon.sourceoecd.org/v1=1960783/cl=12/nw=1/rpsv/cw/vhosts/oecdjournals/1607310x/v1n4/contp1-1.htm |
| Office of chemical safety and pollution prevention | http://www.epa.gov/ocspp/pubs/frs/publications/Test_Guidelines/series870.htm |
| Redbook 2000, guidance for industry and other stakeholders; toxicological principles for the safety assessment of food ingredients | http://www.fda.gov/Food/GuidanceComplianceRegulatory Information/GuidanceDocuments/FoodIngredientsand Packaging/Redbook/default/htm |
| Redbook 2000, biological evaluation of medical devices (ISO 10993 series) | www.iso.org |

## 4. KEY REGULATORY MANDATES

There are other regulatory mandates, in addition to the 21CFR 58 GLP mandates described in the preceding section, that impact conduct of nonclinical studies, including the following.

### 4.1 Animal Welfare

The FDA shares a common concern for the welfare of laboratory animals with other pertinent US regulatory agencies [9]. Thus, a memorandum of understanding was developed among the US Department of Agriculture, the US National Institutes of Health, and the FDA. The agreement creates a framework for those agencies to meet their responsibilities related to laboratory animal care and welfare. The agreement further outlines the responsibilities of the respective agencies, indicates information of mutual concern that will be shared with regard to laboratory animal care, and identifies agency liaisons as part of a pertinent standing committee. Other chapters in this text provide more details about animal welfare-related regulations in the research environment and readers are encouraged to consult those pages for more information.

## 5. KEY PERSONNEL

To understand the roles and responsibilities the various stakeholders have under GLP regulations in a nonclinical research environment, it is helpful to walk through a hypothetical new drug program. Imagine a university professor with a promising compound to be developed. Working through a group such as the Wisconsin Alumni Research Foundation, this individual starts a new virtual company to begin to develop the compound. The goal of this particular company is to submit an IND Application, needed to ship a nonapproved drug across state lines, and proceed to clinical research. To reach this goal, preclinical safety testing must be conducted with the following goal, as summarized by the FDA [10]:

> During a new drug's early preclinical development, the sponsor's primary goal is to determine if the product is reasonably safe for initial use in humans, and if the compound exhibits pharmacological activity that justifies commercial development. When a product is identified as a viable candidate for further development, the sponsor then focuses on collecting the data and information necessary to establish that the product will not expose humans to unreasonable risks when used in limited, early-stage clinical studies.

Because this company is virtual, with no physical testing capabilities, it will need to contract the services of a laboratory to conduct the necessary preclinical/nonclinical testing in order to obtain the data needed to submit the IND. Such laboratories are termed Contract Research Organizations (CROs); the company contracting their services is the *sponsor* of the research. As defined in 21 CFR 58, 58.3(f), "sponsor" in this case means, "A person who initiates and supports, by provision of financial or other resources, a nonclinical laboratory study." Note that subsection 58.3(h) further defines "person" as an "individual, partnership, corporation, association, scientific or academic establishment, government agency, or organizational unit thereof, and any other legal entity"; person can therefore in the context of these regulations more clearly be thought of in most cases as "entity."

The CRO site at which the nonclinical study is conducted is the *testing facility*, defined in subpart 58.3(g) as the entity that "actually uses the test article in a test system." The testing facility has the responsibilities outlined in Section 3.1.2 of this chapter.

Of prime importance in any nonclinical study is the *study director*. This individual, as simply stated in subpart 58.3(m), is "the individual responsible for the overall conduct of a nonclinical laboratory study." This is, quite literally, the most key person of any nonclinical study. The study director must have ultimate control (with one exception described later) over the conduct of the study and is ultimately responsible for the conduct and outcome of the study. The signature of this individual on the final study report verifies that all aspects of the study were in accordance with the US FDA GLPs, Title 21 of the US CFR Part 58 (unless otherwise specifically stated within the compliance section of the report), and that they stand behind all conclusions drawn from the data collected under that study.

To summarize thus far, then, the professor's virtual company is the *sponsor* of the nonclinical study conducted at the CRO under the control of the *study director*. Although the study director is the single point of control on the study, one individual can obviously not conduct the entire study single-handedly. The physical work of the study is conducted by various operational groups; for this sponsor's study, this might include:

- In-life staff, who conduct animal care, dosing, and monitoring (e.g., clinical observations, ophthalmic evaluation, electrocardiographic evaluation) aspects of the study.
- Dose formulations staff members, who dispense dosing formulations, which may include some or all of the following:
  - Preparation of vehicle/control article (for use in preparing test article formulations and/or dosing of control animals).
  - Preparation of doseable formulations from the neat (i.e., undiluted) test article as provided by the sponsor.
  - Transfer of dosing formulations to the appropriate containers for in-life staff (e.g., infusion bags, syringes, vials).

- Collection of samples, including:
  - Reserve samples (described in Section 3.2.6 of this chapter),
  - Dose analysis samples.
- Analytical chemistry staff members, who conduct dose analysis (needed to ensure the uniformity of the mixture and stability of the test and control articles within the mixture as described in section 3.2.6 of this chapter).
- Bioanalytical staff members: analyze biological samples (generally serum or plasma) for test article. (for some study designs, analysis for metabolites, analysis for both prodrug and active compound, analysis for antidrug antibodies, or other types of bioanalysis may be needed.)
- Pathology staff members: conduct clinical pathology (e.g., serum and/or urine chemistry, hematology) and anatomic pathology (e.g., necropsy/macroscopic observations, organ weight measurements) testing.

To be valid, a nonclinical study must demonstrate that the intended dose level was administered to the test system (dose analysis); that exposure to the test article occurred (e.g., the material was not all metabolized to inactive forms and/or excreted—bioanalysis); and that effects of the exposure were characterized appropriately (e.g., in-life monitoring, pathology). The operational groups described carry out the work needed to provide the study director with the data required to demonstrate that these criteria were met, which ultimately results in the hypothetical virtual company having the information needed to submit the IND and move toward clinical testing.

Because a wide array of scientific knowledge is needed to properly evaluate the often vast quantities of data collected under a nonclinical study, specialty expertise is often required. Although the FDA GLP regulations do not specify titles for such personnel, OECD GLP [11] requirements are often used for multisite studies. Per OECD GLP regulations, a *principal investigator* is assigned to act on behalf of the study director and has defined responsibility for a delegated phase in a multisite study. This is a portion of the study conducted at a test site that is a separate location from the site at which the study director is located (test facility). For portions of the study conducted at the test facility (where the study director is located) that require an individual with specialty expertise, the scientist may be considered a contributing scientist or similar title. Regardless of title, however, the FDA GLPs—subpart 58.185(a) (12)—require that the signed and dated reports of each of the individual scientists or other professionals involved in the study be included in the final study report, which the sponsor in this case will use for IND submission.

The primary required mechanisms for coordination of study events and personnel (both operational and scientific) on a GLP nonclinical study include the study protocol (described in Section 3.2.7 of this chapter) and the master schedule. Although the format of the master schedule is not specified in the regulations and has evolved over time, the following general rules apply [12]:

- All studies must be included in the schedule.
- A change control procedure is in place to reflect shifts in dates and workload.
- Time-consuming activities such as protocol review and report preparation should also be included.
- The schedule is "official" (i.e., there should not be two or more competing systems for the same purpose).

- The system is described in an approved SOP.
- Responsibilities for maintenance and updating of the master schedule are defined by management.
- Various versions of the master schedule are approved and maintained in the archive as data.
- Distribution is adequate and key responsibilities are identified.

Test facility management and QAU personnel are also key to conducting a nonclinical study. Duties required of these personnel are outlined in Section 3.2.2 of this chapter.

Overall, then, the *sponsor* has contracted with a CRO to conduct a nonclinical study at the test facility. *Test facility management* must assign a *study director* at the facility (this individual has ultimate responsibility for ensuring the GLP compliance of the study) and ensure the other study aspects outlined in section 3.2.2 of this chapter. The *study director* then, via the master schedule and protocol, must communicate the study conduct requirements to the study team, consisting of *operational groups* and *contributing scientists* (who may be titled *principal investigators* for work conducted at study phases conducted at test sites, apart from the test facility). The entire study process (including review of data, reports, and master schedule, as well as study activity and facility audits) is overseen from a quality standpoint by the *quality assurance unit* of the test facility and, if applicable, of associated test sites.

## 6. COMMON COMPLIANCE CHALLENGES

An advantage new or existing test facilities have is the wealth of regulatory history and inspection results. The information can be used to establish business, procedural, regulatory, and resource priorities for the business. Typically, specific compliance history information provides the greatest and most useful information, as the "feedback" originates from regulatory authorities. This section of the chapter discusses common compliance challenges observed across the drug development industry, options to address gaps (proactively and retrospectively), and potential areas of risk.

Training files are often viewed as easy, straightforward document types when in reality they are complex, always changing, and key to determining if staff and study conduct were completed appropriately. Common training file gaps include the following:

- Outdated documents
- Curriculum vitae (CV) that are missing, outdated, or inaccurate
- Position descriptions (PD) that are outdated, inaccurate, or not maintained
- Missing training certificates (job functions or regulatory training)
- Lack of, or insufficient, SOP training
- Missing or unavailable training files
- Training files not properly archived.

To address these general categories, test facility management and operational staff members must both be accountable for maintaining training files in a regulatory readiness state. The following items or suggestions should be considered when remediating or establishing a training file system.

The CVs of individuals who are involved in the study should be reviewed on a periodic basis by both the individual and management. Accuracy of position requirements, responsibilities, training required matching PD requirements, and-up-to date regulatory training should be confirmed. Where gaps exist, immediate corrective action should be taken and documentation of these actions completed and retained with the training file.

The PDs of individuals who are involved in the study should be reviewed on a periodic basis by both the individual and management to confirm accuracy and ensure that the minimal job requirements are covered in existing training records. Confirmation that the employee meets the minimal position requirements can be confirmed against the CV. Historical PDs should be maintained either as facility records or individually in training files because they contain previous position requirement information that may not be available in current PDs.

Missing certificates of training should be regenerated. If training can or cannot be recreated, documentation should be added to the training file explaining the situation, missing information, and missing records.

Consultants or subcontractors supporting study activities should have training files maintained locally that support the expertise they bring to a study or facility (e.g., CV, accreditation) and documented training on local procedures.

Insufficient (timely) SOP reading represents another common challenge for test facilities. SOP reading represents the most frequent type of training documented and is something every visiting auditor or regulator will check while on site. Care should be taken when developing a training program to ensure SOP training is completed before the individual completes a revised procedure BUT does not unnecessarily drive non-value-added activities (constant reading of existing procedures).

Quality control (QC), or lack thereof, represents another common challenge for test facilities, especially for small operations where resources are generally tight. A robust QC process ensures that documentation misses are addressed in a timely manner, data are reconstructible, and errors are addressed before external party review. Investment in QC can cover not only study data but also facility records, training files, reports, or any other record required by regulatory agencies. QC should be completed by trained individuals who have not participated in generation of the data under review. QA should occur soon after the data have been generated as the opportunity to correct error diminishes farther out.

The generation of robust written procedures, commonly referred to as SOPs, is essential for operating within a regulated environment as they ensure a consistent approach is taken across and within studies. SOPs should be authored by a subject matter expert and approved by management. As SOPs are updated, a revision history should be maintained with the document to ensure changes over time are visible. Upon retiring a procedure, the current document and all versions should be archived such that the procedure can be referenced in future audits. Documentation of training on SOPs should be incorporated in the training file or a department training document.

Section 58.81 of 21 CFR Part 58 details the foundational SOP required to meet GLP compliance. Most test facilities have many more procedures than those listed because of the complex nature of such studies and the importance of consistency and standardization.

It cannot be emphasized enough the importance of consistent, robust documentation practices. These practices should be defined in a local SOP and follow the principles found in Section 58.130 of 21 CFR 50, Good Laboratory Regulations [8]. Gaps in documentation should be specifically noted and impact addressed. Regular training on documentation practices should occur at least annually. Such training should include consultants or subcontractors who generate data locally.

Storage units for reagents and test and control articles should ensure such materials do not degrade and function appropriately for the given task and do not impact integrity of the data generated. Procedures addressing labeling, the assignment of expiration dates, and control of material in the laboratory should be in place. In general, storage conditions are defined by the manufacturer or the study sponsor. Controlled storage environments with proper monitoring systems and alarms should be in place, described in an SOP and tested routinely. Controlled access for certain materials may be required based on classification. Vendors supplying common materials and reagents should be assessed routinely and approved by management. Impact of improperly stored material ranges from no impact to being of such significance that the study must be repeated.

Existence of adequate personnel, including those filling critical roles such as a Study Director, is routinely evaluated by FDA investigators. As noted in the FDA inspection manual [13], the Study Director workload is evaluated using the Master Schedule report. Management should be able to explain workload metrics, general study volume limits, and any variances. Often, study workload is separated into two categories: ongoing studies (active procedures taking place) and those in the reporting phases where much less oversight is required.

During facility tours, the FDA will evaluate staffing levels and equipment availability. This could include interviews with staff, availability of equipment during procedures, or general feel of the pace of ongoing procedures in the laboratory. Following samples or test article from receipt to analysis to reporting is a common approach requested by inspectors. Ensuring staff members are properly trained on interactions with the FDA is something that should be covered in initial GLP training as well as refresher training. Notification that the FDA is on site with reminders about interactions and proper conduct should be sent to all staff members when an inspection begins.

Increasingly, GLP studies are expanded to collect more data and data that require special training or knowledge to generate and/or evaluate. Appropriate specialists may be sourced from the test facility, the sponsor, or third-party consultants, although in all cases the test facility management and/or Study Director need to confirm that the following are addressed:

- Individuals have completed and documented GLP training.
- Any equipment used during the collection or analysis of data/specimens is calibrated and validated and records are available for review during an inspection.
- Data collected meet GLP expectations.
- Phase of study is covered by a QAU that ensures the procedures, data, and associated contributing report are inspected.
- Standard procedures are approved by management.
- Contracts ensure consultants to maintain confidentiality of data and studies.
- Procedures address timely archival of study records.

Mechanisms to confirm these requirements could include subcontractor audits, confirmation the facility/individual participates in a regulatory monitoring program, prestudy communications that confirm agreement to follow GLP, and confirmation of general communications which typically take place during study conduct (e.g., sharing of test site inspection reports with the Study Director) are in place. If gaps are identified, the type and degree of follow-up and impact to the study would be dictated by the issues themselves. In summary, the inspectors use general compliance requirements as a framework for organizing their inspections and focusing on compliance gaps. Facility tours provide a view of the laboratory, staff members, and procedures and are then brought back to SOP and data. Such an approach is very effective.

## 6.1 Inspections

Inspections of facilities conducting GLP studies are typically unannounced because the FDA compliance manual specifically directs for unannounced inspections. Each test facility should have a procedure that discusses responsibilities, actions, and communications associated with inspections. The following items would typically be covered.

- Reception of FDA and confirmation of credentials
- Notification of the QAU (responsible for hosting FDA inspections)
- Internal communication plan
- Client/sponsor notification process and frequency of updates
- Documents that can be provided to the FDA
- Documentation of records that were provided to the FDA and copies of records collected by the FDA
- Documentation of items or issues that require additional research
- Inspection close-outs/debriefs
- Inspection responses.

A general announcement should be sent to the facility when an inspection begins. The announcement should remind people of proper conduct, how to answer questions, and generally give everyone a heads-up that the agency is on site. Staff hosting or participating in inspections should be proficient in the area being inspected, confident, and effective communicators. Maintaining calm under questioning is also critical. Staff members should never guess at an answer; rather, the uncertainty should be stated and follow-up promised. All staff members must be trained on GLP regulations as interactions may occur during tours or phase inspections.

Inspectors should be escorted on all tours, interviews, or other activities taking place at the test facility. A dedicated room with enough space for the investigators, test facility staff members, and data should be obtained. Access to electronic systems used to generate data should be secured for the duration of the inspection. Typically, quality assurance representatives host regulatory visits. Scientific staff members provide a study overview, access to data, and address science-based questions. A cooperative relationship between all parties is critical to success.

During inspections, the FDA will typically request copies of data, reports, and facility records to act as exhibits for their reports. In most instances, the requested documents should be provided; however, copies or records of any document the agency takes with them are important in the event the results of the inspection escalate. It is also important to complete such requests in a timely manner because a delay could cause concern or slow down the pace of the inspection. Tracking the requests and completions is a best practice because it avoids disagreement regarding timeliness of request and level of cooperation.

## 7. ADDRESSING NONCOMPLIANCE

It is not uncommon that during an inspection the FDA will identify a noncompliance item. Based on the severity and frequency of the issue, it may be formally identified on a Form 483 (a record that documents findings of FDA inspections), which is then issued to management of the test facility. It is an expectation that test facilities formally respond to items noted on a Form 483[1] within 15 business days. Activities addressing the items of noncompliance do not necessarily have to be completed at the time the letter is sent but a detailed action plan should be discussed. If possible, immediate corrective and preventive actions would be completed before close of the inspection. Though not eliminating the need for a response letter, completing these actions with urgency provides a tangible example of the importance placed upon compliance at the test facility. For example, if a missing protocol deviation was identified during an inspection, a record could be generated documenting the deviation and the report amended while the inspection is still occurring. By taking immediate action, the importance of quality and compliance is clear to the inspectors.

Typical inspections close out with a debrief. Debriefs are valuable because they provide test facility management an opportunity to review findings or comments from investigators, ensure understanding, and discuss any differences of opinions. Respectful discussion is a must, even in situations in which findings may be disputed. Disagreements and specific actions taken or not taken can be resolved in the response letter. In addition, the same FDA staff members often inspect the same facility, which heightens the need to establish a good working relationship.

It is not uncommon for FDA to issue a Form 483 at the conclusion of an inspection. The responses should be approved by management and include both corrective and preventive actions. Not all actions have to be completed before the letter is sent. Typically, at the time of the next inspection, the agency will follow-up on previous issues and promised actions. When a promised action has not been completed, additional regulatory scrutiny may occur. This could include the issue being included on another Form 483 or issuing of a warning letter.[2] Were a test facility to receive a warning letter, management and legal counsel should be immediately notified.

In summary, the goal of test facilities and the regulatory bodies is to ensure safe and effective drugs/products are available to mankind. Compliance with the various regulations ensures that the data generated to make such assessments are trustworthy. When struggling with compliance issues, associated cost, and value of the requirements, it is important to keep in mind the final objective and importance of the work to mankind.

---

[1] Form 483 is the document issued at the conclusion of an investigation and details objectionable conditions identified during an inspection. Officially the agency indicates responses are encouraged though not responding within 15 business days may result in additional agency attention.

[2] Warning letters are issued when the FDA feels significant issues have been identified, compliance history includes repeat violations, or lack of effective corrective action. Warning letters serve as official notification to management that immediate corrective actions are needed. The goal of a warning letter is to drive voluntary compliance.

# References

[1] United States Food and Drug Administration. How drugs are developed and approved. http://www.fda.gov/Drugs/DevelopmentApprovalProcess/HowDrugsareDevelopedandApproved/default.htm [accessed 13.12.13].

[2] United States Food and Drug Administration. History. http://www.fda.gov/AboutFDA/WhatWeDo/History/default.htm [accessed 24.12.13].

[3] United States Food and Drug Administration. Milestones in U.S. Food and drug law history. http://www.fda.gov/AboutFDA/WhatWeDo/History/Milestones/ucm128305.htm [accessed 24.12.13].

[4] Karki L. Review of FDA law related to pharmaceuticals: the Hatch-Waxman act, regulatory amendments and implications for drug patent enforcement. J Patent Trademark Office Soc 2005;87:602–20.

[5] Scientific Working Group on GLP issues, World Health Organization. Good laboratory practice. Handbook: quality practices for regulated non-clinical research and development Geneva: World Health Organization; 2009. pp. 1–309.

[6] Seiler JP. In: Mager T, editor. Good laboratory practice—the why and the how. 2nd ed. Berlin: Springer; 2005.

[7] United States Food and Drug Administration website. www.fda.gov [accessed 17.02.14].

[8] United States Food and Drug Administration. Code of federal regulations title 21, Part 58 (21CFR58): good laboratory practices for nonclinical laboratory studies.

[9] United States Department of Health and Human Services, National institutes of health, office of laboratory animal welfare. Memorandum of Understanding among USDA, FDA and NIH. http://grants.nih.gov/grants/olaw/references/finalmou.htm [accessed 27.02.14].

[10] United States Food and Drug Administration website: http://www.fda.gov/drugs/developmentapprovalprocess/howdrugsaredevelopedandapproved/approvalapplications/investigationalnewdrugindapplication/default.htm [accessed 20.02.14].

[11] Organisation for Economic Co-operation and Development (OECD) Principles of Good Laboratory Practice, ENV/MC/CHEM (98) 17 (Revised in 1997, Issued January 1998). Paris: Organization for Economic Cooperation and Development.

[12] Special Programme for Research and Training in Tropical Diseases, World Health Organization. Good laboratory practice training manual for the trainee: a tool for training and promoting good laboratory practice (GLP) concepts in disease endemic countries. 2nd ed. Geneva: World Health Organization; 2008.

[13] United States Food and Drug Administration. Compliance program manual. 2001. [Chapter 48]. Bioresearch Monitoring, Program 7348.808.

# Human Embryonic Stem Cell Research Oversight: A Confluence of Voluntary Self-Regulation and Shifting Policy Initiatives

*Melinda Abelman[1], Melissa Lopes[2], P. Pearl O'Rourke[1]*

[1]Partners HealthCare System, Boston, MA, USA; [2]Harvard University, Cambridge, MA, USA

## 1. INTRODUCTION

The oversight of pluripotent stem cell research in the United States has developed largely in a piecemeal way through a patchwork combination of policy statements, successive executive orders, funding restrictions, voluntary professional guidance, and state-based initiatives. The uneven development of research policy in this area has lent itself to a lack of uniformity and, at times, a lack of clarity for researchers and research institutions conducting this research.

To trace the development of oversight, it is important to trace the early developments in the science and the attendant political and ethical debates surrounding the same. When the derivation of human embryonic stem cells (hESCs) was first reported, the discussion immediately focused on the fact that an embryo was destroyed in the process of derivation. From the start, this area of research has been forced to evolve in the very sensitive and polarized arena of reproductive technologies and specifically the moral status of the embryo, thus contributing to rather convoluted and complicated oversight.

The oversight of hESC research must be considered in the context of the oversight processes for research in general that are informed by laws (federal, state and local), agreed-upon best practices, conditions of grant award, and public opinion. The relevant federal laws in the area of research oversight include the Food and Drug Administration (FDA) regulations that pertain to research on any product regulated by the FDA and the Common Rule that addresses the oversight of research involving human subjects [1,2].

*Research Regulatory Compliance*
http://dx.doi.org/10.1016/B978-0-12-420058-6.00012-5

Research in which hESCs were derived from human blastocysts fell into a relative gap between US research regulations—neither the Common Rule nor FDA regulations were triggered. There was no FDA-regulated product, and because neither human blastocysts nor derived hESCs are considered human subjects, the Common Rule was not triggered for the derivation itself. The only component of this research that was affected by the Common Rule was the "donation" of gametes or embryos that would be used in the research—and the adequacy of the informed consent of the gamete donors was the primary focus.

Even in the absence of statutory mandate, conditions for receiving federal grant awards can result in "nonregulatory" oversight. This was, and remains, the case with hESC research. From the beginning, efforts to provide funding guidelines for hESC research were stymied by political opposition to the research itself and by the Dickey–Wicker Amendment (DWA), a 1995 amendment to an appropriations bill (described in detail later) [3]. The DWA, which prohibits the use of federal funds for most embryo research activities, would cast a long shadow over federal funding of hESC research for years to come. As a result, federal funding of stem cell research became the lever to either foster or restrict this research at the federal level.

Although the first hESC derivation used embryos initially created for in vitro fertilization (IVF), there was interest in creating embryos specifically for hESC derivation. This included a method used in cloning, called somatic cell nuclear transfer (SCNT), by which a blastocyst is created by inserting a somatic cell nucleus into an enucleated human egg. SCNT presented not only the concern of blastocyst creation and destruction, but also issues of cloning and the challenges of access to human eggs for research. This fueled debate regarding the commodification of human gametes, specifically ova.

Although the DWA made it clear that no federal funds could be used to derive hESCs, the next question was whether federal monies could be used for research using hESCs that were derived using private funds. The answer to this depended on the scope of the DWA, and whether it encompassed hESCs themselves. The question was resolved, not through legislation or regulation, but through a formal legal opinion that hESCs are outside the scope of the DWA. This opinion cleared the way for federal funding of research using hESCs derived with private funds.

Given the sensitivity and public scrutiny of this research, a need arose for the National Institutes of Health (NIH) to develop guidelines for the federal funding of hESC research. Development and implementation of these guidelines had several starts and stops temporally associated with changes in political leadership. In the end, the NIH Guidelines, although not a regulatory mandate, most certainly inform the oversight of this research.

Even with the NIH Guidelines for the federal funding of research involving hESCs in place, there remained a need for oversight/guidance surrounding the derivation of hESCs. At the national level, leadership was assumed by the National Academy of Sciences (NAS), which developed an hESC Committee to analyze the ethical issues and to develop national guidelines [4].

Building upon the work of the NAS hESC Committee and seeking to fill the void left by the federal government in the oversight of stem cell research, a number of state-specific statues also came into play. Some offered reinterpretations of old statutes to clear the way for hESC research within their state, some drafted specific new laws, and others created directed funding initiatives specific to stem cell research. These are described later in this chapter.

The absence of federal regulation beyond funding guidelines combined with the interplay of voluntary guidelines, and varying state-specific laws created a perfect storm for interstate research. Questions of appropriate oversight for stem cell research as well as of the applicability of state mandates across jurisdictions arose as a result. Such questions did, and continue to, challenge the field.

The discovery of induced pluripotent stem cells (iPSCs) in 2007 spawned new discussion [5]. The derivation of iPSCs did not involve the manipulation or use of a blastocyst; this removed the myriad concerns associated with the destruction of an embryo in hESC derivation. With iPSCs, the somatic cell donor became the focus. As with any other tissue donation, if that donation was made specifically for research uses or if the specimen itself was identifiable, then the donor was considered a human subject triggering the Common Rule requirements. The US Department of Health and Human Services (DHHS) Office for Human Research Protections (OHRP) opined that iPSC research should not be "exceptionalized" and the somatic cell donors could be treated the same as the donor of any tissue for biomedical research [6].

Beyond derivation of lines, there has also been considerable debate regarding the uses of hESCs and iPSCs. The extreme plasticity of these stem cells raised several questions, one of which relative to both iPSCs and hESCs is whether, with their degree of plasticity, the cells could in fact, "overhumanize" a laboratory animal. The two specific concerns being integration into the central nervous system or germ line: concerns that are multiplied when the recipient animal is in early gestation [7]. Both the NAS and NIH Guidelines touch upon these concerns; albeit, with little in the way of guidance for the oversight of such research.

Even though the challenges of appropriate oversight for basic hESC and iPSC research remain, new challenges are on the immediate horizon as the next step is the clinical application of hESC and iPSCs as well as derived products.

## 2. HISTORICAL PERSPECTIVES

As stated previously, federal oversight of stem cell research has been confined to the decidedly nonregulatory sphere of funding authorization. In particular, the defining question has centered on whether hESC research is eligible for federal funding and under what conditions. The answer to this question has varied across presidential administrations. The development of policy surrounding the federal funding of hESC research can be analyzed by reference to three eras: the Clinton Era, the Bush Era, and the Obama Era. Across these, a variety of nonregulatory measures such as establishment of commissions, Congressional amendments to appropriations bills, executive orders, and the issuance of subregulatory guidelines were used to establish or further federal policy in this area.

### 2.1 The Clinton Era: The Long Shadow of Dickey–Wicker is Cast

When President William Clinton signed the DHHS appropriations bill for fiscal year 1996, two years before the first successful hESC derivation, he could not have anticipated the extent to which the DWA would serve to frustrate later efforts to establish clear guidelines, facilitating the funding of hESC research. The DWA disallows federal funding for the "creation of a human embryo, or embryos for research purposes or research in which a human embryo or embryos are destroyed, discarded..." [3]. This means that no federal funds should be used for the derivation of hESCs from a blastocyst. This limitation applies to the derivation of hESCs from the existing blastocysts created for IVF that were donated for research when no longer needed for clinical care as well as to the creation of a blastocyst specifically for research. The DWA has been reenacted every year since its initial passage and has become the backbone of US federal policy on hESC research.

The 1997 landmark announcement of the birth of Dolly [8], a cloned sheep, also predated the first successful derivation of hESCs and would prove to fuel additional controversy surrounding hESC research [9]. As noted previously, there are several ways to obtaining embryos for stem cell derivation. One is to use the excess embryos created for IVF; another is to create an embryo in vitro using donor gametes (oocyte and sperm); and a third way is to create an embryo in vitro using a donor oocyte and a donor somatic cell. This last method, called SCNT, is the method that was used to create Dolly, the sheep which was the first cloned mammal. SCNT, also called therapeutic cloning, is the process by which a somatic cell is fused with an enucleated oocyte. The nucleus of the somatic cell provides the genetic information, whereas the donor oocyte provides the nutrients and other energy-producing materials. SCNT, although controversial because it involves a form a cloning, was considered a promising option because it uses a patient's own somatic cell to provide the genetic information for the embryo. As a result, any cellular therapy developed from SCNT hESCs would be immunologically compatible to the donor and theoretically would eliminate the possibility of rejection. And, perhaps more important, this provided a way to create disease-specific hESCs for research. The Clinton administration recognized that many were troubled that this advancement might lead down a slippery slope toward the actual cloning of living human beings. As a result, the Clinton administration sought to allay these concerns by placing a federal ban on funding for cloning research and requesting that private companies also place a temporary moratorium on such research in 1997 [10].

In 1998, Wisconsin biologist James Thomson reported the first successful derivation of hESCs [11]. These cells were shown to have two unique and important characteristics. They were pluripotent, which means that they had the ability to become any kind of the different cell types in the body and they were self-renewing—able to grow continuously under laboratory conditions for over two years without losing their ability to renew themselves or to become any kind of human cell.

Less than one month after Dr Thomson's publication, Dr Harold Varmus, then the Director of NIH, addressed a Senate hearing and proclaimed, "It is not too unrealistic to say that this research has the potential to revolutionize the practice of medicine and improve the quality and length of life... There is almost no realm of medicine that might not be touched by this innovation" [12]. hESC research captured the imagination of many; some welcomed the prospect for a new era of research and possible cures, whereas others expressed concern or deemed the research unethical.

The Clinton administration, generally supportive of hESC research, sought to clarify federal policy in the wake of this new scientific advancement. In particular, it sought to eliminate any obstacles, perceived or actual, posed by the DWA. The NIH requested a legal opinion from the DHHS as to whether federal funds could be used to support hESC research. In a letter to then-NIH Director Harold Varmus dated January 15, 1999, HHS General Counsel

Harriet Rabb interpreted hESCs as outside the scope of the DWA, stating that "pluripotent stem cells cannot be considered human embryos consistent with the commonly accepted or scientific understanding of the term" [13]. This opinion ushered in the Clinton stem cell policy, establishing that although the creation of embryos for research purposes and the derivation of hESCs would be ineligible for federal funding, the use of hESCs derived from embryos created for IVF purposes in excess of clinical need would be eligible for federal funding under certain circumstances. Pursuant to this policy, the *National Institutes of Health Guidelines for Research Using Human Pluripotent Stem Cells* was published in the *Federal Register* in August 2000 [14]. Although these guidelines set a thoughtful standard that would allow for federal funding of pluripotent stem cell research derived from human embryos, no funding was ever awarded pursuant to them. Within 3 months of the Guidelines' publication, George W. Bush was elected President.

## 2.2 The Bush Era: A Solomonic Compromise Ushers in an Era of Limited Funding

After setting aside the Clinton Administration guidelines for the funding of hESC research, President Bush announced his stem cell policy via prime time television on August 9, 2001. The Bush policy led to the first actual implementation of hESC federal funding guidelines. Federal funding pursuant to the Bush policy was limited by the following parameters: federal funds could not be used to support research on embryonic stem cells that had been derived after the date of his August 2001 announcement; the stem cells must have been derived from an embryo that had been created for reproductive purposes and was no longer needed; informed consent must have been obtained from the donor of the embryo; and no financial inducements had been made to the donor [15].

The Bush policy did not prohibit private or state funding for hESC research, but limited the use of federal funds to cells that fulfilled the aforementioned criteria and, as such, were listed on a new NIH Registry of hESC lines. This new Registry only listed 64 hESC lines that had already been derived as of August 9, 2001. Cells derived after that date would not be eligible. By 2004, hESC researchers felt that the original 64 stem cell lines available for federal research had been overestimated and that many of the cell lines were unsuitable for research [14].

Bush appointed the President's Council on Bioethics, which issued three reports in 2004 and 2005, examining the complexity of stem cell research as well as the associated ethical and public policy debates. A 2005 Council White Paper proposed that alternative promising technologies such as the use of adult stem cells should be pursued instead of the more controversial hESC technology [16]. However, it was not until 2007 that human iPSCs derived from nonembryonic sources boasting similar qualities as hESCs were first derived, providing a realistic alternative [5].

These gaps in oversight, the absence of a central regulatory authority, and the desire for additional ethical guidance spurred the creation of a special NAS Committee and the growth and development of state hESC regulatory regimes.

As its first order of business, the NAS hESC Committee of experts from a variety of disciplines took on the development of guidance so that the field of embryonic stem cell research could move forward in the disjointed regulatory environment that existed. The NAS committee issued voluntary guidelines in 2005, followed in 2006, 2007, 2008, and 2010 by updated guidelines. These guidelines address issues such as ethical procurement of the blastocysts, SCNT, gamete donation, implantation of hESCs into animals, and banking of hESCs [4].

In the absence of formal regulation, the wholly voluntary NAS hESC guidelines took on the mantle of regulation. In fact, several states based their state statutory language on, or specifically referenced, the NAS hESC guidelines. It is also the NAS hESC guidelines that first recommended the development of Embryonic Stem Cell Research Oversight (ESCRO) Committees as a vehicle for providing on-going oversight of this research.

Concurrent with the development of the NAS hESC Committee's voluntary guidelines was the development of state laws seeking to support and/or regulate the research. Although federal funding was allowed for a limited scope of hESC research, some states sought to facilitate or constrain such research activity through a clear mandate. States took different paths in achieving this goal, as will be explored in greater depth later in this chapter.

## 2.3 The Obama Era: Fits and Starts in the Wake of Judicial Challenge

During his presidential campaign, candidate Obama pledged to expand federal funding of hESC research [17]. Upon election in 2008, President Obama issued a new directive to overturn President Bush's policy. In March 2009, President Obama signed an executive order allowing federal funding of research using newly derived hESCs [18]. A few months later, new NIH guidelines for human stem cell research [19] were promulgated, opening the door to an expanded NIH Registry of hESC lines eligible for federal funding and a corresponding expansion of federal funding opportunities. One month after these new guidelines went into effect, their implementation was stalled by a federal court challenge, threatening the future of federal hESC funding.

To fully appreciate the instability of the federal regulatory environment surrounding stem cell research, one need to look no further than the federal funding rollercoaster traced by the case of *Sherley v. Sebelius*. The course of this lawsuit, which involved a challenge to the federal funding of hESC research, provides a condensed synopsis of the ups and downs historically faced by institutions and researchers conducting such research. The challenge to the NIH Guidelines, brought by two stem cell researchers along with six other plaintiffs, was couched in an interpretation that the DWA prohibits the federal government from funding hESC research. Originally dismissed for lack of standing, the suit found new life when standing was reinstated for the two stem cell researchers only and the case was allowed to proceed [20].

The central question turned on an interpretation of the DWA. That the interpretation of the DWA was reopened by this case highlights the vulnerability of policies and regulations to legal challenges as well as changes in administration. This was further evidence of the unpredictable nature of regulation in this area. The interpretation of the DWA had remained consistent through three successive administrations. The Rabb memorandum, issued by the DHHS General Counsel during the Clinton Administration, distinguished between embryos and hESCs and determined that hESCs are not embryos subject to the DWA. Federal funding of hESC research during the Bush administration, though limited, was grounded in the Rabb determination that hESCs were not embryos. The Obama Administration continued to build upon the foundation of the Rabb determination and implicitly endorsed by the Bush administration, through executive order and the issuance of its own federal funding guidelines.

Of note, the Congressional Record during the Bush and Obama Administrations demonstrated support for the Rabb determination (passage of two bills in support of federal funding of hESC research and a committee report supporting the Obama executive order) [21].

During the course of this case, which traveled up to the appeals court and eventually to the Supreme Court, hESC researchers were placed in limbo as the NIH Guidelines ricocheted back and forth between valid and invalid. Access to federal funding for embryonic stem cell researchers waxed and waned accordingly. The tailspin began on August 23, 2010, when the Federal District Court determined that NIH funding of hESC research violated the DWA and enjoined NIH from funding the research. Neither NIH nor the researchers seeking funding from the NIH knew conclusively whether the District Court's injunction applied to ongoing funding pursuant to the previous Bush-era guidelines and/or new funding initiatives pursuant to the 2009 Guidelines. Seven days later, NIH issued a notice to suspend all hESC funding activities [22]. DHHS filed an emergency motion to stay the preliminary injunction, and on September 7, Judge Lambreth of the federal district court denied this motion and suggested that the preliminary injunction did not extend to the so-called Bush lines or previously funded research. The NIH funding suspension remained in place until the Appeals Court imposed a stay of the federal court injunction on September 9, 2010, a stay made durable for the course of the litigation later in the same month. Although funding pursuant to the guidelines was allowed to proceed during the course of the litigation, the seeds of uncertainty had been sown and plagued the research community until the court eventually determined that NIH's interpretation of the DWA was reasonable. In January 2013, the Supreme Court refused to review the challenge to the guidelines. As *Sherley vs. Sebelius* aptly encapsulates, researchers and research institutions have historically navigated a less than fixed or predictable regulatory route in this area.

# 3. RELEVANT REGULATORY AGENCIES AND OVERSIGHT LAWS, REGULATIONS, AND GUIDANCE DOCUMENTS IN EFFECT TODAY

## 3.1 International Regulatory Environment

According to an analysis of world stem cell policies by the Hinxton Group, more than 40 countries representing more than half the world's population have adopted permissive policies for conducting hESC research [23]. Although it is beyond the scope of this chapter to discuss the standards and regulations adopted in other countries, it is important to note the significant role played by the International Society of Stem Cell Research (ISSCR) in developing a fundamental ethical framework and guiding principles to promote international collaboration. The Society's *2006 Guidelines for the Conduct of Human Embryonic Stem Cell Research*, written by a committee of researchers, ethicists, and lawyers from 14 countries including the United States, provided guidance by which they agreed to abide. The Society has also been integral in facilitating international collaboration through its conferences and publications [24].

The International Stem Cell Forum is a group of funders of stem cell research that aims to promote international collaboration and global good practices [25]. The International Stem Cell Forum's working groups on ethics, intellectual property, standards for deriving stem cells, and for banking address harmonization in these challenging areas. Another group, the Hinxton Group, comprising well-respected scientists and ethicists from around the world, has authored several consensus reports on issues that challenge transnational collaboration. The reports can be found on their Website [26].

## 3.2 Federal Legislation, Regulations, and Guidance

Although it is true that aside from the NIH funding guidelines there are no federal statutes or regulations specifically applicable to hESC research, it does not mean that there is no federal oversight of this research. Many of the activities involved in hESC research are governed by existing federal regulations applicable to other types of research. An understanding of the regulations that affect hESC research and knowledge of how institutions implement these regulations are essential. This section outlines these regulations in addition to voluntary guidelines that are specific to hESC research.

### 3.2.1 Dickey-Wicker Amendment (DWA) of the DHHS Appropriations Bill

This amendment, described previously, was authored by Representatives Jay Dickey and Roger Wicker as a rider for the budget: Balanced Budget Downpayment Act, I, Public Law No 104-99, §128, 110 Stat. 26, 34 [3]. It has been reenacted each year and continues to disallow the use of federal funds for the derivation of hESCs as well as the creation of a human embryo by any means for this research.

### 3.2.2 2009 NIH Guidelines on Human Stem Cell Research [19]

These guidelines, issued to implement President Barack Obama's *Executive Order 13505: Removing Barriers to Responsible Scientific Research Involving Human Stem Cells* [18], outline the current conditions under which federal funds may be expended to conduct research using hESCs. The guidelines are based on the premise that hESCs are not embryos and outline the criteria and mechanisms for establishing eligibility to be listed on a new *NIH Embryonic Stem Cell Registry* (NIH Registry).

### 3.2.3 NIH Human Embryonic Stem Cell Registry [27]

Although its genesis and purpose have been described in the previous paragraph, the importance of this web-based resource for compliance with current federal policy merits its listing as a separate document. As of January 9, 2015, 303 hESC lines had been listed as eligible for federal funding.

### 3.2.4 Final Report of the National Academy's Human Embryonic Stem Cell Research Advisory Committee and 2010 Amendments to the National Academies' Guidelines for Human Embryonic Stem Cell Research [28]

The NAS Guidelines, when initially issued in April 2005, were received by research institutions and researchers as a meaningful guide bridging a policy abyss. Major research institutions almost immediately adopted these voluntary guidelines either fully or in part. The recommendations offered in the guidelines carried significant weight in the development of research oversight policies and offered institutions a starting point in the consideration of embryonic stem cell research proposals. Additionally, as discussed previously, the guidelines have also been incorporated by reference into several state laws. As titled, the 2010 guidelines represent the final report of the NAS hESC task force. Originally, the NAS committee recommended that a national board be established to periodically assess the adequacy of the guidelines. No such board currently exists.

The NAS, one of four of the National Academies, is neither a regulatory body nor a governmental agency with any authority to enforce compliance. Although the NAS does not have any regulatory authority, there are precedents [29] in scientific self-regulation, such as, the 1975 Asilomar conference that introduced guidelines to safeguard recombinant DNA work, ultimately leading to the creation of the NIH Recombinant DNA Advisory Committee and guidelines for federally funded recombinant DNA.

Unlike the NIH Guidelines, the NAS Guidelines cover all types of derivation of hESC lines and all research that uses hESCs derived from blastocysts: (1) made for reproductive purposes and later obtained for research from IVF clinics, (2) made specifically for research using IVF, and (3) made via SCNT. hESC lines may also be derived from morulae (an earlier stage of embryo development than the blastocyst), parthenogenesis, or androgenesis.

The guidelines were framed around the following major areas:

1. Establishing an institutional ESCRO committee.
2. Ethical procurement of gametes, blastocysts, or somatic cells for hESC generation. About half of the committee's recommendations relate to embryo procurement and consenting of donors.
3. Derivation of hESC lines.
4. Research use of hESC lines.
5. Banking of hESC lines.
6. International collaboration: If a US-based investigator collaborates with an investigator in another country, the ESCRO committee may determine that the procedures prescribed by the foreign institution afford protections consistent with these guidelines, and the ESCRO committee may approve the substitution of some of or all of the foreign procedures for its own.

Although ESCROs were given protocol review responsibilities, the report stressed that the ESCRO committee should not duplicate or interfere with the operations of other existing institutional committees. ESCROs should assist investigators in assessing which regulations might apply to proposed research activities, and in identifying the types and levels of review for each protocol including review by an Institutional Review Board (IRB), an Institutional Animal Care and Use Committee (IACUC), an Institutional Biosafety Committee (IBC), and/or radiation safety committee, as appropriate.

If hESC research involves potential clinical applications, such as development of products to be tested in humans, all applicable FDA regulations must be followed. The guidelines also suggest that FDA Good Laboratory Practices be followed in hESC labs, so that the research results will be eligible for FDA submission.

The NAS, like the NIH, also delineates prohibitions, or "research that should not be permitted at this time" [4]. These include (1) a prohibition of research involving in vitro culture of any intact human embryo, regardless of derivation method, for longer than 14 days or until formation of the primitive streak begins, whichever occurs first; (2) a prohibition of research in which hESCs are introduced into nonhuman primate blastocysts or in which any embryonic stem cells are introduced into human blastocysts (addressing how far scientists should go in mixing human and animal cells to create so-called chimeras); and (3) a prohibition of breeding any animal into which hESCs have been introduced such that they could contribute to the germ line. The categories listed as prohibited make it clear that the NAS committee wanted guidelines that would allow for most stem cell research, including the creation of new cell lines by nuclear transfer (cloning) and the creation of animal–human chimeras—both of which are banned in some countries and many states. With this as the goal, the guidelines offer ways of responding to concerns about the conduct of embryonic stem cell research without preventing the research from taking place.

### 3.2.5 Federal Human Subject Protection Regulation and Guidance

The FDA and DHHS human subject regulations and guidance documents [1,2,30], well described elsewhere in this book, come into play when procuring gametes, somatic cells, and embryos from human donors to derive hESCs and when using identifiable hESCs. Both the NAS Guidelines and the NIH Guidelines for hESC research are clear on the need to comply with these federally mandated regulations.

Of note, in 2002, the DHHS' OHRP issued a guidance that describes the circumstances under which "research activities involving hESCs, hESCs derived from fetal tissue, or hESC- or germ cell-derived test articles are considered human subjects research" and what regulatory controls apply to that research. The guidance is essentially a clarification seeking to avoid the "exceptionalization" of the use of these tissues.

According to the DHHS guidance, stem cells and preimplantation embryos are not human subjects, and the donors of the stem cells or embryos and/or the treated patients may be considered research subjects if identifiable private data are linked to them or can be readily ascertained, or if pertinent data are obtained through direct intervention or interaction with a living human as part of a research protocol.

### 3.2.6 US Food and Drug Administration [2]

The FDA has jurisdiction over cell-based therapies using hESCs or their derivatives. In 2010, Geron's hESC-derived product to treat spinal cord-injured subjects became the first such product granted an investigational new drug application (IND) by the FDA. Transplantation of hESCs or tissues developed from hESCs is subject to the regulations of the Center for Biologics Evaluation and Research branch of the FDA, and the product is classified and regulated either as a drug or as a device depending on its mode of action according to the Food, Drug, and Cosmetic Act and its amendments. The regulations describe a product approval path based on safety and efficacy data.

In addition, as biologics, hESC-derived products are also subject to precautions related to control of the transmission of infectious diseases, based on the *Public Health Service Act, Title 42 Chapter 6a, Subchapter II Part F—Licensing of Biological Products and Clinical Laboratories; §262. Regulation of Biological Products* [31]. The Code of Federal Regulations CFR 21 has several parts that apply to the Biological Licensing process and to the IND process, including Parts 312, 314, 58, and 201 [2].

*FDA Regulation 21 CFR Part 58* applies to the management of laboratories where products are being developed that might be introduced into humans. The regulations were developed to ensure a high quality of data in preclinical in vitro or in vivo nonhuman safety studies. Although noncompliance is not unlawful, any data collected out of compliance are not usable in support of an IND application. In other words, companies and institutions that are conducting preclinical research using hESC technology to support an IND application should be fully versed in Good Laboratory Practices regulations.

*FDA Regulation 21 CFR 1271* was brought about in 1997 because the FDA, in recognition that the human cellular and tissue-based products industry is confronted with a disjointed collection of governmental regulation, announced a "Tissue Action Plan" that called for the development of a comprehensive regulatory system to ensure product safety without imposing unnecessary restrictions. As a result of this plan, three rules, which compose FDA Regulation 21 CFR 1271, were implemented to regulate the methods, facilities, and controls used in the manufacture of these products. These new Good Current Tissue Practices regulations, which apply to institutions that derive hESCs for transplantation into humans, are to supplement, and not replace, current good manufacturing practice and quality systems regulations that apply to drugs and devices. To summarize, the regulations call for:

- Registration of establishments
- Testing for donor suitability, and tracking mechanism to link donor with tissue
- Good Tissue Practices
- Labeling
- FDA inspection of establishments; FDA enforcement of compliance.

*FDA Regulation 21 CFR Parts 210 and 211—Current Good Manufacturing Practice in Manufacturing, Processing, Packing, or Holding of Drugs; General and Current Good Manufacturing Practice For Finished Pharmaceuticals*—were revised in 2006 to reference the new tissue regulations. In a sense, the tissue regulations are a subset of the Good Manufacturing Practices that assure the quality and consistency of the cellular or tissue product.

Of note, the FDA has asserted its jurisdiction over clinical research using cloning technology, and indicated that such research would require an IND application. It also stated that until safety issues are resolved research would be placed on "clinical hold" and not allowed to proceed. This was asserted in a letter, issued October 26, 1998, to IRBs. In March 2001, the FDA sent a letter to associations involved in cloning research to remind them of FDA's jurisdiction and the need for submission of an IND to FDA's Center for Biologics Evaluation and Research. In that year, Dr Kathryn C. Zoon, Director, Center for Biologics Evaluation and Research, gave testimony before the Subcommittee on Oversight and Investigations Committee on Energy and Commerce, US House of Representatives, regarding FDA oversight of cloning technology to clone a human being and the consensus on scientific concerns in this area.

### 3.2.7 NIH and Uniform Biological Materials Transfer Agreements

The federal legislation that mandates and defines the government's technology transfer activities applies to stem cell research funded by NIH. The two primary pieces of legislation are the *Federal Technology Transfer Act of 1986* [32] and the *National Technology Transfer and Advancement Act of 1995* [33]. In 1999, the NIH issued a pertinent guidance: *Principals and Guidelines for Recipients of NIH Research Grants and Contracts on Obtaining and Disseminating Biomedical Research Resources* [34]. The purpose is to assure dissemination of resources developed using NIH funds and to minimize administrative impediments to academic research.

Although the stem cell lines listed in the NIH Stem Cell Registry remain the property of the individual stem cell providers, researchers can negotiate a material transfer agreement with the cell providers to specify rights and responsibilities concerning resulting data, publications, and potential patents.

### 3.2.8 US Patent and Licensing Laws

Embryonic stem cells, the process of their derivation and culture, and their uses are also subject to federal patent protection laws. Many patents have been filed relating to hESC research on technology developed both by private and federally funded research. The Bayh–Dole Act made it possible for academic research centers to own intellectual property and to grant exclusive rights to these patents to the private sector.

Maria Friere, former Director, Office of Technology Transfer, in a speech before the Senate Appropriations Committee regarding intellectual property considerations and stem cell research, used the University of Wisconsin as an example of how the Bayh–Dole Act is implemented:

> Early work by Dr Thomson on non-human primates, such as Rhesus monkeys, was federally funded and therefore, the patent obtained on stem cells arising from this work is governed by this Act. In accordance with the law, the invention was disclosed to the NIH, a patent application was filed by the University, through the Wisconsin Alumni Research Foundation (WARF), and WARF licensed the technology to a small company (Geron). Because federal funds were used for this non-human primate work, the government has a non-exclusive, royalty-free right to use the patented cells by or on behalf of the government. This would allow the government laboratories and contractors the right to use the patented cells for further research. In addition, in handling this invention the University must ensure that the goals of the Bayh–Dole Act—utilization, commercialization, and public availability—are implemented. [35]

There has been a long history of opposition to patenting human material [36, 37]. As stem cell technologies are coming closer to commercial application, it is important for institutions to be mindful of evolving patent laws in the United States and internationally. The European Union ban on patenting stem cells was challenged in 2013 and is currently in the court system [38]. The US Consumer Watchdog, a nonprofit advocacy group, has been waging a six-year battle to invalidate the Wisconsin Alumni Research Foundation patent. Interest has been renewed since the US Supreme Court ruled in June 2013 that certain human genetic material is not patentable [39].

### 3.2.9 Health Insurance Portability and Accountability Act Privacy Rule and Research Uses of Medical Record Information

Research organizations and researchers involved in hESC may or may not be covered by the Privacy Rule of The Health Insurance Portability and Accountability Act (HIPAA) [40]. If a research organization is a "covered entity," it may not use or disclose protected health information unless either a prior authorization by the research participant or a waiver of authorization from an IRB or Privacy Board is obtained.

Researchers in a HIPAA-covered entity who collect, store, and/or share identifiable information about gamete donors or somatic cell donors need to consider when this would trigger the need to comply with HIPAA regulations as well as the regulations associated with human subject protections previously described.

### 3.2.10  Recombinant DNA Research, Gene Therapy, and hESC

The NIH has defined recombinant DNA as molecules that are constructed outside living cells by joining natural or synthetic DNA segments to DNA molecules that can replicate in a living cell, or synthetic DNA molecules that result from the replication of these molecules. Because a great deal of the research being done on hESC lines will involve this kind of genetic manipulation, research institutions are responsible for ensuring compliance with the NIH Guidelines for Research Involving Recombinant DNA Molecules regardless of the source of funding. An article by King Lee, "Comparison of Additional Regulatory Requirements for Conducting Clinical Trials on Genetically-Modified Micro-Organisms and Recombinant DNA in Europe, the United States and Canada," provides an outline of these often "cumbersome requirements"[41]. Key requirements are:

* Review of the research by an IBC. IBCs, registered with the NIH, are mandated under the NIH Guidelines for Research Involving Recombinant DNA Molecules to provide local, institutional oversight of research involving recombinant DNA. IBC review focuses on safety only, not on compliance with other aspects of state and federal law regarding ethical conduct of scientific research.
* In 1978, the NIH established the Recombinant DNA Advisory Committee to review policies related to this research. An important role of this committee is to oversee all human gene transfer research that is NIH-funded. It has also evolved to oversee privately funded research under FDA jurisdiction, and FDA requires Recombinant DNA Advisory Committee review of any procedures submitted to it that involve recombinant DNA research.

### 3.2.11  Creation of Chimeras and Human Embryonic Stem Cell Research

hESC research involving the creation of transgenic or chimeric animals is subject to animal welfare protections including the US Department of Agriculture's Animal Welfare Act ensures humane treatment of animals used in research, and the NIH Public Health Service Policy on Human Care and Use of Laboratory Animals [42]. Institutions must have an IACUC the responsibilities of which are outlined in the Public Health Service Policy.

### 3.2.12  Importation of Cell Lines or Derived Tissues for Clinical Use

Researchers who plan to import hESC lines from outside of the United States for clinical use should follow FDA's new tissue regulations (CFR 21 Part 1271.420), which regulate this importation and require approval by the FDA [43]. The purpose of these FDA regulations is to prevent transmission of communicable diseases. Researchers should assure that imported cell lines are properly transported, under quarantine if necessary, and accompanied by the proper documentation to be reviewed by the FDA for suitability to enter the country. Also, it may be necessary to determine whether there are other tissue regulations in the country from which the lines are imported.

### 3.2.13  Clinical Research Involving Xenotransplantation

According to the FDA definition, any procedure that involves the transplantation of human body fluids, cells, tissues, or organs that have had ex vivo contact with live nonhuman animal cells, tissues, or organs is considered to be xenotransplantation and is subject to additional review because of the potential for cross-species infection by retroviruses. Both the DHHS and the FDA have committees to oversee this research and set policies with special attention to the issues raised by xenotransplantation. hESC researchers developing products for human transplantation should take this under consideration [44].

## 3.3 State Agencies, Regulation, and Guidance

As noted previously, states, through legislation and funding initiatives, sought to fill the existing federal level gaps in the oversight and support of stem cell research. State laws can generally be characterized as permissive, flexible, or restrictive [45]. Permissive states focused on rolling back laws that could be interpreted as posing barriers to such research, and/or establishing state policies specifically supporting stem cell research, through statute or state funding initiative. Restrictive states, on the other hand, sought to go beyond the federal funding restrictions to clearly prohibit the conduct of certain types of research ineligible for federal research funding or to strengthen or extend previous embryo research restrictions to specifically apply to hESC research.

Approaches to some specific areas of hESC research are similar across states broadly designated as permissive or restrictive. For example, as of March 2005, when the NAS issued its first set of hESC Guidelines, restrictive states including Arkansas, Iowa, Michigan, North Dakota, and South Dakota had laws that clearly prohibited nuclear transfer for research purposes. Similarly, under Maryland's permissive state funding initiative, research involving nuclear transfer is deemed to be ineligible for state funding. However, Maryland law does not otherwise prohibit nuclear transfer. Another example can be seen with restrictions on the procurement of research tissues, specifically the prohibition against compensating oocyte donors. Permissive states such as Massachusetts, California, and Connecticut all contain this restriction, which can have measurable impacts on research collaborations across states. This issue will be explored in more depth later in this chapter.

Beyond the permissive/restrictive distinction, states also chose different modes of regulating stem cell research. In some states, much like at the federal level, the funding of stem cell research drove the oversight, creating restrictions that were not strictly regulatory in nature. Other states established enabling statutes empowering a state agency to regulate the conduct of research. Generally, the former are based on economic development initiatives whereas the latter arise from the state's authority to regulate public health and safety. The regulatory authority accompanying funding statutes are narrowly circumscribed to state-funded research, whereas state public health and safety statutes have broader applicability.

California initiated the largest state stem cell funding initiative. In November 2004, California voters passed Prop 71, the California Stem Cell Research and Cures Initiative, which authorized $3 billion for stem cell research funding in California and established the California Institute for Regenerative Medicine (CIRM). CIRM has developed and adopted one of the most comprehensive sets of regulations in the United States including ethical standards, grants administration policy, and intellectual property management rules that apply to its grantees. Because CIRM is such a major funder of stem cell research, both within California and nationally, the CIRM regulations are rather influential in driving institutional research compliance and standards.

Other states that developed stem cell funding initiatives include New Jersey, Connecticut, Maryland, and New York. In Connecticut, An Act Permitting Stem Cell Research and Banning the Cloning of Human Beings was approved by the General Assembly and signed by Governor M. Jodi Rell on June 15, 2005. Passage of the legislation positioned Connecticut as the third state in the nation to provide public funding in support of human embryonic and adult stem cell research. Maryland's Stem Cell Act created the Maryland Stem Cell Research Commission as an independent body whose members include the Attorney General or designee, patient advocates, individuals with experience in biotechnology, scientists from the University System of Maryland and Johns Hopkins University, and bioethicists. The Commission adopts regulations that ensure that adult stem cell and stem cell research financed by the state fund complies with state law and develops criteria, standards, and requirements for the submission and review of grant applications.

In New York, both public and private funding initiatives have largely influenced stem cell policy and regulation. The New York Stem Cell Foundation, funded entirely by private philanthropy, was founded in 2005 and was deeply involved in establishing the state policies that emerged through the state funding program. State funding was ushered in with the Enactment of Public Health Law Title5-A in 2007, which established the NYSTEM stem cell research funding program and the Empire State Stem Cell Research Fund and Board. The Board consists of two committees, the funding committee and the ethics committee, which provide standards and guidelines for the conduct of research.

Another state particularly influential in the emergence of state policy, the Commonwealth of Massachusetts, represents the type of state with an enabling statute, Massachusetts General Laws, Chapter 111L. The frame of the statute is largely supportive of hESC research, but with certain restrictions on research. The opening salvo of Chapter 111L states that "it shall be the policy of the commonwealth to actively foster research and therapies... by permitting research and clinical applications involving SCNT, placental and umbilical cord cells and human adult stem cells and other methods to create embryonic stem cells" [46]. On the other hand, the statute includes a number of restrictions such as the prohibition against compensating research donors cited earlier in this chapter, violations of which subject regulated parties to criminal penalties. Massachusetts also promulgated a $1.25 billion life sciences initiative in 2007. Although not directed solely at stem cell research, but at the broader category of life sciences, this initiative sought to establish a stem cell bank in Massachusetts and was seen as a move to expand opportunities for the funding of such research.

Much like at the federal level, changes in state stem cell policy often reflect changes in the State Administration. For example, Massachusetts Chapter 111L was passed by a largely democratic state Congress, through the override of then-Governor Mitt Romney's veto. Massachusetts Department of Public Health regulations promulgated by the Romney Administration contained an interpretation of Chapter 111L that further restricted the use of hESCs. In 2007, The Massachusetts Department of Public Health rescinded this Romney-era restriction pursuant to one of the first official acts of the Governor Deval Patrick Administration [47].

## 4. KEY REGULATORY MANDATES

### 4.1 Federal

There is no federal mandate to establish an ESCRO committee or any other ancillary institutional committee to oversee human stem cell research. Such committees are purely voluntary except where mandated by state law.

The current federal mandates specific to hESC research reflect *Obama's executive order and the 2009 NIH Guidelines*. They include:

1. Federal funding grantees may use any hESC lines listed on the NIH Registry and must name the lines used in the grant. If the NIH Registry lists any limitations for use in the Details section for a cell line, federal funding will only be provided within the limitations. For example, the early HUES stem cell lines derived at Harvard University have such limitations based on language in the IRB-approved consent forms signed by the gamete donors.

2. To submit an application for hESCs to be listed on the NIH Registry, institutions must include documentation that hESCs were derived from IVF embryos created for reproductive purposes and in excess of clinical need. In addition, specific criteria for the ethical procurement of the embryos must be met including written informed consent from the embryo donor(s) and confirmation that no payments were offered to the embryo donor/s.

3. Federal funds may *not* be used for (1) derivation of new hESC lines by any means, (2) research using hESCs that are not listed on the NIH Stem Cell Registry, (3) research involving the breeding of animals where the introduction of hESCs (even if the hESCs are NIH-registered) or other human pluripotent stem cells may contribute to the germ line, and (4) research in which hESCs (even if from the hESCs are NIH-registered) or other human pluripotent stem cells are introduced into nonhuman primate blastocysts.

Other federal regulatory mandates are not specific to hESC research, but relate to human tissue research in general.

### 4.2 State

As described previously, several states entered into the stem cell regulatory space with their own legislation and funding-based restrictions. Although not ideal from the perspective of ensuring consistency nationally in the oversight of such research, state legislation did provide a vehicle for formalizing voluntary guidelines in this area. As referenced earlier in this chapter, many states incorporated by reference, either explicitly or implicitly, the NAS hESC Guidelines. The Connecticut stem cell law specifically references the NAS hESC Guidelines at a number of points; importing the concept of "acceptably derived" from the NAS hESC Guidelines; requiring ESCRO committees, as defined by the guidelines; and requiring informed consent in conformance with the NAS hESC Guidelines. New York also specifically references the NAS hESC Guidelines in its contracts for state funding requiring ESCRO committee review and thus imbuing such requirement with the weight of law [48]. Other states, such as California, incorporated many of the concepts and language of the NAS hESC Guidelines without specifically referencing the guidelines themselves. For example, the CIRM Guidelines incorporate the concept established by the NAS hESC Guidelines that stem cell research be subject to review by an ESCRO or, as the CIRM guidelines term it, an "SCRO" (Stem Cell Research Oversight).

# 5. KEY PERSONNEL AND UNIVERSITY COMMITTEES DESIGNATED TO IMPLEMENT REGULATORY MANDATES

Accountable conduct of hESC research includes a number of tasks and responsibilities. Each institution must clearly delegate roles and not simply assume that the ESCRO committee will meet them. The following describes the components that should be considered and how this might be structured.

## 5.1 Institutional Official

An institutional official designated to oversee research programs is key to establishing and implementing policies. Within a University system, or an academic medical center, this may be the Vice Provost for Research, the Chief Compliance Officer, or a Research Dean.

## 5.2 ESCRO Committee/SCRO Committee

ESCRO committees have been widely, if not consistently, implemented in academic institutions. However, some institutions choose not to create ESCROs. Institutions that conduct a small amount of fairly straightforward in vitro hESC research may decide that no additional oversight is needed as long as their state laws do not mandate more. The use of a reliance agreement with an established ESCRO or SCRO is an alternative, but requires due diligence to ascertain that the relying institutions research policies and standards are met.

For institutions that do establish their own ESCRO committee, there are a number of logistics to consider. The ESCRO committee must have a clear charge in terms of its authority and clear identification regarding to whom it reports. Who will select members? Who will have the authority to develop and/or approve policy? How will the Committee be structured? How will it operate? The scope of review may vary from institution to institution because the scope of such committees is not clearly defined, even within states where law mandates the creation of such a committee. An informal 2011 survey of 30 Committees posted on the website of the Interstate Alliance for Stem Cell Research (IASCR) demonstrates this diversity. It is unclear from the survey whether this diversity stems from State requirements.

The ESCRO Chair and/or ESCRO Administrator should be responsible for keeping abreast of advances in this research, changing attitudes and the evolving political framework that may impact the scope of local oversight.

## 5.3 Ancillary Committees

As previously described, the IRB, the IACUC, and the IBC each have a role in reviewing human stem cell research. Although focused review of protocols involving the derivation and use of hESCs is the role of the ESCRO committee itself, reviews by other relevant committees must be coordinated and care must be taken not to overburden investigators with unnecessary duplicative reviews. With all these distinct committees, how does an institution ensure that information is shared across committees to ensure compliance and the ethical conduct of research? Institutions have begun to struggle with these issues, sometimes collapsing the ESCRO committee into the IRB, or otherwise ensuring coordination through overlapping membership on both committees, and/or designing formal reporting mechanisms across oversight committees. There are a number of benefits to the combined IRB/ESCRO approach. Benefits include: (1) experienced staff with expertise in regulatory issues and day-to-day operations of institutional research oversight; (2) ready communication regarding the many intertwined issues affecting IRB and ESCRO Committee oversight; (3) ease of scheduling parallel or concurrent protocol review; and (4) and easy access to IRB resources such as information technology tools and staff, investigator education programs, and compliance mechanisms.

## 5.4 Compliance Office

This office may be involved in oversight of conflicts of interest, research integrity, and audits.

## 5.5 Grants and Contracts Department

Myriad conditions of grants awards from various funding entities must be carefully reviewed. Investigators must be kept informed of notices issued regarding grant requirements.

## 5.6 Office of Technology Transfer

This office will consider intellectual property issues such as licenses and material transfer agreements.

## 5.7 Office of General Counsel

The patchwork of international as well as state law requires ongoing and informed legal expertise.

## 5.8 Public Relations Office

Because hESC research is a topic of great public interest, institutions should anticipate and be prepared to involve their public relations office to address queries from the press as well as the public.

## 6. COMMON COMPLIANCE CHALLENGES

### 6.1 Uneven Regulatory Landscape

As highlighted in previous sections, the stem cell research regulatory landscape has been uneven at best, marked by nonregulatory measures at the federal level, a lack of central oversight authority, a lack of uniformity or coordination among state policies, political reversals, and legal challenge. That there is no federal policy specifically addressing the unique issues associated with stem cell research activities in this area lends an air of uncertainty for research institutions seeking to develop and maintain robust compliance programs. The NIH issued national guidelines for stem cell research in 2009, but these guidelines only apply to determine which hESC lines are eligible for federal funding. The NAS Human Embryonic Stem Cell Research Advisory Committee convened experts from across the country to develop guidelines for the ethical conduct of stem cell research, but the committee was disbanded in 2010 and no longer issues interpretative guidance for the field. After the dismantling of the NAS Advisory Committee, there has been no national body to provide guidance and encourage uniformity across state policies. State law mandates exist, but the lack of uniformity across states in their approach to regulation of stem cell research only compounds the compliance challenges. Thus, little guidance is provided for establishing institutional policy for the oversight of stem cell research. This is particularly challenging for institutions seeking to develop guidance with respect to collaborations across institutions, particularly when the institutions are subject to different state or international laws.

## 6.2 Divergent State Laws Present Unique Compliance Challenges

The development of state laws and funding programs served to fill in the gaps left by the absence of federal regulation but created a complex patchwork of oversight for the conduct of stem cell research. Scientific research and discovery is often conducted through collaboration, among researchers, laboratories, and institutions, across states and countries. The piecemeal approach to stem cell regulation in the United States, based largely in the uncertainty bred by federal policy, posed and continues to pose unique challenges for research collaboration. The Interstate Alliance for Stem Cell Research (IASCR), a voluntary body of state policymakers, was formed in 2007 by organizers of Connecticut's Stem Cell Research International Symposium [49]. The IASCR was initially convened to advance stem cell research by fostering effective interstate collaboration, assisting states in developing research programs, and by promoting efficient and responsible use of public funds for stem cell research. The IASCR brought together regulatory and policy people from states seeking to advance stem cell research, such as California, Massachusetts, New York, Connecticut, Rhode Island, Maryland, and Wisconsin. Representatives from Canada, the United Kingdom, NAS, and ISSCR also participated in the convened discussions of the IASCR. The convening of such meetings of various state and international representatives working in the area of stem cell research policy and ethics provided a valuable forum for the sharing of state experiences and expertise in the development of stem cell policy and regulation. Although the group still has a Website and provides resources to stakeholders, it has not convened regular meetings of the state representatives since its funding ran out in early 2010.

One of the issues discussed in-depth by members of the IASCR was the issue of compensation of human gamete, and specifically egg, donors. The first successful derivation of lines from human embryos created through SCNT in May of 2013, an advancement hailed as a contender for Breakthrough of the Year in the December 2013 issue of *Science* [50], brought this issue to the fore once again.

The SCNT lines described previously were derived in Oregon pursuant to a state law allowing for the compensation of egg donors to research. Questions were raised as to whether the resultant lines could be used by researchers in Massachusetts or California, both of which prohibit compensation of egg donors beyond reimbursement of out-of-pocket costs. Such questions are emblematic of questions facing institutions conducting interstate and collaborative stem cell research. Where the state law is unclear, this may require requesting an advisory ruling from the state regulatory agency or proceeding based on a legal opinion and defending the decision in court if the action is later challenged.

Compensation of Egg Donors by State/Voluntary Guidance

| State/guideline | No prohibition | Prohibits compensation | Allows reimbursement of out-of-pocket costs only |
|---|---|---|---|
| California | | √[a] | √ |
| Connecticut | | √ | √ |
| Massachusetts | | √ | √ |
| Maryland | √ | | |
| New York | √ | | |
| New Jersey | √ | | |
| Oregon | √ | | |
| NAS | | | √ |
| ISSCR | √[b] | | |

[a]California considered a bill to allow for compensation of egg donors in June of 2013. See http://www.nature.com/news/california-bill-poised-to-lift-restrictions-on-egg-donation-1.13218.
[b]The ISSCR guidelines do however counsel against the offering of financial compensation based on the number or quality of the oocytes provided for research.
Lomax G, Stayn S. Similarities and differences among stem cell research policies: opportunities for policymakers, patients and researchers. BNA Medical Research Law & Policy Report, Vol 7, No. 21 (May 11, 2008), Table 3, p. 698; New York Allows Payment for Egg Donors, http://www.nytimes.com/2009/06/26/nyregion/26stemcell.html?_r=0, National Academy of Sciences (NAS) Committee on Guidelines for Human Embryonic Stem Cell Research 2005). "Guidelines for Human Embryonic Stem Cell Research", National Academies Press, Washington, D.C. Available at: http://www.nap.edu/ books/0309096537/html/ [accessed 02.10.14], ISSCR hESC Guidelines, http://www.isscr.org/docs/default-source/hesc-guidelines/isscrhescguidelines2006.pdf [accessed 02.10.14].

# 7. ADDRESSING NONCOMPLIANCE AND ANTICIPATING EMERGING COMPLIANCE ISSUES

Institutions conducting stem cell research must thoughtfully construct compliance programs largely in the absence of clear federal or state guidance. Such compliance programs need to consider not only policies, procedures, and oversight mechanisms, but also enforcement of noncompliance and regular review of the adequacy of oversight mechanisms. There should be procedures for suspending research approvals in cases of noncompliance and audits of the review process to ensure compliance with institutional policies and conditions of approval. Without effective enforcement and audit mechanisms, an institution's capacity to address noncompliance is severely limited.

Beyond enforcement and audit capabilities, a robust compliance program must also anticipate and address emerging regulatory frameworks and emerging ethical issues as the research progresses. It is difficult to predict what regulatory frameworks may be constructed or deconstructed in the future. For instance, a question arises as to what may happen to the regulatory oversight borne of state funding initiatives when the state funding runs out. Will the conditions of state funding be otherwise converted into state law/regulation? And, if so, will opening these oversight mechanisms to the political process result in far more stringent regulation of the research? A 2010 study found that states, not the federal government, funded the majority of hESC research [51]. This trend may have slowed significantly in recent years, as states struggle with budget shortfalls. New Jersey, one of the first states to appropriate funds for stem cell research, cut funding by 75% to close a budget shortfall in 2009 [52]. State funding of a stem cell bank in Massachusetts came to an abrupt end in 2012 in response to state budget constraints. Institutional compliance programs must be nimble enough to ensure compliance with potentially shifting legislative and regulatory mandates.

Institutional compliance programs must also be aware of ancillary laws that may affect the conduct of this research. At times, state legislation directed at broader issues may impose additional regulatory restrictions on stem cell research. Measures directed at regulating reproductive health or outlawing abortion, such as the so-called "Personhood Amendments", are particularly likely to directly or indirectly impact the research. These ballot initiatives, Acts, or proposed amendments to state constitutions, have proliferated in recent years and seek to grant fertilized eggs the same rights as adult humans. Aimed primarily at outlawing abortions, these measures also have regulatory implications for IVF, stem cell research, and birth control. In recent years, personhood amendments have been considered in 10 states, but only one, North Dakota, has adopted the same. Colorado considered passage of a Personhood Amendment for the third time in 2014 [53]. The implications of these emerging measures must be also be examined and understood.

The field of stem cell research is not static and any institutional compliance program must regularly and critically reevaluate the oversight mechanisms implemented. As described earlier in this chapter, ESCROs developed as voluntary oversight bodies pursuant to equally voluntary national guidelines. Although some states have converted the voluntary requirement of ESCRO committee review to a mandatory one with the force of state law, the 2009 NIH Stem Cell Guidelines do not require ESCRO review as a condition of federal funding. As new ethical issues emerge for both federally funded and nonfederally funded research, the question has arisen as to the future role and authority of ESCRO committees [54].

Several leaders in the field focused on precisely this question in the January 2013 issue of the *American Journal of Bioethics*. Hank Greely, in his "Assessing ESCROs: Yesterday and Tomorrow" [55], both recognizes the unique and important role played by ESCRO committees in the early developments of the science and posits whether the time has come to sunset such special review committees. It is a question institutions must face: is there a continuing need for such committees? Although some of the early thorny ethical and compliance issues have been addressed and perhaps the work of such committees has become rote in some ways as intimated by Greely, the science is still evolving, bringing with it new ethical issues. In the main, stem cell research has historically been self-regulated. The voluntary guidelines developed by NAS predated many state regulations. Voluntary self-regulation pursuant to the NAS Guidelines has opened the door to expanded funding opportunities and has influenced formal state regulation.

Some institutions may choose to maintain the expertise of such committees as developed over time to inform oversight of new ethical issues brought on by future developments in the science. Reviews of ethical issues and the sharing of experiences across ESCROs may develop a voluntary case law of how to handle potential compliance issues. It is not easy to predict the next big discovery, or where and how the political process may again step in to regulate such research—but informed and experienced internal mechanisms for oversight and review might help to inform any regulatory process. The successful derivation of lines using SCNT may reinvigorate the debate regarding payment of donors. There is evidence it already has: in July of 2013, CIRM requested a reevaluation of its prohibition against compensation of donors in light of this development [56]. Additionally, the potential to derive human gametes from iPSC and the ongoing issues of moral status raised by the implantation of neural iPS cells into animals suggest that oversight and guidance to ensure, and reassure, that the science is proceeding ethically, is needed.

# References

[1] Code of Federal Regulations (45 CFR 46). http://www.hhs.gov/ohrp/humansubjects/guidance/45cfr46.html [accessed 22.02.14].

[2] Code of Federal Regulations, Title 21. http://www.accessdata.fda.gov/scripts/cdrh/cfdocs/cfcfr/cfrsearch.cfm [accessed 03.03.14].

[3] Balanced Budget Downpayment Act, I, Public Law No. 104-99, §128, 110 Stat. 26, 34. http://www.gpo.gov/fdsys/pkg/PLAW-104publ99/pdf/PLAW-104publ99.pdf [accessed 12.02.14].

[4] National Academy of Sciences (NAS) Committee on Guidelines for Human Embryonic Stem Cell Research. Guidelines for human embryonic stem cell research. Washington, DC: National Academies Press; 2005. Available at: http://www.nap.edu/books/0309096537/html/. [accessed 10.02.14].

[5] Takahashi K, Tanabe K, Ohnuki M, et al. Induction of pluripotent stem cells from adult human fibroblasts by defined factor. Cell 2007;131:861–72.

[6] Office for Human Research Protections (OHRP), Department of Health and Human Services (DHHS). Guidance for investigators and institutional review boards regarding research involving human embryonic stem cells, germ cells and stem cell-derived test articles. March 19, 2002. http://www.hhs.gov/ohrp/policy/stemcell.pdf. [accessed 12.02.14].

[7] Abelman M, O'Rourke P, Sonntag K. Part-human animal research: the imperative to move beyond a philosophical debate. Am J Bioethics 2012;12:26–8.

[8] Wilmut I, Schnicke AE, McWhir J, Kind AJ, Campbell RH. Viable offspring derived from fetal and adult mammalian cells. Nature 1997;385:810–3.

[9] Wadman M. Dolly: a decade on. Nature 2007;445:800–1.

[10] The White House. Memorandum for the Heads of executive Departments and Agencies: Prohibition on federal funding for cloning of human beings. http://grants.nih.gov/grants/policy/cloning_directive.htm [accessed 12.02.14].

[11] Thomson J, Itskovitz-Eldor J, Shapiro SS, et al. Embryonic stem cell lines derived from human blastocysts. Science 1998;282:1145–7.

[12] NIH Director's statement on research using stem Cells—12/02/98. http://stemcells.nih.gov/policy/statements/pages/120298.aspx [accessed 09.03.14].

[13] Letter from Rabb HS. General counsel, department of health and human services to Harold varmus, MD, director, NIH titled federal funding for research involving human pluripotent stem cells. dated January 15, 1999 https://m.repository.library.georgetown.edu/bitstream/handle/10822/534826/rabbmemo.pdf?sequence=1 [accessed 12.02.14].

[14] Federal Register. 65 FR 51976. National Institutes of Health. Guidelines for research using human pluripotent stem cells. August 2000. http://stemcells.nih.gov/news/newsarchives/pages/stemcellguidelines.aspx. [accessed 12.02.14].

[15] National Institute of Health (NIH). Stem cell information. http://stemcells.nih.gov/policy/pages/2001policy.aspx [accessed 12.02.14].

[16] President's Council on Bioethics (PCBE). https://bioethicsarchive.georgetown.edu/pcbe/reports/past_commissions/ [accessed 12.02.14].

[17] Religion and Politics. The candidates on the issues. 2008. http://www.pewforum.org/2008/11/04/religion-and-politics-08-the-candidates-on-the-issues/. [accessed 27.02.14].

[18] Executive Order 13505: removing barriers to responsible scientific research involving human stem cells. http://www.whitehouse.gov/the_press_office/Removing-Barriers-to-Responsible-Scientific-Research-Involving-Human-Stem-Cell [accessed 01.03.14].

[19] National Institutes of Health Guidelines on Human Stem Cell Research at http://stemcells.nih.gov/policy/pages/2009guidelines.aspx [accessed 27.02.14].

[20] Sebelius Sherley v. U.S. Court of Appeals for the District of Columbia Circuit. August 24, 2012.

[21] Concurrent House and Senate reports in 2001 contained language explicitly stating that the Dickey–Wicker amendment "should not be construed to limit federal support for research involving hESCs listed on an NIH Registry and carried out in accordance with the policy outlined by the President." See H.R. Rep. No. 107-229 @ 180 (October 9, 2001). Under the Bush Administration, the Stem Cell Research Acts of 2005 and 2007, which explicitly provided for the federal funding of hESC research, passed both houses of Congress, but neither had enough votes to override President Bush's veto. See Stem Cell Research Act of 2005, H.R. 810, 109th Congress (2005–2006).

[22] NIH Notice NOT-OD-10-126 issued August 30, 2001. http://grants.nih.gov/grants/guide/notice-files/NOT-OD-10-126.html [accessed 09.03.14].

[23] Hinxton Group. http://www.hinxtongroup.org/wp_am_map.html [accessed 21.12.12].

[24] International Society for Stem Cell Research (ISSCR). http://www.isscr.org/home/publications/guide-clintrans [accessed 27.02.14].

[25] International Stem Cell Initiative. http://www.stem-cell-forum.net/initiatives/ [accessed 09.03.14].

[26] The Hinxton Group. http://www.hinxtongroup.org/au.html [accessed 09.03.14].

[27] NIH Human Embryonic Stem Cell Registry. http://grants.nih.gov/stem_cells/registry/current.htm [accessed 02.03.14].

[28] National Research Council. Final report of the national academies' human embryonic stem cell research advisory committee and 2010 amendments to the national academies' guidelines for human embryonic stem cell research. Washington, DC: The National Academies Press; 2010.

[29] See also, the Joint Commission for the Accreditation of Health Care Organizations—failure to meet its standards can result in the loss of Medicare reimbursement; and in the field of assisted reproduction, the lack of government funding has resulted in professional efforts to generate standards, such as those promulgated by the American Society for Reproductive Medicine (ASRM) and the Society for Assisted Reproductive Technologies.

[30] OHRP Guidance. http://www.hhs.gov/ohrp/policy/biodata/index.html [accessed 09.03.14].

[31] Title 42 Chapter 6a - Subchapter II Part F—Licensing of Biological Products and Clinical Laboratories; Sec. 262. Regulation of biological products. http://www.fda.gov/RegulatoryInformation/Legislation/ucm149278.htm [accessed 09.03.14].

[32] PHS Federal Technology Transfer Act of 1986. http://history.nih.gov/research/downloads/PL99-502.pdf [accessed 09.03.14].

[33] National Technology Transfer and Advancement Act of 1995. http://www.gpo.gov/fdsys/pkg/PLAW-104publ113/pdf/PLAW-104publ113.pdf [accessed 09.03.2014].

[34] Recipients of NIH Research Grants and Contracts on Obtaining and Disseminating Biomedical Research Resources. http://grants.nih.gov/grants/intell-property_64FR72090.pdf [accessed 09.03.14].

[35] Stem Cell Research: Patenting and health implications: testimony of Maria C. Freire, Ph.D., Director, national institutes of health office of technology Transfer [Hearing of the subcommittee on Labor, health and human service, and education, committee on appropriations, U.S. Senate. January 26, 1999]. https://repository.library.georgetown.edu/handle/10822/534912 [accessed 06.03.14].

[36] Loring JF, Campbell C. Intellectual property and human embryonic stem cell research. Science 2006;311:1716–7.

[37] Bahadur G, Morrison M. Patenting human pluripotent cells: balancing commercial, academic and ethical interests. Hum Reprod 2010;25:14–21.

[38] Stem cell patents and the European Court of Justice. http://www.eurostemcell.org/stem-cell-patents [accessed 12.02.14].

[39] Gene Patent Case Fuels U.S. Court Test of Stem Cell Right. http://www.bloomberg.com/news/2014-01-06/gene-patent-case-fuels-u-s-court-test-of-stem-cell-right.html [accessed 06.03.14].

[40] U.S. Department of Health and Human Services. The privacy rule. http://www.hhs.gov/ocr/privacy/hipaa/administrative/privacyrule/ [accessed 02.03.14].

[41] Lee KC. Comparison of additional regulatory requirements for conducting clinical trials on genetically-modified microorganisms and recombinant DNA in Europe, the United States, and Canada. Drug Information J 2002;36:379–86.

[42] http://www.neavs.org/research/laws [accessed 06.03.14].

[43] CFR 21 Part 1271.420. http://www.accessdata.fda.gov/scripts/cdrh/cfdocs/cfcfr/CFRSearch.cfm?fr=1271.420 [accessed 06.03.14].

[44] FDA Xenotransplantation Guidance. http://www.fda.gov/BiologicsBloodVaccines/GuidanceComplianceRegulatoryInformation/Guidances/Xenotransplantation/default.htm [accessed 06.03.14].

[45] See Minnesota Biomedical and Bioscience Network Map on Human Embryonic Stem Cell Research at: http://www.mbbnet.umn.edu/scmap.html [accessed 09.03.14].

[46] Massachusetts Biotechnology statute, Mass. Gen. Laws. Ann. Ch. 111L, §1(c) at https://malegislature.gov/Laws/GeneralLaws/PartI/TitleXVI/Chapter111l [accessed 27.02.14].

[47] Massachusetts Biotechnology regulations, 105 CMR 960.00. 2007. Available at. http://www.lawlib.state.ma.us/source/mass/cmr/cmrtext/105CMR960.pdf. [accessed 27.02.14].

[48] In the NY Stem Cell Board's Comment Letter to NIH, it specifically endorsed the NAS Guidelines and in particular, the establishment and use of ESCRO committees. See http://stemcell.ny.gov/sites/default/files/documents/files/ESSCB_letter_may-26-2009.pdf [accessed 10.06.14].

[49] See Policy Harmonization through Collaboration: the Interstate Alliance for Stem Cell Research, World Stem Cell Report. 2010. http://nas-sites.org/iascr/files/2013/01/Lomax_IASCR_2010_publication.pdf. [accessed 27.02.14].

[50] See Breakthrough of the Year 2013. Science December 20, 2013;342(6165):1436–7.

[51] Levine, A. States now fund the majority of human embryonic stem cell research at http://www.news.gatech.edu/2010/12/09/states-now-fund-majority-human-embryonic-stem-cell-research [accessed 27.02.14].

[52] Wagner J, Helderman R. Renewed federal funding for stem cell studies could make cash-strapped states think twice about spending their own money. March 10, 2009. The Washington Post http://www.washingtonpost.com/wp-dyn/content/article/2009/03/09/AR2009030902616.html. [accessed 27.02.14].

[53] Wilson R. Colorado will vote on a personhood amendment. October 15, 2014. The Washington Post http://www.washingtonpost.com/blogs/govbeat/wp/2013/10/15/colorado-will-vote-on-personhood-amendment/. [accessed 27.02.14].

[54] The January 2013 edition of The American Journal of Bioethics contained a series of articles focusing on the future of ESCRO committees:
[a] Master Z, Resnik DB. Promoting public trust: ESCROs won't fix the problem of stem cell tourism.
[b] Lomax G. The great ESCRO experiment: there is still value to be gained.
[c] Chapman AR. Evaluating ESCROs: Perspectives from the university of Connecticut.
[d] Devereaux M, Kalichman M. ESCRO committees—not dead yet.
[e] Aultman J. Dissolution of ESCROs and evolution of a national ethics committee for scientific advancement.
[f] Ellison B. Making ESCRO committees work in New York.
[g] Brewer CD, DeGrote H. Justifying tomorrow's ESCROs.
[h] Robert JS. Stem cell research oversight: personal reflections and public reasoning.

[55] Greely HT. Assessing ESCROs: yesterday and tomorrow. Am J Bioethics 2013;13:44–52.

[56] Memo to the CIRM Medical Ethics and Standards Working Group entitled Consideration of Exception for Covered Stem Cell Lines. July 1, 2013. Available at. http://www.cirm.ca.gov/sites/default/files/files/agenda/130701_SWG%20Briefing%20Memo%20%2800200980-2%29.pdf. [accessed 27.02.14].

# Index

*Note:* Page numbers followed by "f" and "t" indicate figures and tables respectively.

## A

AAALAC. *See* Association for Assessment and Accreditation of Laboratory Animal Care International

AAHRPP. *See* Association for Accreditation of Human Research Protection Programs

AAMC. *See* Association of American Medical Colleges

AAU. *See* Association of American Universities

Abbreviated new drug application (ANDA), 28–29

Absorbed dose (AD), 115, 151

AD. *See* Absorbed dose

Advance notice of proposed rulemaking (ANPRM), 17–18

AEA. *See* Atomic Energy Act

AEC. *See* Atomic Energy Commission

AECA. *See* Arms Export Control Act

ALARA principle. *See* As low as reasonably achievable principle

Alfred P. Sloan Foundation, 219–220

Alternate responsible officials (AROs), 102

American Schools and Hospitals Abroad, 217

American Veterinary Medical Association (AVMA), 47–48

Ancillary Committees, 313–314

ANDA. *See* Abbreviated new drug application

Animal and Plant Health Inspection Service (APHIS), 80

Animal and Plant Health Inspection Service/Animal Care Policies (APHIS/AC), 45

Animal welfare, 287
  assurance, 47

Animal Welfare Act (AWA), 43–45

ANPRM. *See* Advance notice of proposed rulemaking

Antiboycott Regimes, 199

APHIS. *See* Animal and Plant Health Inspection Service

APHIS/AC. *See* Animal and Plant Health Inspection Service/Animal Care Policies

Approval period, 18

Arms Export Control Act (AECA), 188

AROs. *See* Alternate responsible officials

As low as reasonably achievable principle (ALARA principle), 118

Association for Assessment and Accreditation of Laboratory Animal Care International (AAALAC), 59, 159–160

Association for Accreditation of Human Research Protection Programs (AAHRPP), 2

Association of American Medical Colleges (AAMC), 258

Association of American Universities (AAU), 258

Association of Research Integrity Officers, 236

Atomic Energy Act (AEA), 121–122

Atomic Energy Commission (AEC), 121–122

Attending veterinarian (AV), 45, 62

Authorized user (AU), 134–136, 141–142

AV. *See* Attending veterinarian

AVMA. *See* American Veterinary Medical Association

AWA. *See* Animal Welfare Act

## B

Bayh-Dole Act, 255

BBP. *See* Bloodborne pathogen standard

BEAR. *See* Biological Effects of Atomic Radiation

BEIR committee. *See* Biological Effects of Ionizing Radiation committee

Belmont Report, 2–3

Beneficence, 4

Biennial inventory, 172

BIO. *See* Biological Sciences Directorate

Biologic licensing application (BLA), 28–29

Biological Effects of Atomic Radiation (BEAR), 122

Biological Effects of Ionizing Radiation committee (BEIR committee), 122

Biological hazards, 79. *See also* Radiological hazards
  addressing noncompliance, 108
  compliance challenges
    CDC and USDA APHIS IPPs, 105–106
    dangerous goods shipping, 106
    Federal Select Agent Program, 103–105
    NIH Guidelines, 103
    Occupational Safety and Health Administration Bloodborne Pathogen Standard, 106–108
  department of health and human services, 85–89
  historical perspectives, 79–84

Biological hazards (*Continued*)
  personnel and university committees
    BSO, 101
    IBC, 100–101
  regulatory mandates
    CDC IPP, 95–96
    dangerous goods shipping regulations, 96–99
    federal select agent and toxin program, 93–95
    NIH guidelines, 89–92
    OSHA BBP, 99–100
    OSHA PPE standard, 100
    USDA APHIS, 96
  select agents and toxins list, 82t–84t
Biological safety, 79–80
Biological safety officer (BSO), 92, 101
Biological Sciences Directorate (BIO), 213
Biosafety in Microbiological and Biomedical
  Laboratories (BMBL), 80
BIS Lists, 198
BLA. *See* Biologic licensing application
Bloodborne pathogen standard (BBP), 81
Bloodborne pathogens, 87–88
BMBL. *See* Biosafety in Microbiological and Biomedical
  Laboratories
BMD. *See* Bureau of Medical Devices
BRH. *See* Bureau of Radiological Health
BSO. *See* Biological safety officer
Bureau of Export Administration (BXA), 193
Bureau of Medical Devices (BMD), 123
Bureau of Radiological Health (BRH), 123
Bush lines, 303

**C**

California Institute for Regenerative Medicine (CIRM),
  310–311
CBER. *See* Center for Biologics Evaluation and
  Research
CBP. *See* Customs and Border Protection
CCL. *See* Commerce Control List
CDC. *See* Centers for Disease Control and Prevention
CDER. *See* Center for Drug Evaluation and Research
CDRH. *See* Center for Devices and Radiological Health
Cell-lines importation, 309
Center for Biologics Evaluation and Research (CBER), 23
Center for Devices and Radiological Health (CDRH),
  29–30, 123
Center for Drug Evaluation and Research (CDER), 23
Conference of Radiation Control Program Directors
  (CRCPD), 123–124
Centers for Disease Control and Prevention (CDC),
  80–81, 220
  IPP, 95–96
Centers for Medicare and Medicaid Services (CMS),
  260–261
Central Intelligence Agency (CIA), 189

CFR. *See* Code of Federal Regulations
cGMP. *See* current good manufacturing practice
Chief Information Officer, 215
Chimeras, 305–306, 309
CIA. *See* Central Intelligence Agency
CIRM. *See* California Institute for Regenerative Medicine
CISE Directorate. *See* Computer and Information
  Sciences and Engineering Directorate
Climate and Environmental Sciences Division, 216
Clinical trials, 22
  networks, 274
CMS. *See* Centers for Medicare and Medicaid Services
Code of Federal Regulations (CFR), 159–160, 277
Code of Federal Regulations and Subparts (Title 21), 282
Code of Federal Regulations 45 Part 46 (45 CFR 46), 7
COI. *See* Conflict of interest
Collaborative IRB review, 19–20
Commerce Control List (CCL), 188
Committee on Science, Engineering, and Public Policy
  (COSEPUP), 191
Common rule, 7–12, 298
  examples, 10–11
  guidelines for informed consent, 12
  IRB, 10
  minimal risk, 10
  OHRP, 8
  research, 8–9
Comprehensive Methamphetamine Control Act (1996),
  165
Computer and Information Sciences and Engineering
  Directorate (CISE Directorate), 214
Conference of Radiation Control Program Directors
  (CRCPD), 127
Confidentiality, 229, 232
Conflict of interest (COI), 249–250, 254
  academic–industry relationships growth, 254–256
  addressing noncompliance, 274–275
  committee, 270
  compliance challenges, 272–274
  emergence of regulation and guidance, 256–257
  guidance documents, 261–263
  in human subject research, 257
  institutional, 261
  key personnel, 269–270
  PHS regulation (2011), 263–269
  Physician Payments Sunshine Act, 260–261
  related committees and offices, 270–272
  relevant regulatory/oversight agencies, regulations,
    261–263, 262t–263t
  responsibilities, 257–259
  scandals of 2000s, 259–260
  stringent federal regulations, 260
  power of attorney, 174–175
Contract Research Organizations (CROs), 288
Controlled substances, 159–160

addressing noncompliance, 184
compliance program development, 181
  institutional compliance policies alignment, 183
  institutional controlled substance policy
    development, 181–182
  licensing and registration compliance, 182
  security practices establishment, 183–184
DEA, 171–175
disposal, 176
federal controlled substance regulations, 166–167
  DEA organization, 167
  FDA, 167–168
  Schedule I Controlled Substances, 168
historical perspectives
  Combat Methamphetamine Act of 2005, 165
  Comprehensive Methamphetamine Control Act
    (1996), 165
  Controlled Substances Act of 1970, 163–164
  Drug Abuse Control Amendments of 1965, 163
  Food and Drug Act (1906), 160–161
  Food, Drug, and Cosmetic Act (1938), 161–162
  Harrison Tax Act of 1914, 161
  International treaties, 164
  Kefauver–Harris Amendments of 1962, 162–163
  list chemicals, 165–166
  Omnibus Drug Act (1988), 165
personnel and university committees
  department chairs and unit directors, 180
  department of public safety or local law
    enforcement, 180–181
  IACUC, 178
  institutional health care center or hospital
    pharmacy, 180
  laboratory animal care veterinarians, 178–179
  office of clinical regulatory affairs and general
    counsel, 179–180
  office of research compliance, 177–178
  OSEH, 178
  state and federal regulating agencies, 181
security, 175
  controls, 175
  theft and loss, 176
state controlled substance licensing, 171
state controlled substance regulations, 166
Title 21 CFR, Chapter II—DEA, Department of
  Justice, 168–169
  drug enforcement administaration registration, 169
  drug enforcement administration registration
    exemptions, 171
  registration for independent and coincident
    activities, 170
  schedule I controlled substance registration, 170–171
  separate registrations for separate locations, 169–170
Controlled Substances Ordering System (CSOS), 174
Convention on Psychotropic Substances of 1971, 164

COSEPUP. *See* Committee on Science, Engineering,
  and Public Policy
CRCPD. *See* Center for Radiation Control Program
  Directors; Conference of Radiation Control
  Program Directors
CROs. *See* Contract Research Organizations
Cs-137 source, 130
CSOS. *See* Controlled Substances Ordering System
current good manufacturing practice (cGMP), 27
Customs and Border Protection (CBP), 195

D
Dangerous Goods Regulations (DGR), 86, 87t
Dangerous goods shipping, 106
  regulations, 96–99
Data
  access, 229
  acquisition and management, 221
  analysis, 212
  collection, 211
  ownership, 230
  protection, 212
  reporting, 212
  retention, 228–229
  sharing, 212, 229, 232
    policy, 218
  storage, 212
  transfer, 229
  usage, 228
Data management, 209, 211
  addressing noncompliance
    appeals, 240
    case summaries, 240
    initial allegations, 238
    initial assessment, 238
    inquiry phase, 238–239
    institutional decision, 239–240
    investigation phase, 239
    ORI oversight, 240
    parties, 236–238
    research integrity, 235
    research misconduct, 235–236
  CDC, 220
  compliance challenges, 227
    communication, 233–234
    creating internal policies, 227–230
    data sharing, 232
    data types, 231
    financial requirements, 232–233
    leadership, 234
    managing conflicts, 234–235
    project needs, 230–231
    project-based data management plans, 230
    standards for data and metadata, 231–232
  current changes in federal agencies, 210–211

Data management (*Continued*)
DoD, 220
IMLS, 219
NASA, 218–219
National Endowment for Humanities, 219
National Institute of Standards and Technology, 220–221
NIH, 215
NIJ, 220
NOAA, 218
NSF, 213–214
ORI, 221–222
personnel and university committees, 225
  IRB, 226–227
  libraries, 225
  outside parties, 227
  PIs, 225–226
  research compliance, 226
  research office, 226
  responsible conduct of research committee, 226
  sponsored projects, 226
  university libraries, 227
regulatory mandates, 222–225
regulatory/oversight agencies, 212
US Department of Agriculture, 221
US Department of Education, 216–217
US Department of Energy, 215–216
USAID, 217
USEPA, 217
DEA. *See* Drug Enforcement Administration
Deciding official (DO), 236–237
Deemed Export Rule, Creation of, 193
Deemed exports, 188, 196–197
Department of Defense (DoD), 190, 220
Department of Energy (DOE), 123–124
Department of Environmental Health, 102–103
Department of public safety or local law enforcement, 180–181
Department of Transportation (DOT), 86
Designated member review (DMR), 51
Device, 13
DGR. *See* Dangerous Goods Regulations
DHHS. *See* US Department of Health and Human Services
Dickey-Wicker Amendment (DWA), 298
Dietary Supplement Health and Education Act, 23
Digital data, 233
Disclosure review committee, 270
Discovery research, 277
Divergent state laws, 315–316
Diversion, 160
DMR. *See* Designated member review
DO. *See* Deciding official
DoD. *See* Department of Defense

DOE. *See* Department of Energy
DOJ. *See* US Department of Justice
DOT. *See* Department of Transportation
Drug Abuse Control Amendments of 1965, 163
Drug Enforcement Administration (DEA), 160, 167, 171
continuing records, 173–175
  ordering and purchasing, 174
  power of attorney, 174–175
inspections, 176–177
inventory criteria, 172–173
inventory records, 171–172
  biennial inventory, 172
  initial inventory, 172
  new classification inventory, 172
Drug safety, 280
responsibilities related to, 281
Drugs and biologics, 24t
clinical laboratory practice requirements, 28
clinical practice requirements, 28
components, 26–27
FDA approval for commercial marketing, 28–29
FDA guidance documents, 28
manufacturing and labeling requirements, 27
pertinent investigational drug and biologic guidance documents, 29t
requirements for submission of investigational new drug application, 23–26
responsible FDA entities, 23
Durham–Humphrey Amendment, 22
DWA. *See* Dickey-Wicker Amendment

**E**
E2C2. *See* Export Enforcement Coordination Center
EAA. *See* Export Administration Act
EAR. *See* Export Administration Regulations
Earth Science Missions, 218
ECO. *See* Export control officer
ED. *See* Effective dose
EDE. *See* Effective dose equivalent
Educating clinical research staff, 221
Educating investigators, 272
Education and Human Resources Directorate, 214
Effective dose (ED), 118
Effective dose equivalent (EDE), 118
Embryonic Stem Cell Research Oversight (ESCRO), 302
Committee, 313
Empowered official (EO), 201
Energy Policy Act, 124–125
Energy Research and Development Administration (ERDA), 123–124
Engineering Directorate, 213
Entity List, 198
Environmental Protection Agency (EPA), 88, 122

EO. *See* Empowered official
EPA. *See* Environmental Protection Agency
Equity Management Committee, 247–248
Equivalent dose, 115
ERDA. *See* Energy Research and Development
    Administration
ESCRO. *See* Embryonic Stem Cell Research Oversight
Exempt radioactive material, 128
Exemption, 188
Export Administration Act (EAA), 193
Export Administration Regulations (EAR), 187
Export control officer (ECO), 200
Export controls, 187–188
    addressing noncompliance, 204–206
    antiboycott regimes, 199
    BIS lists, 198
    compliance challenges, 203
        decentralization, 204
        faculty travel, 203
        global research, 204
        misapplication of FRE, 203
    historical perspectives, 188–194
        constitutional challenges and escalating
            government action, 189–191
        development of national policy and regulatory
            changes, 191
        NSDD-189, 191–194
    personnel and university committees, 199–200
        EO, 201
        International Travel Office, 201–202
        offices and resources, 202–203
        sponsored programs, 200
        University Export Control Committee, 201
        university export control officer, 200
    prohibited end use, 199
    regulatory mandates, 195–196
        deemed exports, 196–197
        defense services, 197
        office of foreign assets control sanctions, 198
        physical exports, 196
    regulatory/oversight agencies, regulations, and
        guidance documents, 195
    restricted parties, 198
    state department lists, 198–199
Export Enforcement Coordination Center (E2C2), 195
Export Enforcement Coordination Fusion Center, 195

**F**

FACR. *See* Foreign Assets Control Regulations
FBI. *See* Federal Bureau of Investigation
FCOI. *See* Financial conflicts of interest
FCR. *See* Full committee review
FD&C Act. *See* Food, Drug and Cosmetic Act
FDA. *See* US Food and Drug Administration

Federal Bureau of Investigation (FBI), 139
Federal controlled substance regulations, 166–167.
        *See also* State controlled substance regulations
    DEA organization, 167
    FDA, 167–168
Federal Food, Drug, and Cosmetic Act, 282
Federal Hazardous Materials Regulations (FHMR), 86
Federal Human Subject Protection Regulation and
    Guidance, 306
Federal legislation, regulations, and guidance, 304
    Amendments (2010), 304–306
    cell-lines importation, 309
    chimeras creation, 309
    DWA of DHHS appropriations bill, 304
    FDA, 306–307
    Federal Human Subject Protection Regulation and
        Guidance, 306
    Final Report of National Academy's hESCs Research
        Advisory Committee, 304–306
    gene therapy, 309
    hESC, 309
    HIPAA, 308
    NIH and uniform biological materials transfer
        agreements, 307–308
    NIH Guidelines on hESCs research (2009), 304
    NIH hESCs registry, 304
    recombinant DNA research, 309
    US Patent and Licensing Laws, 308
    xenotransplantation, 309–310
Federal Radiation Council (FRC), 122
Federal regulatory mandates, 312
Federal Select Agent Program (FSAP), 81–84
Federal Select Agent Program, 103–105
Federal Wide Assurance (FWA), 7, 13
FHCRC. *See* Fred Hutchinson Cancer Research Center
FHMR. *See* Federal Hazardous Materials Regulations
Financial conflicts of interest (FCOI), 254, 257, 266.
        *See also* Conflict of interest (COI)
    managing, 267–268
    public reporting, 268–269
510k. *See* Premarket notification
Food and Drug Act (1906), 160–161
Food, Drug and Cosmetic Act (FD&C Act), 22, 161–162
Foreign Assets Control Regulations (FACR), 187, 195
Foreign national, 188
Foreign Quarantine Program, 96
45 CFR 46. *See* Code of Federal Regulations 45 Part 46
FRC. *See* Federal Radiation Council
FRE. *See* Fundamental research exemption or exclusion
FSAP. *See* Federal Select Agent Program
Full committee review (FCR), 50–51
Fundamental research, 188
Fundamental research exemption or exclusion (FRE), 203
FWA. *See* Federal Wide Assurance

**G**

GAO. *See* US Government Accountability Office
GCP. *See* Good clinical practice
Gene therapy, 309
General counsel, office of, 314
General Duty Clause, 87
Geosciences Directorate, 214
GLSP. *See* Good large-scale practice
Good clinical practice (GCP), 28, 33, 277
   addressing noncompliance, 294
   compliance challenges, 290
      GLP studies, 292
      inspections, 293
      QC, 291
   drug development process map, 278f
   FDA origins, 279
      laws and regulations, 282
      place in US government, 281
      responsibilities related to drug safety, 281
   personnel, 287–290
   regulations
      conduct of nonclinical laboratory study, 285
      disqualification of testing facilities, 286
      equipment, 284
      facilities, 283–284
      guidance documents, 286, 287t
      organization and personnel, 282–283
      protocol for, 285
      provisions, 282
      records and reports, 285–286
      test and control articles, 285
      testing facilities operation, 284–285
   regulatory mandates, 287
   requirements, 33
Good large-scale practice (GLSP), 92
Guide for Affiliate Research Awards, 219
Guidelines for Responsible Data Management in
     Scientific Research, 221

**H**

Harrison Tax Act of 1914, 161
Health and Human Services (HHS), 81–84, 123. *See also*
     US Department of Health and Human Services
     (DHHS)
Health Insurance Portability and Accountability Act
     (HIPAA), 14, 308
hESCs. *See* human embryonic stem cells
HHS. *See* Health and Human Services
HIPAA. *See* Health Insurance Portability and
     Accountability Act
HPA. *See* Human protections administrator
HRPP. *See* Human research protection program
human embryonic stem cells (hESCs), 297

addressing noncompliance, 316–317
compliance challenges
   divergent state laws, 315–316
   uneven regulatory landscape, 314–315
historical perspectives, 299
   Bush era, 301–302
   Clinton era, 299–301
   Obama era, 302–303
NIH Guidelines, 298
personnel and university committees, 313
   Ancillary Committees, 313–314
   compliance office, 314
   ESCRO Committee, 313
   general counsel office, 314
   grants and contracts department, 314
   institutional official, 313
   public relations office, 314
   SCRO Committee, 313
   TTO, 314
regulatory agencies and oversight laws, regulations
   federal legislation, regulations, and guidance,
     304–310
   international regulatory environment, 303–304
   state agencies, regulation, and guidance,
     310–311
regulatory mandates
   federal, 312
   state, 312–313
Human gene transfer, 90, 100, 102
Human immunodeficiency virus (HIV), 87–88
Human protections administrator (HPA), 13
Human research protection program (HRPP), 2
   agencies, 7–8
   challenges, 14
      addressing noncompliance, 16–17
      education of research community, 14
      FDA compliance, 15–16
      identification of research, 15
      mission creep, 15
   historical perspectives
      recognition of need, 2–4
      unethical research, 4–7
   influences, 17
      collaborative IRB review, 19–20
      flexibility, 17–19
   regulations
      common rule, 8–12
      FDA regulations, 12–13
      FWA, 13
      HIPAA, 14
Human subject research, 144
   COI in, 257
   FDA regulations, 144–145

HUSC, 144
protections, 2
research protocols
  evaluation or research use, 145–146
  use of standard procedures, 144–145
Human use subcommittee (HUSC), 144

## I

IACUC. *See* Institutional Animal Care and Use
    Committee
IASCR. *See* Interstate Alliance for Stem Cell Research
IATA. *See* International Air Transport Association
IBC. *See* Institutional Biosafety Committee
IC. *See* Increased controls
ICAO. *See* International Civil Aviation Organization
ICH. *See* International Commission on Harmonization
ICOI. *See* Institutional conflict of interest
ICRP. *See* International Commission on Radiological
    Protection
ICRU. *See* International Commission on Radiation
    Units and Measurements
IDE. *See* Investigational device exemption
IEEPA. *See* International Emergency Economic
    Powers Act
IES. *See* Institute for Education Science
IMLS. *See* Institute of Museum and Library Services
Import permit (IP), 95
Import Permit Program (IPP), 86
In vitro diagnostic device (IVD), 31
In vitro fertilization (IVF), 298
Increased controls (IC), 139
IND. *See* Investigational new drug
induced pluripotent stem cells (iPSCs), 299
Information technology (IT), 273
Initial inventory, 172
Inquiry committee, 238–239
Institute for Education Science (IES), 216–217
Institute of Museum and Library Services (IMLS), 219
Institutional Animal Care and Use Committee
    (IACUC), 41–42, 159–160, 178, 265, 305
  AAALAC, 59
  addressing noncompliance
    initial responses, 71–72
    investigating allegations of noncompliance, 72–73
    using postapproval monitoring, 74–75
    subsequent actions, 73–74
  compliance challenges, 65–66
  members or consultants, 65
  other committees, 58–59
  personnel
    general comments, 59–61
    institutional animal care and use committee chair,
     61–62

member with primary concerns in nonscientific
    area, 63–64
scientist having experience in research involving
    animals, 63
unaffiliated with institution, 64–65
protocol form, 48–49
regulatory and oversight laws, regulations, and
    guidance documents
  Animal Welfare Act, 44–45
  Animal Welfare Act Regulations, 45
  Animal Welfare Assurance, 47
  guide for care and use of agricultural animals,
    48–49
  PHS policy, 46–47
  Program of Veterinary Care, 45
regulatory history, 42–43
  AWA, 43
  national protections for animals, 43–44
  NIH policy, 44
  USDA, 44
regulatory mandates, 49–50
veterinarian, 62–63
Institutional Biosafety Committee (IBC), 58–59, 89,
    100–101, 305
Institutional conflict of interest (ICOI), 257–258
Institutional culture, 69–70
Institutional decision, 239–240
Institutional official (IO), 52, 313
Institutional resources, 108
Institutional review board (IRB), 2, 90, 134, 214,
    226–227, 258, 270–271, 305
Intellectual property (IP), 243
  addressing noncompliance, 250–251
  assignment of rights to, 249
  COI, 249–250
  compliance challenges, 248
  failure to disclosing IP creation, 248–249
  inappropriate sharing, 250
  personnel and university committees, 243–244
    Equity Management Committee, 247–248
    financial services, 246–247
    Office of Legal Counsel, 247
    ORS, 245–246
    TTO, 244–245
Interactive data management module, 221–222
Internal policies creation, 227–230
Internal Revenue Service (IRS), 247
International Air Transport Association (IATA), 86
  proper shipping names, 98t
International Civil Aviation Organization (ICAO), 99
International Commission on Harmonization (ICH), 28
International Commission on Radiation Units and
    Measurements (ICRU), 121

International Commission on Radiological Protection (ICRP), 118
International Emergency Economic Powers Act (IEEPA), 195
International regulatory environment, 303
International Society of Stem Cell Research (ISSCR), 303
International Stem Cell Forum, 303–304
International Travel Office, 201–202
International treaties
    convention on psychotropic substances (1971), 164
    single convention on narcotic drugs (1961), 164
    United Nations convention against illicit traffic in narcotic drugs and psychotropic substances (1988), 164
Interstate Alliance for Stem Cell Research (IASCR), 315
Inventory records, 171–172
    biennial inventory, 172
    initial inventory, 172
    new classification inventory, 172
Investigational device exemption (IDE), 30–32, 145
    components, 32–33
Investigational new drug (IND), 137, 277–279
    application, 7, 23, 306
    compliance challenges, 39
    drugs and biologics, 24t
        components, 26–27
        FDA approval for commercial marketing, 28–29
        FDA guidance documents, 28
        good clinical laboratory practice requirements, 28
        good clinical practice requirements, 28
        manufacturing and labeling requirements, 27
        pertinent investigational drug and biologic guidance documents, 29t
        requirements for submission of investigational new drug application, 23–26
        responsible FDA entities, 23
    historical perspectives, 21
        Durham–Humphrey Amendment, 22
        FD&C Act, 22
        FDA, 22
        Medical Device Amendments, 23
    medical devices
        FDA approval for commercial marketing, 34–35
        FDA guidance documents, 33
        good clinical laboratory practice requirements, 33
        good clinical practice requirements, 33
        IDE applications, 30–32
        manufacturing requirements, 33
        pertinent investigational medical device guidance documents, 34t
        responsible FDA entity, 29–30
    noncompliance, addressing, 39–40
    personnel and university committees, 38–39
    regulatory mandates, 35

investigator responsibilities, 37–38
sponsor responsibilities, 35–37
Investigator
    monitoring investigator compliance, 273
    responsibilities, 37–38
IO. *See* Institutional official
Ionizing radiation, 113. *See also* Nonionizing radiation
    exposure
        health effects, 117
        sources, 116–117, 116f
    producing machines regulation, 130
    types and uses of sources
        radiation producing equipment, 115
        radioactive material, 113–115
IP. *See* Import permit; Intellectual property
IPP. *See* Import Permit Program
iPSCs. *See* induced pluripotent stem cells
IRB. *See* Institutional review board
IRS. *See* Internal Revenue Service
ISSCR. *See* International Society of Stem Cell Research
IT. *See* Information technology
IVD. *See* In vitro diagnostic device
IVF. *See* In vitro fertilization

**J**
Justice principle, 4

**K**
Kefauver–Harris Amendment, 22, 162–163

**L**
Laboratory acquired infection (LAI), 79
LAI. *See* Laboratory acquired infection
Lasers, 146–147
Legal office, 271–272
LET. *See* Linear energy transfer
License exception, 188
Linear, no-threshold model (LNT model), 125
Linear energy transfer (LET), 116
LNT model. *See* Linear, no-threshold model

**M**
Magnetic resonance imaging (MRI), 267
Managing conflicts, 234–235
Mathematical and Physical Sciences Directorate, 214
Maximum permissible dose (MPD), 122
Media relations, 272
Medical and infectious waste handling regulations, 89
Medical Device Amendments, 23
Medical device classification panels, 34–35
Medical event, 155
Metadata, 231
Minimal risk, 10
Mission creep, 15

MPD. *See* Maximum permissible dose
MRI. *See* Magnetic resonance imaging
Multiagency Task Force, 210–211

# N

NABP®. *See* National Association Boards of Pharmacy
NARM. *See* Naturally occurring radioactive material
NARSTO. *See* North American Research Strategy for Tropospheric Ozone
NAS. *See* National Academy of Sciences
NAS/NRC. *See* National Academy of Sciences–National Research Council
NASA. *See* National Aeronautics and Space Administration
National Academy of Sciences (NAS), 298
National Academy of Sciences–National Research Council (NAS/NRC), 122
National Aeronautics and Space Administration (NASA), 218
  data rights and related issues, 218
  Earth Science Missions, 218
  Heliophysics, 219
National Association Boards of Pharmacy (NABP®), 166, 171
National Committee on Radiation Protection. *See* National Council on Radiation Protection and Measurements (NCRP)
National Council on Radiation Protection and Measurements (NCRP), 117, 120–121
National Endowment for Humanities, 219
National Institute of Drug Abuse (NIDA), 167–168
National Institute of Justice (NIJ), 220
National Institute of Standards and Technology, 220–221
National Institutes of Health (NIH), 18, 42–43, 80, 209–210, 256, 298
  Data Sharing Policy, 215
  guidelines, 89–92, 103, 302, 304
  hESCs registry, 304
  human embryonic stem cell registry, 304
  Public Access Policy, 215
National Nuclear Security Administration (NNSA), 195
National Oceanographic and Atmospheric Administration (NOAA), 218
National Research Act, 2–3
National Science Foundation (NSF), 209, 211, 256
  data management plan requirement, 213
  data sharing requirement, 213
  recommendations, 232
  specific program guidance, 213–214
National Security Decision Directive 189 (NSDD-189), 191–194
  Creation of Deemed Export Rule, 193

US *v.* Roth, 193–194
Naturally occurring radioactive material (NARM), 123–124, 127
NCRP. *See* National Council on Radiation Protection and Measurements
NDA. *See* New Drug Application
New Drug Application (NDA), 28–29, 279
NIDA. *See* National Institute of Drug Abuse
NIH. *See* National Institutes of Health
NIJ. *See* National Institute of Justice
NNSA. *See* National Nuclear Security Administration
NOAA. *See* National Oceanographic and Atmospheric Administration
Nonclinical laboratory study, 285
Nonionizing radiation, 118–119
  producing machines regulation, 131
North American Research Strategy for Tropospheric Ozone (NARSTO), 216
NRC. *See* Nuclear Regulatory Commission
NSDD-189. *See* National Security Decision Directive 189
NSF. *See* National Science Foundation
Nuclear Regulatory Commission (NRC), 123–124
Nuremberg Code, 5

# O

OAS. *See* Organization of Agreement States
OBA. *See* Office of Biotechnology Activities
Occupational safety and environmental health (OSEH), 178
Occupational Safety and Health Administration (OSHA), 81, 127–128
  BBP, 99–100
  PPE standard, 100
Occupational Safety and Health Administration Bloodborne Pathogen Standard, 106–108
Oceanographic Data, 218
OECD. *See* Organization for Economic Cooperation and Development
OEE. *See* Office of Export Enforcement
OFAC. *See* Office of Foreign Assets Control
Office for Human Research Protections (OHRP), 299
Office of Biotechnology Activities (OBA), 90
Office of Digital Humanities, 219
Office of Export Enforcement (OEE), 195
Office of Foreign Assets Control (OFAC), 187–188
Office of Good Clinical Practice, 7
Office of Human Research Protections (OHRP), 7–8
Office of Legal Counsel, 247
Office of Science and Technology Policy, 211
OHRP. *See* Office for Human Research Protections; Office of Human Research Protections
Omnibus Drug Act (1988), 165
Open Government Data Quality Plan, 217

OPIM. *See* Other potentially infectious materials
Organization for Economic Cooperation and Development (OECD), 280
Organization of Agreement States (OAS), 127
ORI. *See* Office of Research Integrity
ORS. *See* Office of research services
OSEH. *See* Occupational safety and environmental health
OSHA. *See* Occupational Safety and Health Administration
OTC. *See* Over-the-counter
Other potentially infectious materials (OPIM), 81
Outside parties, 227
Over-the-counter (OTC), 281

**P**

PAM. *See* Postapproval monitoring
PD. *See* Position descriptions
Personal protective equipment (PPE), 79–80
Personhood Amendments, 317
PET. *See* Positron emission tomography
PHS. *See* Public Health Service; US Public Health Service
PHS Awarding Agency, reporting to, 268
Physical exports, 196
Physician Payments Sunshine Act, 260–261
PI. *See* Principal investigator
Plant protection and quarantine (PPQ), 80
PMA. *See* Premarket approval
Position descriptions (PD), 290
Positron emission tomography (PET), 114
Postapproval monitoring (PAM), 74
PPE. *See* Personal protective equipment
PPQ. *See* Plant protection and quarantine
Premarket approval (PMA), 34–35
Premarket notification, 34–35
Principal investigator (PI), 101–102, 135, 225–226
Program of Veterinary Care, 45
Prohibited End Use, 199
Project-based data management plans, 230
Protocol deviation, 39
Public Health Service (PHS), 43–44, 159–160, 235, 263
    PHS regulation (2011), 263
        disclosure review, 266–267
        investigator determination, 264
        managing FCOIs, 267–268
        policies, 263
        public reporting of FCOIs, 268–269
        reporting to PHS Awarding Agency, 268
        retrospective review, 269
        scope of financial interests, 265–266
        SFIs, 264–265
    policy, 46–47
    regulation, 254

Public member. *See* Unaffiliated member
Public relations office, 314

**Q**

Quality assurance unit (QAU), 283
Quality control (QC), 291

**R**

RAC. *See* Recombinant DNA Advisory Committee
Radiation, 113
    producing equipment, 115
    quantities, 115–116
    risk statement, 151–152
    safety
        audits and surveys, 154
        committee, 140–141
        office, 141
    workers, 142
Radiation dose
    determination, 151
    limits, 117–118, 136–137, 136t–137t, 150–151
Radiation exposure, 115
Radiation protection program (RPP), 119, 132–133
Radiation protection recommendations development, 121–122, 125
    AEC, 123–124
    CRCPD, 124
    Energy Policy Act, 124–125
    EPA, 123
    FRC, 122
    NARM, 123–124
    NRC, 124
    PHS, 123
    political consensus, 122
    radiation exposure, 125
    tolerance dose, 122
Radiation safety officer (RSO), 119, 140
Radioactive drug research committee (RDRC), 26, 136–139, 138t
Radioactive materials, 113–115
    license, 131–132
    regulation, 128
        exempt radioactive material, 128
        general licenses, 128
        specific licenses, 129–130
Radioactivity, 119–120
Radioisotopes, 113–114
Radiological hazards. *See also* Biological hazards
    addressing noncompliance
        inspections of human subject research, 154–155
        institutional inspections, 153–154
        medical event and notification reporting requirements, 155
        radiation safety audits and surveys, 154

compliance challenges
   ethical aspects, 149–150
   human use research, 149
   laboratory use of radioactive materials,
     147–148
   pregnancy, 153
   radiation dose determination, 151
   radiation dose limits, 150–151
   radiation risk statement, 151–152
   research in children, 153
   use of radiation producing machines,
     148–149
health effects of ionizing radiation exposure, 117
historical perspectives
   early recommendations for radiation protection,
     120–121
   radiation protection recommendations
     development, 121–124
   radioactivity, 119–120
   X-rays, 119–120
ionizing radiation, 113–115
   producing machines regulation, 130
nonionizing radiation, 118–119
   producing machines regulation, 131
personnel and university committees, 140
   authorized users, 141–142
   human subject research, 144–146
   lasers, 146–147
   organization structure, 146
   radiation safety committee, 140–141
   radiation safety office, 141
   radiation workers, 142
   RSO, 140
   security requirements, 143
   use of radiation sources with animals, 143
radiation dose limits, 117–118
radiation quantities, 115–116
radioactive materials regulation, 128
   exempt radioactive material, 128
   general licenses, 128
   specific licenses, 129–130
regulatory and oversight agencies
   agreement states, 126–127
   CRCPD, 127
   FDA, 127
   non-agreement states, 127
   OSHA, 127–128
   US nuclear regulatory commission, 126
regulatory mandates, 131
   AU, 134–136
   IC, 139
   radiation dose limits, 136–137
   radiation protection program, 132–133
   radioactive materials license, 131–132

   registration of ionizing radiation producing
     equipment, 133
   research involving human subjects, 134
   RPP, 119
   sources of ionizing radiation exposure, 116–117
RCR. *See* Responsible conduct of research
rDNA. *See* Recombinant DNA
RDRC. *See* Radioactive drug research committee
REC. *See* Research ethics committee
Recombinant DNA (rDNA), 80–81
   research, 309
Research, 8–9
   data custody, 228
   integrity, 235
   misconduct, 235–236
   office, 226
Research and Sponsored Programs, 225
Research ethics committee (REC), 2
Research Integrity Officer (RIO), 236
Responsible conduct of research (RCR), 209
Responsible official (RO), 93, 102
Restricted parties, 198
Retaliation, 237
RIO. *See* Research Integrity Officer
RO. *See* Responsible official
RPP. *See* Radiation protection program
RSO. *See* Radiation safety officer

**S**
Sanctions, 187–188
Schedule I controlled substance registration, 170–171
Schedule I Controlled Substances, 168
SCNT. *See* Somatic cell nuclear transfer
SCRO Committee. *See* Stem Cell Research Oversight
   Committee
SDN. *See* Specially Designated Nationals
SESIPs. *See* Sharps with engineered sharps injury
   protection
SFIs. *See* Significant financial interests
Sharps with engineered sharps injury protection
   (SESIPs), 81
SI unit. *See* System international unit
Significant financial interests (SFIs), 264–265. *See also*
   Conflict of interest (COI)
Single Convention on Narcotic Drugs of 1961, 164
Single photon emission computed tomography
   (SPECT), 114
Social, Behavioral, and Economic Science Directorate, 214
Somatic cell nuclear transfer (SCNT), 298, 300
SOP. *See* Standard operating procedure
Specially Designated Nationals (SDN), 198
SPECT. *See* Single photon emission computed
   tomography
Sponsor responsibilities, 35–37

Sponsored programs, 200
Sponsored projects, 226
    office, 271
SSRCR. *See* Suggested State Regulations for Control of Radiation
Standard clinical care, 145
Standard operating procedure (SOP), 284, 291
Standards for data and metadata, 231–232
State controlled substance
    licensing, 171
    regulations, 166
State regulatory mandates, 312–313
Stem Cell Research Oversight Committee (SCRO Committee), 312–313
Subrecipients, 273–274
Suggested State Regulations for Control of Radiation (SSRCR), 124

**T**
Technology control plan, 188
Technology transfer office (TTO), 243–245, 271, 314
Therapeutic cloning, 300
Tolerance dose, 122
TTO. *See* Technology transfer office
Tuskegee syphilis study, 3–4

**U**
U.S. Munitions List (USML), 197
UBTI. *See* Unrelated business taxable income
Unaffiliated member, 64
Unethical research, 4–7
United Nations (UN)
    convention, 164
    number, 98
United States export controls, 187
Uniting and Strengthening America by Providing Appropriate Tools Required to Intercept and Obstruct Terrorism Act (USA PATRIOT Act), 81–84
University Export Control Committee, 201
University export control officer, 200
Unrelated business taxable income (UBTI), 249
UPU. *See* Universal Postal Union
US Agency for International Development (USAID), 217
US Citizenship and Immigration Service (USCIS), 202–203
US Department of Agriculture (USDA), 43, 80
    APHIS, 96

US Department of Education, 216–217
US Department of Energy, 215–216
US Department of Health and Human Services (DHHS), 7, 167, 227, 257–258, 299
US Department of Justice (DOJ), 189
US Environmental Protection Agency (USEPA), 217
US Food and Drug Administration (FDA), 7, 22, 123, 257, 277, 297
    clinical translation and approval of investigational drug, 21
    compliance, 15–16
    DHHS and, 167–168
    jurisdiction
    over cell-based therapies, 306–307
    over manufacturer and installation of electronic products, 127
    regulations, 12–13
US Government Accountability Office (GAO), 199–200
US munitions list (USML), 188
US nuclear regulatory commission, 126
US Patent and Licensing Laws, 308
US Pharmacopoeia (USP), 160–161
US Public Health Service (PHS), 123
USA PATRIOT Act. *See* Uniting and Strengthening America by Providing Appropriate Tools Required to Intercept and Obstruct Terrorism Act
USAID. *See* US Agency for International Development
USCIS. *See* US Citizenship and Immigration Service
USDA. *See* US Department of Agriculture
USEPA. *See* US Environmental Protection Agency
USML. *See* U.S. Munitions List; US munitions list
USP. *See* US Pharmacopoeia

**V**
Veterans Administration (VA), 7
Veterinary services (VS), 80
Vice president for research (VPR), 243–244
Vulnerable populations, 3

**W**
Whistleblower, 237

**X**
X-rays, 119–120
Xenotransplantation, 309–310

' in the United States

masters